LEARN HOW YOU CAN . . .

- Cure shingles pain with a hot chili pepper cream   [476]
- Ease the pain of a broken leg with a 40-watt bulb   [542]
- Use acupressure for eyestrain   [143-44]
- Get rid of gas with charcoal   [34]
- Soothe a migraine by imagining your hands
  in hot water   [221]
- Prevent swimmer's ear with alcohol   [119]
- Relieve arthritis with evening primrose oil   [248]
- Ease menstrual cramps with a belly dance
  visualization   [367]
- Laugh at a pet and feel less pain   [563]
- Keep a diary to spot your own pain triggers   [520-21]

Plus, discover . . .

- How to pick a chiropractor
- The best technique for giving a massage
- The importance of support groups and how to find
  the right one for you

**IT'S ALL IN
THE *PREVENTION* PAIN RELIEF SYSTEM**
from the editors of *Prevention* magazine, America's leading health
magazine

D0126650

THE *PREVENTION*

PAIN-RELIEF SYSTEM

A TOTAL PROGRAM FOR RELIEVING ANY PAIN IN YOUR BODY

By the editors of
Prevention Magazine Health Books

Edited by Alice Feinstein

BANTAM BOOKS
New York Toronto London Sydney Auckland

This edition contains the complete text
of the original hardcover edition.
NOT ONE WORD HAS BEEN OMITTED.

THE *PREVENTION* PAIN-RELIEF SYSTEM
A Bantam Book / published by arrangement
with Rodale Press, Inc.

PUBLISHING HISTORY
Rodale Press edition published 1992
Bantam edition / May 1994

Prevention is a registered trademark of Rodale Press, Inc.

ISBN 0-553-56491-9

Published simultaneously in the United States and Canada

Bantam Books are published by Bantam Books, a division of Bantam
Doubleday Dell Publishing Group, Inc. Its trademark, consisting of the
words "Bantam Books" and the portrayal of a rooster, is Registered in
U.S. Patent and Trademark Office and in other countries. Marca
Registrada, Bantam Books, 1540 Broadway, New York, New York 10036.

PRINTED IN THE UNITED STATES OF AMERICA

OPM   0 9 8 7 6 5 4 3 2 1

BOARD OF MEDICAL REVIEWERS FOR PAIN-FINDER CHARTS

Larry Millikan, M.D., professor and chairman of dermatology, Tulane University Medical School, New Orleans, Louisiana

Lawrence A. Pottenger, M.D., Ph.D., associate professor of orthopedic surgery and rehabilitation medicine, University of Chicago, Chicago, Illinois

Paul Vinger, M.D., associate clinical professor of ophthalmology, Tufts University School of Medicine, Boston, Massachusetts and assistant clinical professor of ophthalmology, Harvard Medical School, Cambridge, Massachusetts

Chart coordinator: Anne Imhoff

THE *PREVENTION* PAIN-RELIEF SYSTEM

Editors of *Prevention* Magazine Health Books:
Claudia Allen, Gale Maleskey, Ellen Michaud,
Hank Nuwer, Lyn Votava, Russell Wild

Other Contributors: *Peggy Jo Donahue, Claire Gerus*

Copy Editor: *Barbara Webb*

Illustrator: *Jean Gardener*

Research Chief: *Ann Gossy*

Senior Reserach Associates: *Christine Dreisbach,
Paris Mihely-Muchanic*

Research Associates: *Anne Imhoff, Anna Crawford,
Cynthia Nickerson*

Research Associate Trainees: *Jewel Flegal, Deborah Pedron,
Michele Toth*

CONTENTS

To use the chart, start with the question in the upper left corner of the first page. By answering yes or no to each question and following the appropriate arrows, in short order you'll land on a box that gives you a possible cause of your pain. The box will either advise you to consult your physician or give you a page number. Turn to the appropriate page to find out how to relieve your pain.

Of course, if you already know the cause of your pain or you've been diagnosed by a physician, you can skip the

HOW TO USE THIS BOOK

When you hurt, you want relief—and you want it *fast*.

The Prevention *Pain-Relief System* is designed to put you in touch with the best possible means of dealing with *your* pain. There are countless techniques for eliminating pain—medications, meditations, exercises, high-tech electronic therapies, and so forth. This book looks at the entire universe of pain-relieving techniques, from something as simple as sipping a cup of herbal tea to something as complex as radical surgical intervention.

Pain is a highly individualized experience, however. Even people who have the same disease or injury may not feel pain in quite the same way. Relief of pain is also unique to each person. What works for one person may not work for the next. For that reason this book offers a wide variety of pain-relief techniques. You may have to try more than one, or even (with the blessing of your physician) several at the same time.

To find appropriate pain relief for *you*, it helps to know the cause of your pain. To help you make that determination, we have provided diagnostic charts. They appear at the beginning of each chapter in Part 1 of this book. Turn to the chapter that deals with the area of the body that hurts. First review the list of symptoms that indicate the need to see a physician, and then move on to the diagnostic chart.

To use the chart, start with the question in the upper left corner of the first page. By answering yes or no to each question and following the appropriate arrows, in short order you'll land on a box that will give you a possible cause of your pain. The box will either advise you to consult your physician or give you a page number. Turn to the appropriate page to find out how to relieve your pain.

Of course, if you already know the cause of your pain or you've been diagnosed by a physician, you can skip the chart and simply look up your condition in the table of contents or the index.

Each chapter in Part 1 features sections on the major causes of pain in a particular area of the body. Because we know your main concern is with relief, we've included a section called "Instant Relief" for each condition. It features treatments you can use *right now* to feel better. In most cases there are several actions you do take to find quick relief.

Following each "Instant Relief" section, you'll find a plan for long-term relief called the "Prevention Pain-Relief Program." It gives you long-term strategies for alleviating your pain and preventing its return.

Part 2 of this book presents a detailed description of numerous ways to relieve pain. Techniques like biofeedback or acupuncture, for example, can help relieve the pain of so many different conditions that each deserves a chapter of its own.

The Prevention Pain-Relief System offers a number of avenues for relief. Use this book as a tool to help you talk to your doctor, to help you find resources to eliminate pain, and to help you get on with living a healthy, satisfying life.

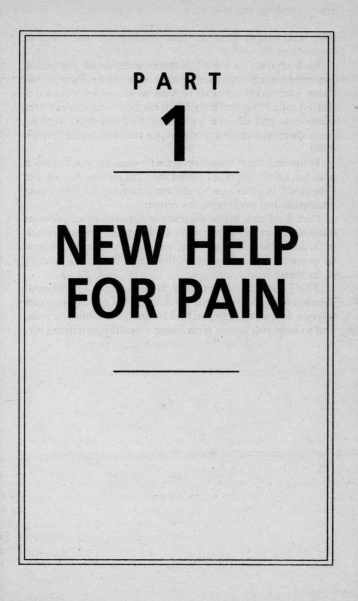

P A R T
1

NEW HELP
FOR PAIN

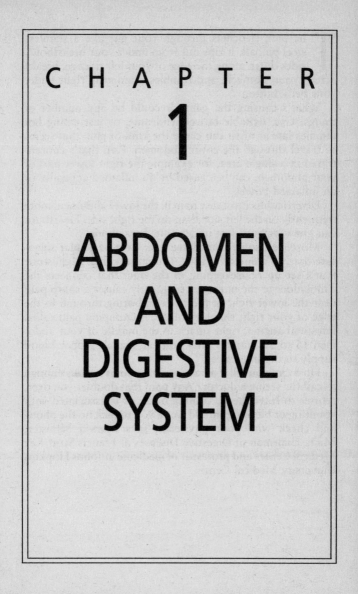

C H A P T E R

1

ABDOMEN
AND
DIGESTIVE
SYSTEM

The pain ricochets through your gut like a stainless steel pinball. It zips out from under your breastbone, rides down along the edge of your left ribcage, breaks across your stomach, and rumbles ominously right under your belly button.

What's causing the pain? It could be any number of things. Gas, irritable bowel syndrome, or just eating hot tamales late at night can cause the kind of pain that seems to travel through the entire abdomen. Pain that's concentrated in a single area, for example the right lower part of your abdomen, can be caused by an inflamed appendix or an inflamed bowel.

Diverticulitis can cause pain in the lower abdomen, more frequently on the left side than on the right side. Heartburn can gnaw or burn just under your breastbone.

Moreover, some pains have their own particular signature that, to a doctor at least, is unmistakable. A gallstone that's set up housekeeping in the duct that connects the gallbladder to the intestines frequently causes a sharp pain near the lower right of the ribcage, boring through to the edge of your right shoulder blade. A cramping pain called intestinal angina, right smack in the middle of your abdomen 15 to 30 minutes after you eat, signals a poor blood supply to the intestines.

How can you tell if an abdominal pain is serious enough to call for seeing a doctor? Any pain that doubles you over, refuses to leave, keeps coming back, or is associated with vomiting or bleeding should cause you to pick up the phone and check with your physician, says Marvin Schuster, M.D., chairman of Digestive Diseases at Francis Scott Key Medical Center and professor of medicine at Johns Hopkins University Medical Center.

GET PROFESSIONAL HELP IF:

- You have extreme abdominal pain that doubles you over
- You have diarrhea for more than one or two days
- You have chronic pain, weight loss, or narrowing of stools
- Your stools have become very dark and tarry looking or blood is present
- You have a dull ache in your upper abdomen, your urine has become dark, and/or the whites of your eyes or your skin appears yellowish

PAIN-FINDER CHART FOR THE ABDOMEN AND DIGESTIVE SYSTEM

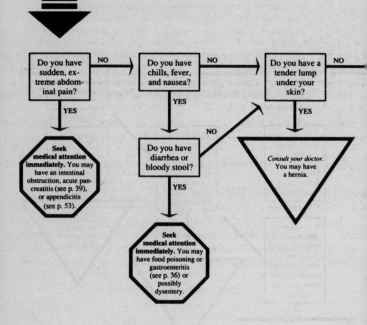

Do you have sudden, extreme abdominal pain? — NO → Do you have chills, fever, and nausea? — NO → Do you have a tender lump under your skin? — NO

YES ↓

Seek medical attention immediately. You may have an intestinal obstruction, acute pancreatitis (see p. 39), or appendicitis (see p. 53).

YES ↓ (from chills, fever, and nausea)

Do you have diarrhea or bloody stool? — NO → (to tender lump)

YES ↓

Seek medical attention immediately. You may have food poisoning or gastroenteritis (see p. 36) or possibly dysentery.

YES ↓ (from tender lump)

Consult your doctor. You may have a hernia.

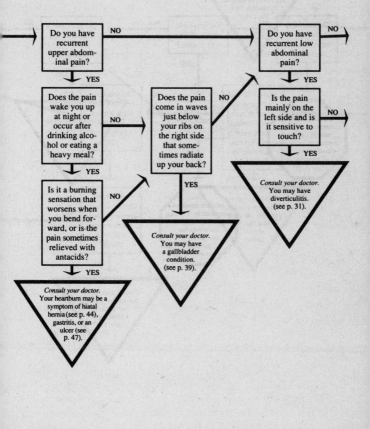

Do you have recurrent upper abdominal pain? — **NO** →

Do you have recurrent low abdominal pain? — **NO** →

↓ **YES**

Does the pain wake you up at night or occur after drinking alcohol or eating a heavy meal? — **NO** → Does the pain come in waves just below your ribs on the right side that sometimes radiate up your back? — **NO** → Is the pain mainly on the left side and is it sensitive to touch? — **NO** →

↓ **YES** (upper pain)   ↓ **YES** (right side)   ↓ **YES** (left side)

Is it a burning sensation that worsens when you bend forward, or is the pain sometimes relieved with antacids? — **NO** ↗

↓ **YES**

Consult your doctor. Your heartburn may be a symptom of hiatal hernia (see p. 44), gastritis, or an ulcer (see p. 47).

Consult your doctor. You may have a gallbladder condition. (see p. 39).

Consult your doctor. You may have diverticulitis. (see p. 31).

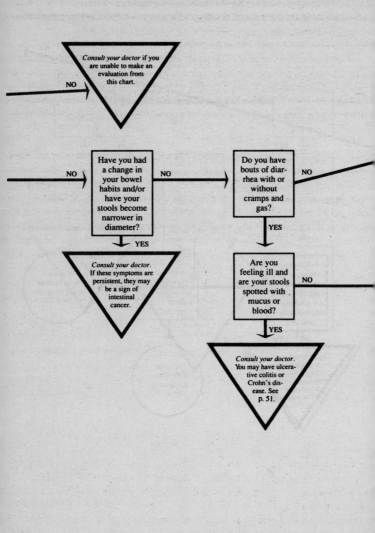

NO

Consult your doctor if you are unable to make an evaluation from this chart.

NO → Have you had a change in your bowel habits and/or have your stools become narrower in diameter?

NO → Do you have bouts of diarrhea with or without cramps and gas?

NO

YES

Consult your doctor. If these symptoms are persistent, they may be a sign of intestinal cancer.

YES

Are you feeling ill and are your stools spotted with mucus or blood?

NO

YES

Consult your doctor. You may have ulcerative colitis or Crohn's disease. See p. 51.

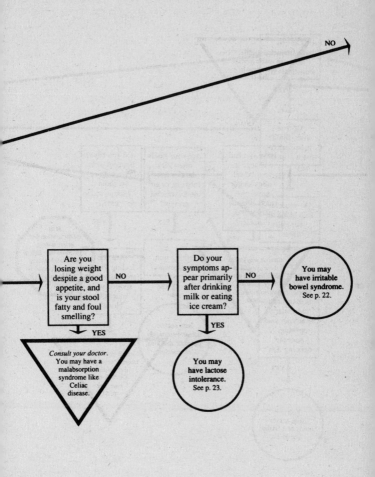

NO

Are you losing weight despite a good appetite, and is your stool fatty and foul smelling?

NO

Do your symptoms appear primarily after drinking milk or eating ice cream?

NO

You may have irritable bowel syndrome. See p. 22.

YES

Consult your doctor. You may have a malabsorption syndrome like Celiac disease.

YES

You may have lactose intolerance. See p. 23.

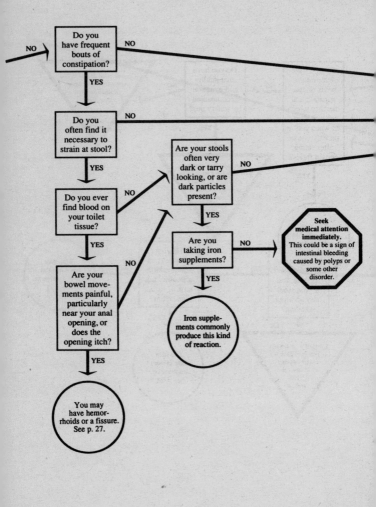

NO →

Do you have frequent bouts of constipation?

NO →

↓ YES

Do you often find it necessary to strain at stool?

NO →

↓ YES

Do you ever find blood on your toilet tissue?

NO →

↓ YES

Are your bowel movements painful, particularly near your anal opening, or does the opening itch?

NO →

↓ YES

You may have hemorrhoids or a fissure. See p. 27.

Are your stools often very dark or tarry looking, or are dark particles present?

NO →

↓ YES

Are you taking iron supplements?

NO →

↓ YES

Iron supplements commonly produce this kind of reaction.

Seek medical attention immediately. This could be a sign of intestinal bleeding caused by polyps or some other disorder.

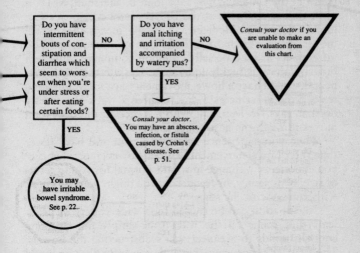

Do you have intermittent bouts of constipation and diarrhea which seem to worsen when you're under stress or after eating certain foods?

NO

Do you have anal itching and irritation accompanied by watery pus?

NO

Consult your doctor if you are unable to make an evaluation from this chart.

YES

YES

Consult your doctor. You may have an abscess, infection, or fistula caused by Crohn's disease. See p. 51.

You may have irritable bowel syndrome. See p. 22..

CONSTIPATION

Constipation is the most common gastrointestinal complaint in the United States, says John B. Marshall, M.D., a professor of medicine at the University of Missouri's Columbia School of Medicine. It usually means that bowel movements are too hard, too small, or too infrequent. "Too infrequent" is an especially common complaint, although bowel activity is highly individual. Despite the myth that people should have a bowel movement once a day, anything from three movements a day to three a week is perfectly normal, says Dr. Marshall, who is a specialist in how food moves through the gastrointestinal tract.

When you experience abdominal pain and have fewer than three bowel movements a week, however, or whenever you experience a change in what's normal for you in terms of size, consistency, or frequency, you might want to check with your doctor, he suggests.

Constipation can be caused by a wide variety of problems that range all the way from simply not drinking enough liquids to a cancer that's obstructing the bowels. The most common causes include too little fiber or liquid in your diet, not going to the bathroom when you feel the urge to defecate, inactivity, taking calcium or iron supplements, or taking certain medications—for allergies, colds, high blood pressure, heart problems, depression, and Parkinson's disease. Even diuretics, antacids, and nonsteroidal anti-inflammatory drugs such as ibuprofen can slow down the bowels.

Chronic constipation is usually caused by more serious conditions such as irritable bowel syndrome (see page 22), a structural problem, or nerve damage from diabetes mellitus, pregnancy, or childbirth.

▶ INSTANT RELIEF

If constipation is a problem, there are a number of things you can do to get things moving.

Use a suppository. A single glycerin suppository from your drugstore may induce defecation within 30 minutes of use, doctors say.

Flush it. An enema may also induce defecation within 30 minutes. Use a single pint of water or salt water, doctors suggest. Avoid over-the-counter enemas containing soapsuds, sodium phosphate, or biphosphate, each of which can irritate and even damage the bowels. An oil-retention enema may be helpful in loosening a hard stool and is available in disposable bottles at your local drugstore. Follow package directions.

Try milk of magnesia or magnesium citrate. Both of these laxatives will jump-start your digestive tract and induce a bowel movement anywhere from 30 minutes to 3 hours after you take them. They work by drawing fluid into the bowels and triggering the release of bowel-activating hormones. Neither, doctors warn, should be used on a regular basis, and they should not be used at all by people with kidney problems. Both should be taken with "an adequate amount of water," which is usually doctor-talk for one to two 8-ounce glasses of water.

▶ PREVENTION PAIN-RELIEF PROGRAM

The best way to both relieve and prevent the cramping pain of constipation is a high-fiber diet, says Dr. Marshall. Although it takes a couple of somewhat gassy weeks to start working, a high-fiber diet will soften your stool and increase its size, cut the amount of time that food takes to work its way through your digestive tract, and reduce the pressures inside your gut that frequently contribute to cramps.

How much fiber should you eat? The standard recommendation is about 30 grams a day, says Dr. Marshall. But you don't have to get hung up on numbers, he adds. Just eat a whole grain cereal such as granola or shredded wheat for breakfast and a whole grain bread with lunch, and add fresh fruits and vegetables to each meal.

The fiber from breads and cereals is particularly safe and

effective because it absorbs water from the intestinal tract and forms jellylike masses that are readily fermented by bowel bacteria. The result is a larger, softer stool that actually lubricates the intestinal wall as it slips easily through the bowels.

Fiber is so important in relieving constipation, says Dr. Marshall, that if you can't get a daily dose—maybe you're traveling or you've decided to skip breakfast, for example—you should take a fiber supplement that contains psyllium. Such preparations—Metamucil is one—are readily available at local drugstores and supermarkets.

And don't forget to drink at least eight glasses of liquid a day when you increase the amount of fiber in your diet. Without lots of liquid—whether it's soup, juice, or water—the extra fiber you've eaten is likely to just sit there and add to your problem instead of moving it out.

FIBER FACTS

Unless you're sitting under an apple tree, fiber isn't likely to simply drop into your lap. The typical American diet provides an average of 11.1 grams per day, while most doctors say that you need to eat approximately 30 grams a day to keep your digestive system in good health.

Why do you need so much? When scientists compare people who eat fiber-rich diets with those who don't, they find that high-fiber eaters are less likely to get such gastrointestinal diseases as constipation, hemorrhoids, irritable bowel syndrome, gallstones, diverticulitis, and colorectal cancer. They have also found that fiber actually relieves many of these diseases.

Fiber—primarily the indigestible stalks and peels of fruits and vegetables and the husks of whole grains—works by reducing the pressures inside your gut that cause pain, increasing the amount of time your small intestine has to grab nutrients out of your food, decreasing the amount of time waste spends hanging around in your colon waiting for excretion, and putting a slippery slope under that waste when it's time for it to move on.

If your diet isn't fiber-rich, start out by adding only a few extra grams of fiber per week. As you increase your fiber intake, remember to drink plenty of water, since fiber soaks up fluid like a sponge. Drink too little water and the fiber can just sit there like a big unmovable plug, causing half the problems it's supposed to solve.

If you want to avoid the gaseous side effects that sometimes accompany increased fiber intake, pick up a bottle of Beano from your local drugstore and use three to eight drops per serving of fiber at each meal. Beano is an enzyme that will help you digest the carbohydrates that normally ferment in your gut and give you gas. It eliminates gas in such champion producers as oats, whole wheat, pistachios, peanuts, corn, and carrots.

Ready to get started? Here's a list of more than 100 fiber-rich foods that will move you toward good health.

Food	Portion	Dietary Fiber (g.)
Breads		
Oatmeal	1 slice	2.4
Cracked wheat	1 slice	1.9
Mixed grain	1 slice	1.9
Pita, whole wheat	1 slice	1.5
Corn bread	1 cube (2")	1.4
Cereals, cold		
All Bran, w/extra fiber	½ cup	13.8
Fiber One	½ cup	11.9
All Bran	⅓ cup	8.6
Heartwise	1 cup	5.7
Raisin Bran	¾ cup	5.3
Benefit	¾ cup	5.0
Oat Bran Crunch	½ cup	4.6
40% Bran Flakes	⅔ cup	4.3
Shredded Wheat	⅔ cup	3.5
Oat Bran Cereal	¾ cup	2.9
Grape-Nuts	¼ cup	2.8
Nutri-Grain Wheat	⅔ cup	2.7
Cheerios	1¼ cup	2.5
Crispy Oats	½ cup	2.4
Wheat Flakes	¾ cup	2.3

Food	Portion	Dietary Fiber (g.)
Cereals, hot		
Corn bran, uncooked	⅓ cup	20.4
Wheat bran, uncooked	⅓ cup	8.2
Rice bran, uncooked	⅓ cup	5.6
Oat bran, uncooked	⅓ cup	4.0
Oatmeal, uncooked	⅓ cup	2.7
Fruits		
Avocado	½	4.8
Guava	1	4.7
Blackberries	¾ cup	3.7
Apricots, w/skin	4	3.5
Raspberries	1 cup	3.3
Figs	2	3.0
Gooseberries	¾ cup	2.9
Mango	½ sm.	2.9
Orange	1 sm.	2.9
Pear, w/skin	1 sm.	2.9
Apple, w/skin	1 sm.	2.8
Pomegranate	½	2.8
Plum, red	2 med.	2.4
Strawberries	1 cup	2.3
Banana	1 sm.	2.2
Applesauce, canned, unsweetened	½ cup	2.0
Peach, w/skin	1 med.	2.0
Rhubarb	1 cup	2.0
Nectarine, w/skin	1	1.8
Kiwifruit	1 lg.	1.7
Prunes	3 med.	1.7
Blueberries	¾ cup	1.4
Grapefruit, yellow	½ med.	1.4
Cantaloupe	1 cup cubes	1.1
Grains		
Wheat germ	3 Tbsp.	3.9
Barley, pearl, uncooked	2 Tbsp.	3.0
Rye flour	2½ Tbsp.	2.6
Whole wheat flour	2½ Tbsp.	2.1
Oat flour	2½ Tbsp.	1.8

Food	Portion	Dietary Fiber (g.)
Legumes		
Butter beans, dried, cooked	½ cup	6.9
Kidney beans, dark red, dried, cooked	½ cup	6.9
Navy beans, dried, cooked	½ cup	6.5
Black beans	½ cup	6.1
Pinto beans, dried, cooked	½ cup	5.9
Cranberry beans, dried, cooked	½ cup	5.4
Pork & beans, w/sauce, canned	½ cup	5.4
Lentils, dried, cooked	½ cup	5.2
Great Northern beans, dried, cooked	½ cup	5.0
Black-eyed peas, canned	½ cup	4.7
Chick-peas, dried, cooked	½ cup	4.3
Split peas, dried, cooked	½ cup	3.1
Nuts and Seeds		
Brazil nuts	¼ cup	2.0
Hazelnuts (filberts)	¼ cup	2.0
Peanut butter, smooth	2 Tbsp.	2.0
Sunflower seeds	¼ cup	2.0
Sesame seeds	2 Tbsp.	1.9
Chestnuts	¼ cup	1.8
Coconut, dried	1½ Tbsp.	1.5
Pasta and Tortillas		
Spaghetti, whole wheat, cooked	½ cup	2.7
Macaroni, whole wheat, cooked	½ cup	2.1
Tortilla, corn	1	1.4
Noodles, spinach, cooked	½ cup	1.1
Snacks		
Popcorn	3 cups	2.0
Whole wheat crackers	4 sm.	2.0

Food	Portion	Dietary Fiber (g.)
Snacks (continued)		
Graham crackers, oat bran	3 (2½″)	1.3
Matzos	1	1.0
Vegetables		
Turnips, cooked	½ cup	4.8
Okra, frozen	½ cup	4.1
Brussels sprouts, cooked	½ cup	3.8
Parsnips, cooked	½ cup	3.3
Celeriac	½ cup	3.1
Green beans, French, cooked	½ cup	2.8
Cabbage, red	1 cup	2.7
Sweet potato, cooked	⅓ cup	2.7
Kale, chopped, frozen	½ cup	2.5
Broccoli, cooked	½ cup	2.4
Corn on the cob, sweet, cooked	1 ear (6″)	2.4
Peas, green, cooked	½ cup	2.4
Carrots	1 (7½″)	2.3
Onion, chopped, cooked	½ cup	2.0
Asparagus, cooked	½ cup	1.8
Beets, cooked	½ cup	1.8
Eggplant	1 cup	1.8
Green pepper, chopped	1 cup	1.7
Bean sprouts	1 cup	1.6
Spinach, cooked	½ cup	1.6
Cabbage, green	1 cup	1.5
Potato	½ cup	1.5
Zucchini	1 cup	1.5
Leeks, sliced, cooked	½ cup	1.3
Endive	1 cup	1.1
Cauliflower, cooked	½ cup	1.0

Use Your Natural Rhythm

Eating lots of fiber may give your bowels the wherewithal to move, but there are a few other things you can do to facilitate their inclination to do so. One is to get some exercise. A sedentary lifestyle slows down the bowels, especially if you've been fairly active and then suddenly spend a lot of time simply sitting around, says Dr. Marshall.

The best time to exercise is when your gut is already moving. Your bowels have a natural rhythm that allows them to move food down through the digestive tract with wavelike propulsion, explains Dr. Marshall. That process takes place at least three times a day, generally right after you eat. It's strongest after breakfast, and if you exercise then, while your gut has this natural inclination to move, you can actually increase your body's propulsive abilities. Even a short walk will do the trick.

If you really want to get your bowels in a productive mode, you should eat breakfast, relax, then sit on the toilet and give those muscles a leisurely opportunity to do what they were made to do, suggests Edward Donatelle, M.D., professor of family medicine at the University of Kansas School of Medicine in Wichita. Yet another way to mobilize your bowels is to sit on the toilet regularly—at the same time every day. Just make sure you don't go for a walk, eat breakfast, and then talk on the phone for 20 minutes. Not heeding your body's own "call" will completely sabotage your efforts. Your bowels will hang up, and pain will be the only message they leave.

The Lowdown on Laxatives

If diet and exercise don't do the trick, you'll probably be tempted to do what Americans do to the tune of $400 million a year—purchase a laxative. Most doctors today discourage the use of laxatives because some kinds, when taken too often, can actually exacerbate constipation and damage the bowels. Regular use of stimulant laxatives, such as castor oil, senna, aloe, rhubarb, and cascara sagrada, can damage the nerves in the bowels and even flatten tiny intestinal structures that help you absorb nutrients from your food.

Fortunately, besides stimulant laxatives there are four other kinds: *bulk-forming* laxatives such as methylcellulose, polycarbophil, and psyllium; *hyperosmotic* laxatives such as lactulose, which is taken orally, and glycerin, which is taken rectally as a suppository; *saline* laxatives such as magnesium citrate, magnesium hydroxide, and mineral water; and *lubricant* laxatives such as mineral oil and stool softeners.

Doctors generally recommend bulk-forming laxatives. They work in the same way as fiber in the diet, and as long as they're taken with water, they're perfectly safe. People with diabetes should be aware that some over-the-counter brands contain up to 50 percent sugar, but others—Sugar-Free Metamucil, Fiberall powder, and Serutan—are available without added sugar. Either with or without sugar, a bulk-forming laxative should induce a bowel movement within 72 hours.

Hyperosmotic laxatives work by increasing water in the stool. Some are composed of nonabsorbable sugars—lactulose and sorbitol, for example—and they are particularly helpful, doctors say, in relieving chronic constipation. Some doctors feel that they are the "treatment of choice" for constipation when you have to stay in bed, and are second only to fiber in effectiveness among people who are up and about. They should induce a bowel movement within 48 hours.

Another kind of hyperosmotic laxative that works well is glycerin, which is used as a suppository. It causes the rectum to retain fluid and induces defecation within 30 minutes.

Saline laxatives also work fairly quickly—they usually bring about a bowel movement within 6 hours—but doctors say people with kidney problems should not use them.

Lubricants such as mineral oil usually take 6 to 8 hours to do the job. They should not be used on a regular basis, as they can prevent absorption of the fat-soluble vitamins

A, D, E, and K. And they should not be used at all, doctors say, by people who are taking anticoagulant (blood-thinning) drugs.

A stool softener may also prove helpful. This type of lubricant causes the stool to absorb an extra measure of water and fat, softening it and making it easier to pass. Be aware, however, that softeners can enhance the absorption of certain drugs you may be taking; doctors caution that the combination of stool softener plus the drug can cause toxic side effects.

Learning to Relax

None of the above is likely to work, however, if you have the kind of chronic constipation that is caused by difficulty in coordinating the pelvic muscles and anal sphincters that physically regulate a bowel movement.

If your doctor tells you that you fit this description, ask him or her about relaxation exercises in conjunction with biofeedback, says Dr. Marshall. In order to defecate, he explains, you must relax the appropriate muscles. If you have difficulty doing that, you may become constipated, but with a little training you may be able to put this problem behind you.

IRRITABLE BOWEL SYNDROME

Think back to the last time you felt grumpy and out of sorts. Maybe the weather was bad and you'd planned on going to the beach. Or perhaps your husband forgot your birthday. Or maybe someone at work said something mean. Whatever the source of your discontent, think about how you *felt*.

Everything kind of got on your nerves, didn't it? And the least little thing could set you off. The dog barked and you jumped out of your skin. Someone honked a horn as you were driving down the street and you almost ran up on a sidewalk.

Actually, the way you feel when you're grumpy and out of sorts is probably not unlike the way your insides feel when you have irritable bowel syndrome (IBS). The bowel is just as jumpy, twitchy, and, well, irritable; just like you, it overreacts to almost anything.

Give it a little extra fructose—the kind of sugar naturally found in fruit—and it twitches. Give it a little extra sorbitol—the sweetener found in everything from chewing gum to diet soda—and it goes into a spasm. Give it a little extra stress and it feels as though all 23 feet of it are trying to do a rumba.

Unfortunately, IBS is not defined only by its pain. It's defined also by the fact that its victims—who are responsible for 40 percent of all abdominal complaints to doctors—also have either diarrhea or constipation, or both.

If you're a woman with IBS, the hormones that trigger your period every month can also trigger diarrhea. Or hormones released while you're ovulating ten days later can cause constipation. Some women manage to hit the jackpot: They get both, plus an extra bonus of gas.

▶ INSTANT RELIEF

When your bowels get irritable and twitchy, there are a number of things you can do to calm them down.

Go to the bathroom. Passing gas or having a bowel movement frequently relieves the pain of IBS.

Relax. Relaxation techniques such as biofeedback can help relieve the pain, says Douglas Drossman, M.D., a professor of medicine and psychiatry in the Division of Digestive Diseases at the University of North Carolina at Chapel Hill.

▶ PREVENTION PAIN-RELIEF PROGRAM

Most people can handle IBS on their own, says Dr. Drossman. The key is to remember exactly what IBS is: a supersensitive gut that overreacts to a lot of different triggers—triggers that affect everybody else only minimally. As Dr. Drossman points out, "Diet, hormones, and stress are all factors that can affect intestinal function in everyone, but IBS people tend to have a greater response."

You need to get a handle on the particular triggers that cause *your* pain.

Put Your Pain in Writing

The first step in controlling IBS, says Dr. Drossman, is to keep a record for a couple of weeks that details when the pain and bowel symptoms occur. Whenever you experience pain, diarrhea, or constipation, jot down what you recently ate, whether or not you were arguing with someone, where you were in the past few hours, if you had just gotten your period—literally anything you suspect might be aggravating your gut.

Pay particular attention to your diet. The kinds of dietary items that frequently trigger IBS are high-fat foods, beans, cabbage, coffee, too much fruit (particularly apples, pears, and peaches), and, for the lactose intolerant, dairy products.

Dairy products should come under particular scrutiny, he adds, because after age 30 or 40, somewhere around 40 percent of the population becomes lactose intolerant. That means their body doesn't make enough of the enzyme (lactase) that digests the sugar found in milk (lactose). So instead of the lactose being speedily processed through the digestive system as happened in the past, it gets broken down in the gut and then just sits there, causing gas, cramps, and diarrhea.

How can you tell if you're lactose intolerant? Drink a glass of milk by itself, suggests Dr. Drossman. If you develop gas, cramps, and diarrhea within 30 minutes, you're intolerant.

Fiber Redirects the Pressures of IBS

The idea behind keeping track of IBS symptoms and related events is to identify the syndrome's triggers so you can eliminate them from your life, where possible, explains Dr. Drossman. That's easy enough to do when the culprits are foods. And if you've developed lactose intolerance, you can either eliminate dairy products from your diet or purchase the missing enzyme—under the name Lactaid—from your local drugstore. Take it right before you indulge in your favorite dairy foods. You can also mix it directly into a quart of milk.

Once you've eliminated dietary provocateurs from your life, though, you should also gradually increase the amount of fiber you eat until it ranges from 20 to 30 grams a day, says Dr. Drossman. How do you do that, exactly? He recommends adding a couple of bowls of all-bran cereal to your diet because its fiber—about 8 grams per serving—will help increase the bulk of your stool to fill the colon.

To understand how fiber prevents the pain and bowel symptoms of IBS, says Dr. Drossman, think of your bowels as a rubber hose. If a hose full of water is squeezed in a couple of places, pressure builds up in the middle until it stretches the walls of the hose itself.

Simple enough, right? That's precisely what happens to the bowels in someone with IBS. A spasm squeezes the bowels and causes the pressure inside to build until eventually the intestinal wall is stretched. When the bowel wall is stretched, it protests the only way it knows how: with wave after wave of pain.

If your intestine contains a large, bulky, fiber-filled stool, however, then the bowel spasm will create enough pressure to push the stool forward rather than stretch the bowels outward. That forward movement relieves the constipation frequently associated with IBS and reduces the pain as well.

Make Some Changes in Your Lifestyle

As any diary of IBS symptoms and related events will show, stress exacerbates the pain and bowel problems of those who have IBS. That's why anyone who has IBS really needs to learn what causes stress in their life and how it can be managed, says Dr. Drossman.

"If you discover a simple and specific stressor, you may want to take a look at it and see how you can change it," he suggests. Or if you're dealing with more of a generalized stress response—everyday hassles on the job make you tense, for example—regular use of relaxation techniques such as biofeedback, hypnosis, and meditation may help prevent it from having an impact on your bowel.

Also keep in mind that people who exercise regularly can tolerate the pain of IBS better than those who don't, adds Dr. Drossman. Exercise may work by simply reducing stress, but there also may be an added effect—the release of naturally occurring chemical painkillers in your brain. If you've just been sitting around with your pain, says Dr. Drossman, even walking for a couple of miles a day should provide some relief.

Help from the Doctor

In the long run, after the doctor has diagnosed your problem, self-generated treatments such as diet, stress relief, and exercise are far better than doctor-generated treatments, emphasizes Dr. Drossman. But once in a while someone with IBS hits a rough spot where the pain or bowel symptoms seem overwhelming. That's when a visit to the doctor is called for. A short-term prescription for a drug that stops spasms can help you over those rough spots and get you back on your feet and in control of both your bowels and your life.

For a small minority of people with IBS whose bowels react to daily stress, however, nothing seems to work. And for that particular group, Dr. Drossman recommends counseling.

There may be a biological reason for the bowels to overreact to diet, hormones, or stress. In addition, it is possible to condition the bowels to overreact to stress. Consider the child who reacts to life with his bowels, Dr. Drossman says. For example: A six-year-old boy is about to go to school for the first time. He's scared, and he's experiencing the same physiological response to fear that anyone might—sweating, cramps, diarrhea.

Should his parents put him to bed or send him to school? Well, if instead of addressing the *fear*, the parents address the *symptoms* and say, "If you have a tummyache, then you can't go to school. You can curl up on the sofa and watch television until you feel better," chances are very good that over a period of time the child will learn to react to anxiety-producing situations with abdominal pain. After all, if abdominal pain got him out of a fearful situation and into a comforting one as a child, why shouldn't it work when he's an adult?

None of this takes place on a conscious level, of course. If it did, people with this type of IBS would make the connection and stop the behavior. That's why Dr. Drossman suggests that people with IBS who find that stress makes their bowels worse may want to see a psychologist who can help them cope with their stress and, possibly, with their pain.

HEMORRHOIDS

Hemorrhoids are no respecters of status. Judges, truck drivers, jockeys—even baseball players and presidents—have all been forced to admit that, yes, they do spend a certain portion of their lives with a certain portion of their anatomy on a certain doughnut-shaped pillow from the drugstore.

"Hemorrhoids have inflicted pain equally on individuals at all levels of society for centuries," says Emmet F. Ferguson, Jr., M.D., a clinical professor of surgery at the University of Florida.

Yet despite their prevalence, no one knows what causes hemorrhoids to appear in the first place. Scientists do suspect, however, that "straining at stool"—pushing too hard when you're trying to have a bowel movement—may combine with certain genetic tendencies to cause the problem.

There are three elastic cushions of fibrous tissue attached to the internal sphincter muscle that act as a "valvelike stopper" at the anal opening, explains Dr. Ferguson. When you strain on the toilet, these cushions grow larger, the fibers attaching them to the sphincter stretch or break, and the cushions slide out of your anus. The *external* sphincter, at the anal orifice, closes behind the protruding cushions, effectively trapping the tissue outside the anus. It is now forever doomed to dangle just beyond safety as a hemorrhoid—pummeled, irritated, and definitely a nuisance.

Hemorrhoids are painful enough on their own. But if the hemorrhoid hasn't made it all the way to the outside and is stuck right between the internal and external sphincters, every once in a while a hard stool comes along and knocks its top off, leaving behind an open sore—a fissure. Fissures announce themselves with pain every time you move your bowels.

▶ INSTANT RELIEF

Most of the time hemorrhoids don't cause any discomfort. When they do, here are a few things you should do.

Apply a hot compress. Grab the nearest clean washcloth, run it under hot water, wring it out, and hold it against the hemorrhoid. The heat and moisture give some relief, says Dr. Ferguson.

Take a sitz bath. Sit in a warm, shallow bath for 15 to 20 minutes.

Reach for the Vaseline. Forget the expensive over-the-counter hemorrhoid medications at your local drugstore, says Dr. Ferguson. Suppositories, which just slip right past where they're needed and lodge in the rectum, are not as effective as cream ointments and petroleum jelly.

"I tell most of my patients that a jar of Vaseline often can accomplish as much as a $15 bottle of cream," says Dr. Ferguson with a chuckle. Just smear it on and wait for relief.

If the pain is accompanied by itching and burning, however, a hydrocortisone cream (like Cortaid) is better. It's only for occasional use, cautions Dr. Ferguson, since long overuse may cause atrophy of the skin.

➡ PREVENTION PAIN-RELIEF PROGRAM

Hemorrhoids have been helped and hurt by a wide variety of treatments down through the ages, says Dr. Ferguson. "Treatments vary all the way from the days of Hippocrates, when doctors applied a brutal hot iron cautery, to the Middle Ages, when the monks poured hot tallow through a hollow reed into the rectum, with some relief and grief."

But don't be too hard on our ancestral doctors, he advises. When the cause of something is not known, it's hard to devise an effective treatment. That's why many hemorrhoid treatments—including some developed by reputable scientists—have joined hot irons and tallow in medical obscurity. "Treatments rendering short-term relief do not necessarily give long-term cures," says Dr. Ferguson.

Keep It Simple

"Most hemorrhoids can be treated simply with diet and office treatments such as injection and banding, rather than surgery," says Dr. Ferguson.

A high-fiber diet may prevent straining at stool, he says, since it produces soft stool that is easily propelled through the rectum. Cultured buttermilk, yogurt, and sweet acidophilus milk added to your diet will encourage stool-softening "friendly" bacteria in the colon.

If hemorrhoids remain painful, injection and banding are two treatments that may eliminate troublesome symptoms, says Dr. Ferguson. In the doctor's office, the hemorrhoid is tied off with a rubber band and then injected with phenol and almond oil, a treatment that prevents the band from slipping off, or with local anesthesia.

The result? In a study of 95 selected adults, all of their hemorrhoids sloughed off and the patients became symptom-free. Five had pain of varying degrees for a few days after the procedure, and one had some bleeding that required another visit to the doctor's office.

A second procedure that doctors sometimes use is infrared coagulation, says Dr. Ferguson. It's probably just as effective as injection and banding, but the procedure itself—in which several infrared beams are aimed inside the anus to burn an internal hemorrhoid—may generate a considerable amount of pain in a certain number of patients.

Outright surgery is a third option, says Dr. Ferguson. It was once used to treat about 50 percent of all hemorrhoids, but today it's usually reserved for those who have hemorrhoids that are far advanced, with severe protrusion, bleeding, irritation, and soilage. Less than 10 percent of patients suffering from hemorrhoids that are seen in a doctor's office require surgery, since banding handles most hemorrhoids effectively.

This type of surgery—usually referred to as a *hemorrhoidectomy*—requires a night in the hospital. It involves some pain and a week or so of mild anal incontinence, says Dr. Ferguson.

Ninety-eight percent of those undergoing the procedure remain free of hemorrhoidal symptoms for the rest of their life. Even with surgery, though, hemorrhoids may return if their owners continue to strain on the toilet.

A word about lasers: The laser is just another tool for

cutting or destroying tissue. It sounds high-tech, but laser hemorrhoidectomies have no advantage over those using electrocautery techniques or other methods of cutting, says Dr. Ferguson.

DIVERTICULITIS

Diverticula are tiny bulges of the inner lining of your intestinal tract that have poked through the intestinal wall to form protuberances along the outside of your colon. Although this state of affairs sounds pretty gruesome, it's usually not even painful.

Around 65 percent of all adults will have many of these protuberances by the time they're 85, says Atilla Ertan, M.D., professor and chief of gastroenterology at Tulane University Medical Center in New Orleans. Although most people remain blissfully ignorant of the fact that their internal topography has undergone a change, between 10 and 25 percent go on to develop *diverticulitis*, a condition in which one of those tiny protuberances becomes inflamed and begins to hurt.

Since most diverticula tend to form on the left side of your colon, the pain is generally felt on the left lower side of your abdomen, says Dr. Ertan. This pain has been known to switch back and forth, however. No one understands exactly what ignites the pain, but scientists who have looked inside the colon during an attack have noticed that the more inflammation they see, the more pain the patient reports.

▶ INSTANT RELIEF

There really is no instant relief for diverticulitis. Once the pain begins, eat nothing, drink only clear liquids, and see your doctor immediately, says Dr. Ertan. Your doctor will probably run a bunch of tests that may include a blood test, x-rays, and a CAT scan. He or she may also want to examine the colon with a long, flexible tube called an endoscope.

▶ PREVENTION PAIN-RELIEF PROGRAM

Just because you've had one attack of diverticulitis doesn't mean you have to have another. "There seems to be a tendency for high-fiber diets to reduce the frequency of recurrence of diverticulitis and its complications," says Dr. Ertan. So once you've recovered from an initial bout of diverticulitis, bulk up your diet with vegetables, fruits, and whole grain breads and cereals.

You also should drink lots of water. "It's a very bad habit in this society, but people don't drink water," adds Dr. Ertan. "They should drink 1½ to 2 liters [about 2 quarts] of water every day." Water and a high-fiber diet lubricate the intestinal tract, he points out, and facilitate defecation. Besides, adding bulk to your diet without water can cause the very problems you're trying to avoid.

Should diverticulitis strike a second time, however, your doctor will put you through your paces with tests once again. If you pass—if the tests reveal that there is no serious infection, abscess, perforation, or bleeding from diverticulitis—you'll probably be told to go home, go to bed, and give your gut a rest for several days. That means no food, only clear liquids to drink, and a prescription for oral antibiotics, says Dr. Ertan.

If you flunk, however—if the tests reveal the presence of a serious infection, an abscess, or any other complication—you'll probably be admitted to the hospital. There doctors will give you intravenous broad-spectrum antibiotics for four to seven days, deny you food or drink, and try to resolve whatever complications that have developed.

Do You Need Surgery?

In some cases such a resolution may require surgery. If you've developed a fistula—a tubelike passageway that causes one section of bowel to stick to another or perhaps even to your bladder—you must have surgery to correct it, says Dr. Ertan. If you've had three or four disabling attacks of diverticulitis within the course of a single year, your doctor may suggest that you have a section of your colon patched or removed.

You may also need surgery if antibiotics and rest don't work, if your diverticula burst—yes, just like an overinflated balloon—or if they've formed an abscess, says Dr. Ertan. In the case of an abscess, however, a new procedure—percutaneous drainage—is being developed that may well replace the need for surgery. In this procedure, explains Dr. Ertan, a large needlelike device is inserted into the abdomen to drain the abscess. The procedure, he cautions, should be performed only by an experienced doctor in a medical center where this type of procedure has been done before.

GAS

Whether your body produces a belch or flatulence is purely a question of geography.

You belch after you swallow air into the upper reaches of your digestive system, says Harris Clearfield, M.D., chief of gastroenterology at Hahnemann Hospital in Philadelphia. Belches consist of oxygen and nitrogen, the same as the air we breathe, and are an unfortunate side effect of drinking carbonated beverages, sucking on hard candies, chewing gum, eating rapidly, or having ill-fitting dentures that force you to keep them in place by sucking them back into line.

Flatulence is an unfortunate side effect of swallowed air plus bacterial action on the food in your colon, specifically the fibrous carbohydrates that were not absorbed earlier in the digestive process. After a while, these undigested leftovers start to ferment. As in any fermentation process, whether it produces beer, bread, or flatulence, the result is gas.

➡ INSTANT RELIEF

One thing is for certain: No matter where gas finds its exit, it may hurt you before it gets there. You may want to reach for relief at the first sign of bubble or gurgle.

Try an antacid. Antacids can reduce the carbon dioxide component of gas that's produced in your upper intestine.

Take it easy. If swallowed air is causing pain, doctors say, eating slowly may be your answer.

Swallow some charcoal. Purified charcoal, a special steam-treated variety that's available at your drugstore, may absorb intestinal gas when taken after a meal. It also absorbs any drugs you may be taking, however, so doctors suggest you don't use it within 2 hours of taking medication.

Reach for the Pink. The active ingredient in Pepto-Bismol is a bacteria-inhibiting agent called bismuth subsalicylate. In the lab—and presumably in your stomach—it prevents bacteria from fermenting foods that ignite your internal gasworks. Doctors say Pepto-Bismol may help shut down production.

➤ PREVENTION PAIN-RELIEF PROGRAM

Getting rid of gas once you have it can prove pretty tricky. The idea is to prevent the formation of gas in the first place, says Dr. Clearfield.

Look at what you're eating and swallowing. If you're drinking three Cokes a day, chewing gum, and (good for you) trying to eat more fiber, it's no wonder you're a one-man band.

There's also the question of what's "normal," he adds. One study demonstrated that a healthy young American male passes gas approximately 14 times a day. So unless you're passing gas more than 18 times a day, says Dr. Clearfield, don't worry about it. If gas pain continues to plague you, see your doctor. He or she should rule out the possibility that some other digestive complaint, irritable bowel syndrome, for example, may be at the root of your problem. Your doctor can also help you figure out where the gas is coming from.

Should you reduce the amount of fibrous carbohydrate in your diet? Probably not, says Dr. Clearfield. Besides, if you've added fiber to your diet gradually rather than trying to down a box of bran within a week, it really shouldn't cause much of a problem. You should, however, avoid gas-forming foods such as cabbage, cauliflower, broccoli, brussels sprouts, and baked beans. Milk can also cause gas in people who are sensitive to it. (See "Fiber Facts" on page 14.)

GASTROENTERITIS

Do your intestines feel like they're processing a pot of Mexican chili . . . and all you had was a bland seafood salad? You may have gastroenteritis.

Gastroenteritis is the $12 word your doctor uses when your stomach and intestines are inflamed, says John R. Montgomery, M.D., an infectious disease specialist and chief of pediatrics at the University of Alabama in Huntsville.

The inflammation is usually ignited by an infection—bacteria, parasites, and viruses are common causes of it—or by medications such as antibiotics, cancer drugs, and aspirin. Even heavy-duty iron supplements can act like an incendiary device, adds Dr. Montgomery.

A particularly notorious cause of inflammation is food contaminated with staphylococci. These bacteria form a toxin in the food, and once you've eaten it, food poisoning is the likely result, explains Dr. Montgomery.

Your body, however, does not take any of these intestinal invaders lying down. While it's processing the contaminated food in a heroic attempt to move the invader out of your body as fast as possible, your entire intestinal tract contracts harder and faster than it ever has before. These contractions cause pain and the unfortunate diarrhea that always seems to go along with it.

If the pain seems to be connected to any medication you may be taking, check with your doctor. He or she should be able to switch medications, thus providing quick relief.

▶ INSTANT RELIEF

Once food poisoning sets your stomach on fire, there's not much you can do to speed healing—your body is already expelling the invading bacteria. There are, however, a few things you can do to make yourself a little more comfortable for the duration.

Seek heat. Curl yourself around a heating pad or hot

water bottle, suggests Dr. Montgomery. The warmth may help minimize the cramping.

Drink plenty of fluids. If the inflammation is mild—and if the pain is mild, the inflammation frequently is—then rest, lots of fluids, and time will take care of gastroenteritis, says Dr. Montgomery. The best fluids to drink are Gatorade, chicken broth, and 7-Up, he adds, because they all contain either potassium or sodium to replenish some of the nutrients that you're losing through diarrhea.

► PREVENTION PAIN-RELIEF PROGRAM

If the inflammation is severe—if you have severe cramping pain in combination with six to ten bowel movements a day, blood in the stool, weight loss, fever, or faintness—then you need to see your doctor, says Dr. Montgomery. Your doctor will run a series of tests—stool cultures and blood tests, for example—to determine the specific cause of the inflammation and then treat you with the medicinal missile designed to eradicate the problem, if one is available. Not all causes have a specific treatment.

If the inflammation is caused, for example, by *E. coli*, common bacteria that frequently thrive on the hands of people who don't wash after using the toilet and in many untreated drinking water supplies, your doctor may prescribe an antibiotic such as Neomycin, says Dr. Montgomery. Or your doctor may suggest a dose of Pepto-Bismol every 30 minutes for no more than eight doses, tops.

In any case, do not take an antidiarrheal medicine without your doctor's approval, adds Dr. Montgomery. Most of these drugs slow the intestine's contractions. That may relieve your pain for the moment, he points out, but since the point of contractions is to eject the invader, stopping them allows the bacteria to remain in place and even multiply. You'll wind up with more inflammation, more pain, and a longer recovery than if you hadn't used the medication.

Watch Your Food

You might also want to avoid fatty foods and dairy products such as milk, ice cream, and cheese when you're having a bout of gastroenteritis, says Dr. Montgomery. High-fat foods trigger the wave-like intestinal contractions necessary for digestion. Normally that's not a problem; but when your intestine is already cramping from gastroenteritis, the increased action may well double you over in agony.

It's not easy to prevent the recurrence of gastroenteritis when you probably aren't even sure which bug caused the flare-up. But simply because food poisoning is so easy to get from your own kitchen, Dr. Montgomery suggests that as a general precaution, you regularly disinfect all kitchen surfaces and cutting boards with bleach. He also suggests that you avoid raw eggs, cook chicken and turkey at high temperatures, and never put cooked meat back on the plate that held it when it was raw. As unbelievable as it sounds, says Dr. Montgomery, failing to follow this third practice is actually a major cause of food poisoning.

GALLSTONES

Most of the time gallstones behave themselves. They sit quietly in the gallbladder or go along for the ride whenever your gallbladder squirts bile into the upper intestine to help you digest some food.

Occasionally, one gets too big for its britches and decides to make a move—and it gets stuck, either near or partway through the duct that connects the gallbladder and intestine. And from that moment until the stone either moves back into the gallbladder, moves forward into the intestine, or is removed by a surgeon, you will experience absolute agony. The pain, which is so specific that doctors find diagnosis a snap, is centered either in the upper right quadrant of the abdomen or, because the pain is referred along a nerve, in the back at the edge of the right shoulder blade.

Gallstones are generally a disorder of cholesterol metabolism, says Hans Fromm, M.D., director of the Gastroenterology Division at George Washington University Medical Center. A genetic predisposition combines with naturally occurring or supplemental estrogen—birth control pills, for example—and too many calories, increasing the secretion of cholesterol from your liver.

The excess cholesterol, which is mixed with the liver's bile and then stored in your gallbladder, forms soft clumps that eventually harden into stones that can be troublesome in the extreme.

Unfortunately, the motion of a stone through the bile duct can also irritate the pancreas and cause pancreatitis, says Dr. Fromm. And since the pancreas and gallbladder empty into the same duct in most of us, on occasion a stone can cause the pancreatic juices, which were on their way to digest your food, to back up in the duct. The result is that they digest your pancreas instead.

➤ INSTANT RELIEF

From a scientific viewpoint, there really is no instant relief, unless your doctor has prescribed a painkiller for a previous attack.

Press and pray. People who have had stones, however, report that when the pain is referred to the shoulder blade, pressing on the spot where it hurts offers a considerable amount of relief.

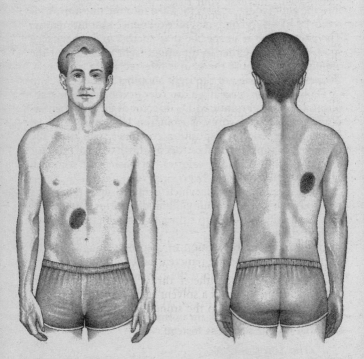

When a gallstone gets stuck in the duct, pain can occur in either of the two shaded areas shown above. Some people report that pressing on the spot on the shoulder blade where it hurts can relieve pain.

▶ PREVENTION PAIN-RELIEF PROGRAM

Once you've got gallstones, you can be comforted by the fact that any attack of pain is transitory, says Dr. Fromm. Complications are uncommon, but the attacks may take anywhere from a few minutes to several hours to subside. You may never have a second attack, although generally, gallstones continue to be a problem until you have them dissolved or removed.

Cholesterol-lowering drugs and dieting may seem like logical treatments, but in some instances, both drugs and diets actually increase your risk of forming stones.

So what are your options?

"Some doctors are not informed and push unnecessary surgery," cautions Dr. Fromm. But "treatment is always the patient's choice," and you should study your options carefully, he notes.

If your stones are small and made of pure cholesterol and you have no other complications, a stone-dissolving drug such as ursodiol (Actigall) may do the trick, says Dr. Fromm. It may take up to a year to dissolve the stones, he adds, but for people who want to avoid surgery and can handle the cost—around $1,300 for a year's supply of the drug—it's an excellent option.

If you have medium-sized stones, lithotripsy—a high-tech procedure that relies on a form of shock waves—can be used with ursodiol to shatter the stones. The fragments then pass into the intestine and out of your body.

If you have large stones, or a lot of smaller ones, your doctor may be able to dissolve them with the direct application of a chemical. Generally, explains Dr. Fromm, the doctor inserts a tiny catheter through the liver into the gallbladder, then applies a solvent such as methyl tertbutyl ether (MTBE) directly to the stones.

The Surgical Option

If you have any complications—jaundice, pancreatitis, or stones that contain calcium salts, for example—you may need to have the gallbladder itself removed, says Dr. Fromm.

The traditional surgery, a cholecystectomy, involves four to six days in the hospital, up to six weeks of recovery time, a 6-inch scar across the upper abdomen, a considerable amount of pain, and a lot of heavy-duty painkillers.

A newer type of surgery—laparoscopic cholecystectomy— involves one day in the hospital, one week of recovery, four small incisions, and perhaps a few days of pain-relief medication.

Which procedure is right for you? There is no definitive answer. Laparoscopic surgery, a procedure in which several thin instruments and needles are inserted into the abdomen and the gallbladder is withdrawn, is being touted as such a revolution in gallstone treatment that at least one medical consultant has said that not only will it become the gallstone "treatment of choice," but surgeons unable to do it will be out of the gallbladder removal business within the year.

But Dr. Fromm feels it needs further study. Laparoscopy is a relatively new technique, he points out, and its safety as a method for gallbladder removal has simply not yet been ascertained. And with reports emerging of complications and fatalities, it has a long way to go before it wins at least his seal of approval.

Preventing a Recurrence

One of the advantages of having your gallbladder removed, by whatever method, is that you'll never have to worry about gallstones again. But with other treatments, you do. For people who have their stones dissolved with ursodiol and then stop taking the drug, for example, the recurrence rate is between 30 and 50 percent.

Fortunately, you may be able to prevent a recurrence by taking ursodiol indefinitely, says Dr. Fromm. The drug is actually a bile acid, and long-term use is unlikely to cause any problems; but doctors generally don't mention this option because of the cost.

Eating more fiber and vegetables may also prevent gallstones, as might—believe it or not—drinking a small amount of alcohol.

A joint study of almost 88,000 nurses by researchers at Brandeis University and the Harvard Medical School suggests that vegetables, fiber, and alcohol may all affect gallstone formation in women by reducing the amount of cholesterol in bile. The study also indicates that contrary to popular thinking, the amount of animal fat and cholesterol in your diet has nothing to do with whether or not you get gallstones.

Scientists are also looking into other strategies that may reduce the odds of recurrence: Anti-inflammatory drugs such as aspirin have prevented the formation of stones in laboratory animals, for example, and at least one study of humans indicates that large daily doses of it—around 1,300 milligrams—may do so in people as well.

Watch That Weight Loss

One of the newest strategies scientists are using to prevent gallstones has to do with the way you diet. Weight loss increases your risk of gallstones so significantly, says Dr. Fromm, that doctors are now recommending that you take ursodiol whenever you go on a diet.

"Even losing a small amount of weight can induce the formation," he adds, and the formation is fairly rapid. In one study, scientists found that 26 percent of those who went on a rapid weight-loss diet developed gallstones within the first three months. Significantly, a second group, which went on the diet *and* took ursodiol, had absolutely none.

HEARTBURN

That "burning sensation" may be the featured player on a series of television commercials, but if it's a featured player in your life, it's no joke, particularly if it occurs after every meal or whenever you lie down.

Heartburn, or gastroesophageal reflux, as doctors like to call it, is the pain you feel as the contents of your stomach back up into your esophagus, says Donald O. Castell, M.D., director of the Division of Gastroenterology and Hepatology at Jefferson Medical College in Philadelphia. The major component of those contents is acid, and if it feels like it can strip bark off a tree, well, that's not too far from the truth.

Cause Unknown

"We don't know exactly what causes the pain," says Dr. Castell. "There are chemically sensitive nerve endings throughout the GI [gastrointestinal] tract, so we postulate that what the acid does is stimulate these chemoreceptors."

What makes your stomach squirt its contents back into the esophagus in the first place? Doctors used to blame a lot of heartburn on a hiatal hernia, a condition in which a part of the stomach accidentally slips through the lower esophageal opening. But today—now that modern radiology has demonstrated that the hernia is present in a lot of people who don't ever get heartburn—doctors are not quite so eager to cite hiatal hernia as a cause.

"In the United States where it's very common, most of this reflux is related to the things that people do," explains Dr. Castell. They eat too much food at one meal, or the meal may contain too much fat. Or they may have a drink before dinner and a cigarette afterward. Or they may lie down after they eat.

Too much food, too much fat, alcohol, cigarette smoke, and lying down all tend to relax the lower esophageal sphincter (LES)—a small ring of muscle that normally acts as a barrier between the stomach and esophagus. And when the LES is relaxed, it's easy for any meal to do an instant replay of its trip down your esophagus—in reverse, of course.

▶ INSTANT RELIEF

Fortunately, there are a lot of things you can do to keep that acid under control and where it belongs.

Swallow. Your saliva contains a naturally occurring bicarbonate that can neutralize the acid that causes heartburn, says Dr. Castell. So just swallowing will help your body smother the flames.

Reach for the algae-covered antacid. All antacids are pretty much the same when it comes to relieving heartburn, says Dr. Castell. But there's a new kid on the block that stands head and shoulders above the rest for relieving daytime heartburn—Gaviscon, an over-the-counter antacid mixed with alginic acid, a derivative of brown algae.

In a small study conducted by Dr. Castell and colleagues at the Bowman Gray School of Medicine in North Carolina, ten volunteers were first fed a heartburn-provoking meal of sausage, egg, and biscuit and then given either Gaviscon or another antacid with equal acid-neutralizing capacity. The volunteers also took the antacids 1 hour later, 2 hours later, and 3 hours later.

The result? The volunteers who took Gaviscon had nearly two-thirds fewer episodes of acid reflux. And the duration of these episodes was a third less than those of the other antacid takers.

▶ PREVENTION PAIN-RELIEF PROGRAM

To get rid of "that burning sensation" for good, says Dr. Castell, make it a practice to eat smaller meals that are low in fat. Keep your weight within normal limits, and avoid both cigarette smoke and alcohol. You should also avoid any particular food—coffee, chocolate, or peppermint, for example—that seems to trigger heartburn.

Nocturnal heartburn, which is frequently not relieved by any antacid, can be avoided by putting 6-inch blocks under the head of your bed. This will elevate the upper portion of your body slightly, allowing gravity to help keep the acidic contents of your stomach down where they belong. You also should not lie down within 3 hours of eating. And when you do lie down, adds Dr. Castell, don't lie on your right side. Preliminary results from his studies indicate that sleeping on your right side may make nocturnal heartburn worse.

If heartburn strikes despite all your precautions, go ahead and reach for an antacid, says Dr. Castell. But if even that doesn't smother your burning esophageal embers, check with your doctor. He or she can prescribe for you a member of the new generation of acid-suppressing drugs—ranitidine (Zantac), for example—that can actually heal your esophagus of past burns while it prevents future fires.

ULCERS

Stressed-out executives often worry that they'll get an ulcer. And sometimes they do. But the fact of the matter is that the ulcer may not have anything to do with being an executive or even with being stressed out.

Nobody has yet figured out what causes ulcers, says David Graham, M.D., a professor of medicine at Baylor College of Medicine in Texas and president of the American College of Gastroenterology.

Some ulcers seem to be induced by the chronic use of nonsteroidal anti-inflammatory drugs (NSAIDs) such as Motrin and aspirin. Others seem to be triggered by an infection from a bacterium such as *Helicobacter pylori*. Still others seem to form when there's too much acid secreted by the stomach—a condition that, in some cases, may be inherited. And smoking aggravates any ulcer, no matter what got it started.

Typically, ulcer pain begins to gnaw at your abdomen 1 to 3 hours after a meal, when the acids secreted by your stomach begin to build up, doctors say. It may also wake you in the early morning hours.

Older folks who have ulcers may have vague pain or no discomfort at all. They should be aware, however, that if the ulcer becomes large, their symptoms may suddenly include vomiting, heartburn, difficulty swallowing, chest pain, or an arthritis-type ache in the left shoulder rather than stomach pain.

▶ INSTANT RELIEF

Relief from ulcer pain really involves keeping stomach acid under control.

Fight the acid. Eat something or take an antacid, doctors suggest.

➡️ PREVENTION PAIN-RELIEF PROGRAM

Getting rid of an ulcer is not terribly difficult for most
people. Two equally effective treatments, says Dr. Graham, are a regimen of antacids and a run of potent acid-
suppressing drugs prescribed by your doctor—with the last
daily dose taken between 6:00 and 8:00 P.M. to control
nighttime corrosion. It usually takes four to six weeks for
the ulcer to heal.

If your ulcer doesn't respond to antacids or acid-
suppressing drugs, however, or if it recurs right after it's
supposed to have been healed, your doctor may suggest
that he or she take a peek inside your stomach using a long,

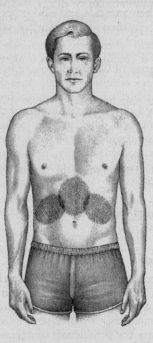

*A gnawing or burning pain in any of these three shaded areas can indicate
an ulcer.*

flexible tube called an endoscope. With the instrument in place, he or she just might take a snippet of tissue from the surrounding area to look at under the microscope.

One of the things for which your doctor will be looking is that obnoxious bug called *Helicobacter pylori*. It is apparently present in 95 percent of ulcers that appear in the duodenum (the upper intestine) and in 70 percent of ulcers that appear in the stomach.

Some researchers feel that this type of bacteria is the single cause for all ulcers that are not triggered by NSAIDs; other researchers feel it causes only a certain percentage. However, an international team of gastroenterologists, including Dr. Graham, has agreed that the bug is likely to be the problem when antacids and acid-suppressing drugs don't seem to be doing their job, particularly when the ulcer is located in the upper intestine.

The gastroenterologists' recommendation, issued at the 1990 World Congress of Gastroenterology, is that doctors prescribe a two-week regimen of triple-drug therapy when this occurs: one tablet of bismuth subsalicylate (Pepto-Bismol) four times a day, 500 milligrams of the antibiotic tetracycline four times a day, and 400 milligrams of the antibacterial metronidazole (Flagyl) three times a day.

A similar drug regimen used by Australian researchers in a large study eradicated the bacteria and cured 94 percent of those with ulcers.

Keeping the Ulcer Away

But even with medicine's biggest guns blasting away, the chances that an ulcer will eventually return are still high. Between 60 and 90 percent recur within one year.

Typically doctors try several approaches to keep the tiny craters from punching out the lining of your stomach or upper intestine a second time. A high-fiber diet, for example, may prove something of a deterrent, as may avoiding foods that stimulate the production of excess acid—cola-type sodas, wine, beer, and both regular and decaffeinated coffee.

Some people also may benefit from learning how to put a positive spin on life. People who have what scientists call a "negative perception of life events" tend to produce more stomach acid. Others may find that learning how to reduce the amount of emotional stress in their lives will help.

And, of course, you should avoid NSAIDs. Not only have they been found to induce the formation of ulcers, but their association with life-threatening complications such as bleeding is, as one researcher concluded, "alarming."

If you've been taking NSAIDs to relieve arthritis pain, then low-dose corticosteroids or an acetaminophen preparation such as Tylenol may provide a short-term alternative, doctors say. If these alternatives don't work and you really need to stay on NSAIDs, your doctor may suggest you take another drug such as misoprostol along with an NSAID to buffer its ulcer-provoking effects.

If your ulcer flares up more than two or three times a year, your doctor may also suggest you stay on a maintenance dose of antacids and acid-suppressing drugs, says Dr. Graham. If ulcers cause only an occasional twinge—as long as you're not elderly or coping with complications—you can just take the medication on an as-needed basis, he says.

INFLAMMATORY BOWEL DISEASE

Imagine pulling out your intestines, shooting them full of holes, drenching them with acid, putting them back inside, and then asking them to digest a six-course meal. That's what people with inflammatory bowel disease (IBD) may well suspect was done with their intestines one dark and stormy night while they were asleep.

A slight exaggeration, right? Maybe. But the fact is that when the inflammation that characterizes IBD sets fire to your gut, the result is craters, abscesses, dead spots, internal bleeding, and swelling so severe that it can interfere with children's growth and set the stage for osteoporosis and cancer in old age.

Unfortunately, no one knows what causes the inflammation of IBD, says Stephan Targan, M.D., director of the Inflammatory Bowel Disease Center at UCLA. Historically, scientists first thought it was one disease and then decided it was two: When the inflammation occurs along a single stretch of colon—the left side in 75 percent of those it affects—it's called ulcerative colitis; when it occurs in patchy segments anywhere along the digestive tract from mouth to anus, it's called Crohn's disease.

But now the emerging concept of IBD is that it's actually several diseases, says Dr. Targan. There may be two kinds of ulcerative colitis, for example, and two kinds of Crohn's. What unites them all, however, is the underlying inflammatory process that, whatever its cause, disrupts people's lives with intense episodes of pain and diarrhea—every time they eat, in some cases.

➡ **INSTANT RELIEF**

There is no instant relief. You'll need to see a doctor to deal with the pain of IBD.

► PREVENTION PAIN-RELIEF PROGRAM

Removing the colon cures ulcerative colitis, says Dr. Targan, but it's such an extreme way to deal with the disease that doctors generally prefer to reserve surgery for dealing with complications like obstructions, adhesions, and perforations. And if a surgeon removes a piece of bowel from someone with Crohn's disease, the inflammation just pops up again somewhere else. That's why relieving the inflammation is a better way to handle IBD, says Dr. Targan.

The initial treatment for mild to moderate IBD is sulfasalazine, a drug that was discovered in the 1940s, he adds. Unfortunately, a full one-third of those who try sulfasalazine can't take the drug because of sensitivity to the drug or allergic reactions to the part of the drug that transports it to the colon. So scientists have recently stripped the allergy-provoking part of the drug away—leaving its active ingredient, 5-aminosalicylic acid, intact. The result is a new drug called olsalazine sodium. And although it's not perfect, a study of 62 people who were intolerant of sulfasalazine revealed that the new drug relieved the symptoms of IBD in 35 percent of those who took it. Its major side effect, diarrhea, can be relieved by not taking the drug on an empty stomach, according to the drug's manufacturer.

This powerful medication can also be applied topically through a retention enema in those who have inflammation limited to the rectum and left side of the colon, says Dr. Targan. In some cases the enemas themselves can trigger a cramping pain, but that can be avoided, says Dr. Targan, by preceding the enema with oral sulfasalazine. Enemas can also be used on a daily basis—maybe even an alternating daily basis—to bank the fires of IBD and prevent a relapse.

If you don't respond to 5-aminosalicylic acid, your doctor may prescribe corticosteroids or an immunosuppressant drug such as 6-mercaptopurine, says Dr. Targan.

Nutritional Support

Although some doctors suggest fasting or eating a low-fiber diet during an active attack of IBD, modifying the diet has never been shown to help reduce the inflammation itself, says Dr. Targan. But some people with IBD seem to have one or more nutritional triggers that set off an incendiary bomb in their gut. If there's a particular food—or even an environmental insult such as stress—that seems to turn up the volume on your IBD symptoms, avoid it as much as possible.

You should also pay particularly close attention to getting adequate amounts of vitamins and minerals in your diet, doctors suggest, since the diarrhea that accompanies IBD—particularly Crohn's disease—can create a deficiency of folate. Sulfasalazine therapy is also associated with folate deficiency.

Check with your doctor to see if your intake is adequate of if you need to take a supplement.

IS IT APPENDICITIS?

The pain in your right side is sharp and hot. And it refuses to go away. Could it be appendicitis?

Even your doctor may have trouble reaching a decision. Studies indicate that between 25 and 50 percent of all diagnoses made primarily on the basis of abdominal pain are incorrect, and between 20 and 30 percent of those who undergo surgery for appendicitis do not have the disease at all.

The problem is not your doctor's competence. It's the difficulty in distinguishing an inch or two of inflamed tissue at a curve in your intestinal tract from any of the myriad other conditions and diseases that can cause similar symptoms, especially in women: heavy periods, pelvic inflammatory disease, ectopic pregnancies, ovarian cysts, diverticulitis, and the onset of Crohn's disease, among others.

The pain of appendicitis can be particularly misleading because its characteristics change over time. It generally comes on gradually around the stomach and above the belly button as the appendix begins to swell. The pain begins mildly, then increases in intensity for about 4 hours. If the appendix bursts and your body walls off the resulting life-threatening infection into a small area, the pain may subside and then localize over the appendix in the right lower part of your abdomen. But if the infection becomes more generalized, the pain can spread across the entire abdomen.

And, of course, this is all assuming that your appendix is where it's supposed to be. In some people, the intestine to which the tiny organ is attached may not be quite where your doctor expects it, and neither is the pain.

Other diagnostic clues: Loss of appetite and nausea usually follow the onset of pain, and on occasion, a low-grade fever will be present.

If you have any reason to suspect your appendix is acting up, check with your doctor. Blood tests, urine tests, x-rays, and CAT scans are some of the tools the doctor may use to figure out what's going on. He or she will also check your abdomen for any lumps or tenderness and probably do a rectal exam as well. If you're a woman, you can count on a pelvic examination, too.

But there are no specific tests or exams that will tell you, "Yes, you've got appendicitis." So once your doctor has ruled out as many other causes of abdominal pain as possible, he or she may suggest a trip to the operating room. No one will know for sure that you have appendicitis until the doctor takes a peek inside your abdomen. And current medical thinking is that you're in far more danger from undiagnosed appendicitis than you are from a relatively safe surgical procedure.

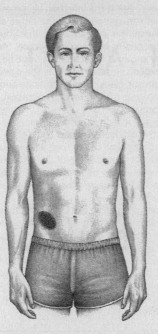

Is that tummyache appendicitis? The pain of appendicitis generally increases in severity over several hours. It generally starts in the area of the belly button. It may then subside and settle in the lower right abdomen.

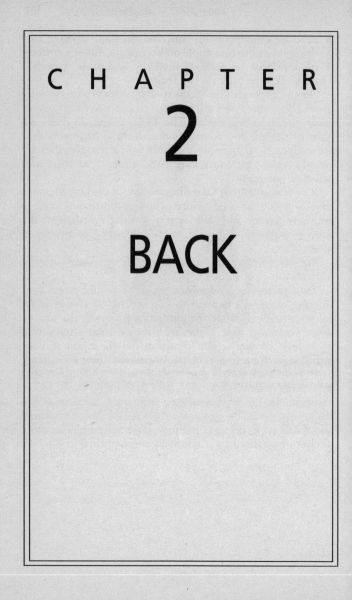

C H A P T E R

2

BACK

saac Newton probably suffered no pain when a tree dropped its historic apple on his noggin. But it's entirely possible that he grabbed his back and said "Yowch!" when he bent to pick up the fruit.

Hardly anybody else seems to escape back pain, so why should Newton? After all, four out of every five backs were made wrong to begin with. The 33 vertebrae, 23 disks, 31 pairs of nerves, and countless muscles and ligaments that are supposed to support the back were put together by genetic codes that must have had "misery" as their first order of business.

It's no wonder that 80 million people in the United States have a back that needs more propping up than a savings and loan association. Nor is it a wonder that half of the adult population is in pain from their back at any given moment.

But poor workmanship in the embryonic shop isn't the only reason your back hurts.

Thoughtlessness is another big reason—like never considering what will happen to you when you shovel snow off your sidewalk after spending an autumn by the fire, or when you bowl nine games in a tournament after sitting at a desk all week. The resulting muscle strain is your punishment for using your back without using your head.

If your back hurts, don't jump to the conclusion that something is seriously wrong, says Richard A. Deyo, M.D., associate professor of medicine and health services at the University of Washington in Seattle. Disks do get ruptured and spinal cords do sustain injury, but back pain is far more likely to be caused by a relatively minor problem.

PAIN-FINDER CHART FOR THE BACK

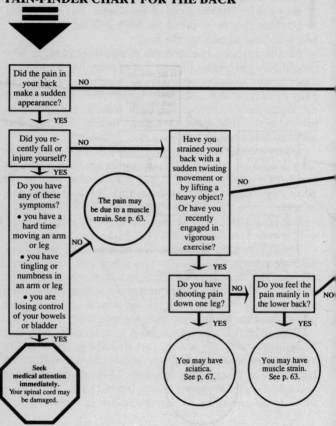

Did the pain in your back make a sudden appearance?

NO →

↓ YES

Did you recently fall or injure yourself?

NO →

↓ YES

Do you have any of these symptoms?
- you have a hard time moving an arm or leg
- you have tingling or numbness in an arm or leg
- you are losing control of your bowels or bladder

NO →

↓ YES

Seek medical attention immediately. Your spinal cord may be damaged.

The pain may be due to a muscle strain. See p. 63.

Have you strained your back with a sudden twisting movement or by lifting a heavy object? Or have you recently engaged in vigorous exercise?

NO →

↓ YES

Do you have shooting pain down one leg?

NO →

↓ YES

You may have sciatica. See p. 67.

Do you feel the pain mainly in the lower back?

NO →

↓ YES

You may have muscle strain. See p. 63.

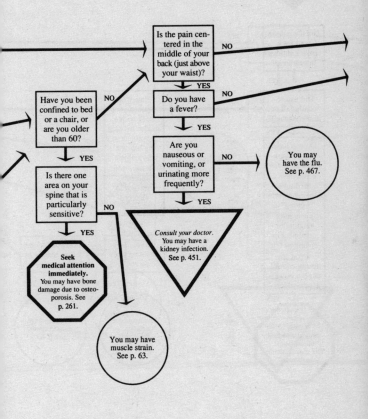

Is the pain centered in the middle of your back (just above your waist)?

NO →

YES ↓

Have you been confined to bed or a chair, or are you older than 60?

NO →

YES ↓

Do you have a fever?

NO →

YES ↓

Is there one area on your spine that is particularly sensitive?

NO →

YES ↓

Are you nauseous or vomiting, or urinating more frequently?

NO →

YES ↓

You may have the flu. See p. 467.

Seek medical attention immediately. You may have bone damage due to osteoporosis. See p. 261.

Consult your doctor. You may have a kidney infection. See p. 451.

You may have muscle strain. See p. 63.

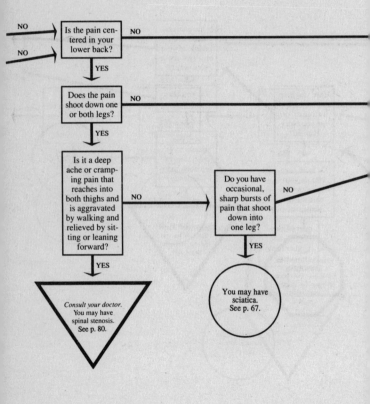

NO → Is the pain centered in your lower back?   NO →

NO →

↓ YES

Does the pain shoot down one or both legs?   NO →

↓ YES

Is it a deep ache or cramping pain that reaches into both thighs and is aggravated by walking and relieved by sitting or leaning forward?   NO →   Do you have occasional, sharp bursts of pain that shoot down into one leg?   NO →

↓ YES   ↓ YES

Consult your doctor. You may have spinal stenosis. See p. 80.

You may have sciatica. See p. 67.

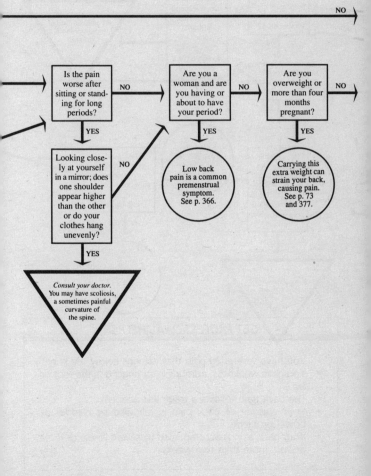

NO →

Is the pain worse after sitting or standing for long periods?

→ NO →

Are you a woman and are you having or about to have your period?

→ NO →

Are you overweight or more than four months pregnant?

→ NO →

YES ↓

Looking closely at yourself in a mirror; does one shoulder appear higher than the other or do your clothes hang unevenly?

NO →

YES ↓

Low back pain is a common premenstrual symptom. See p. 366.

Carrying this extra weight can strain your back, causing pain. See p. 73 and 377.

Consult your doctor. You may have scoliosis, a sometimes painful curvature of the spine.

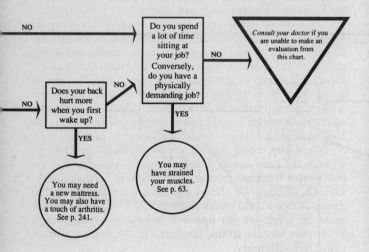

NO →

Do you spend a lot of time sitting at your job? Conversely, do you have a physically demanding job?

NO →

Consult your doctor if you are unable to make an evaluation from this chart.

NO →

Does your back hurt more when you first wake up?

NO →

YES ↓

YES ↓

You may need a new mattress. You may also have a touch of arthritis. See p. 241.

You may have strained your muscles. See p. 63.

GET PROFESSIONAL HELP IF:

- You have severe leg pain that extends below the knee
- You have weakness, numbness, or tingling in the foot or leg
- The back pain follows a traumatic accident
- Your episode of back pain is followed by bladder or bowel problems
- Your back pain is accompanied by severe illness or fever or lasts more than two weeks

MUSCLE STRAIN

When you consider the unceasing demands that all of us make on our back, the amazing thing is not that so many backs go out, but that so many don't.

Think about what your back does, says Augustus A. White III, M.D., professor of orthopedic surgery at Harvard Medical School. First, it supports heavy loads and withstands forces generated by certain activities that can be three or four times the weight of your body. Second, it allows your body to move in all kinds of directions, often while bearing those heavy loads. And third, it protects your spinal cord, which is responsible for transmitting messages back and forth between brain and body.

Thankfully, most muscle strain problems are minor. Usually the pain comes from a group of muscles that go into spasm trying to protect the back from further injury, says Dr. White. We shovel for an hour too long in the garden, catch a child who's about to fall, lift a box of books, tense up when we get upset, or slump too long over a keyboard. Muscle strain, it seems, is the most common cause of back injury.

▶ INSTANT RELIEF

Muscle pain is often so sharp that most people can recall exactly when it first started, says James Wheeler III, M.D., an orthopedic surgeon in Marion, North Carolina. Fortunately, it seldom troubles people long enough to require elaborate treatment. It usually resolves itself in a matter of days or at most several weeks. Here's how to ease the pain when it hits.

Unpack some ice. "I'm a fan of ice for all injuries when they first occur," says Dr. Wheeler. If there's no one around to strap the ice pack on your back with a towel, just put the pack—preferably one made with a gel rather than ice cubes—on a flat surface, cover it with a towel, and gently lie down on it.

Do some gentle stretching. "When you've got stiff, sore muscles, the best thing you can do is loosen them up," says Dr. Wheeler. Gently stretch your back and get it moving. To stretch your lower back, lie on your back with your knees slightly bent. With both hands, gently pull your right knee to your chest. Hold for 15 seconds, lower your leg, then repeat with the other leg. Finish the stretch by pulling both knees to your chest and holding for 15 seconds.

See also:

- Chapter 26, on medications.
- "Rest Easy" on page 65.
- "Healing with Touch" on page 69.
- "Brace Yourself!" on page 81.

▶ PREVENTION PAIN-RELIEF PROGRAM

It's amazing how much pain over-tightening or overstretching a muscle can cause. Fortunately, the pain will usually go away within a day or two, even though it may take your back six weeks to heal itself. If the pain doesn't disappear after a couple of days of taking it easy, go to bed for a couple of days and see if bed rest does the trick, says Dr. White.

In the unlikely event that the pain lasts more than a month, check with your doctor to make sure you don't have some other problem, he adds. If your doctor concurs that the pain is caused by a strain, do some gentle exercise to coax your muscles back into shape. Walking and riding a stationary bicycle are best, or you may want to try swimming.

Don't discount the role that stress may play in your pain. "The varying level of stresses we have all day causes various types of muscle tension. And this tension can equal back pain in varying degrees," says Edward A. Abraham, M.D., orthopedic surgeon at the University of California, Irvine.

If you suspect that tension is causing muscle strain, he adds, learn how to relax your back muscles whenever you feel them tense. A few weeks with a biofeed-back program should do the trick. (For more information on biofeedback, see chapter 17.)

Puppet on a String

One of the most important things you can do to prevent initial or recurring episodes of muscle strain is to improve your posture, says Dr. Abraham. Your back is designed in a particular way to withstand the various physical forces it encounters, he says. If it encounters these forces when it's not properly aligned, then it can't withstand them. It's going to get hurt.

You can improve your posture by standing tall, doctors say. Think of yourself as a puppet on a string. Now imagine that the string is attached to your head and is pulling you upward. Adjust your posture to go with the upward pull: Tilt your pelvis forward and tighten the muscles in your abdomen until you feel your lower back flatten and become longer.

Imagine also that your puppet neck has an eye on it. But for that eye to see, you must pull your head and shoulders back and tuck in your chin until your neck becomes straighter and longer.

Now look in the mirror. See? You're standing straighter already!

Multipurpose Relief

For: Muscle Strain, Disk Problems, Low Back Pain, Spinal Stenosis

REST EASY

If back pain has knocked you down, don't get up. At least not right away.

"I'm enthusiastic about short periods of rest for two or three days," says Augustus A. White III, M.D., professor of orthopedic surgery at Harvard Medical School. When your back hurts, the best action is often no action at all.

A couple of days on a firm mattress or a hard floor is

perfect, agrees Richard A. Deyo, M.D., associate professor of medicine and health services at the University of Washington in Seattle. If your bed is about as firm as a wet noodle, place a board between the box spring and mattress, he advises.

"The most comfortable position usually is lying on your side with your knees bent," says James Wheeler III, M.D., an orthopedic surgeon in Marion, North Carolina. Some people find additional relief by using one pillow to support their head and putting another between their legs.

Just don't lie flat. Whether on your back or your stomach, lying flat puts too much stress on your lower back, says Dr. Wheeler. If you must lie on your back, have your knees propped up by a pillow.

And don't undo a good thing by bopping in and out of bed, cautions Leon Root, M.D., orthopedic surgeon at the Hospital for Special Surgery in New York City. Let someone else get your snacks out of the fridge—especially if you've got a ruptured disk or sciatic pain. And use a bottle or bedpan in which to urinate.

Getting Up
Once you're ready to get up, first consider the mechanics of how to heft a stiff and vulnerable body out of bed, says David Lehrman, M.D., director and founder of the Lehrman Back Center in Miami Beach, Florida.

Lie on your side, stiffen your body, and push yourself into a sitting position with your arms. At the same time, allow your legs to glide to the floor. The momentum of the movement brings you into a sitting position.

After bending forward slightly at the hip and knees, slide one foot ahead of the other and get up, adds Dr. Bassam.

DISK PROBLEMS

Disks are those silver dollar-sized cushions of cartilage that separate your vertebrae. Normally they protect the vertebrae and add to your back's flexibility. But on occasion, an injury or just the normal wear and tear of an active life can cause one of them to slip or rupture. Then the disk itself or its contents start to press against a nerve root right where it emerges from the spinal cord.

As you might expect, pressing on nerves hurts. How badly it hurts depends on how much of the slipped or ruptured disk bulges out against the nerve—and how much extra room you have in your spinal canal to accommodate it. It also depends on which nerve is getting mashed. When it's the sciatic nerve, for example, the resulting discomfort can be an electrifying pain that shoots out from the disk, across the buttock, down the leg, and into the foot.

Many people describe this pain as similar to an electric shock, says Dr. Wheeler. Fortunately, he adds, "Ninety percent or more of sciatica problems resolve themselves."

▶ INSTANT RELIEF

Like most back problems, a slipped or ruptured disk takes time to heal. Here's what you can do to kill the pain until it does.

Stop it cold. If you've been injured, apply ice packs two or three times a day for one or two days, says Bassam A. Bassam, M.D., associate professor of neurology at the University of South Alabama College of Medicine in Mobile. Keep the ice on your back for 15 to 20 minutes each time you use it.

Take a dose of your own medicine. In most cases, you won't have to look any further than your medicine cabinet for relief. Try an analgesic such as Extra-Strength Tylenol or an anti-inflammatory medicine such as aspirin or ibuprofen, says Jean-Jacques Abitbol, M.D., assistant professor of orthopedics at the University of California, San Diego. Not only do these drugs relieve disk pain temporarily, they actually reduce the inflammation in the sciatic nerve, which in turn usually brings longer-term relief.

See also:

- "Rest Easy" on page 65.
- "Healing with Touch" on facing page.
- "Brace Yourself!" on page 81.

➡ PREVENTION PAIN-RELIEF PROGRAM

Eight out of ten people recover from disk problems within six weeks, doctors say. A day or two of bed rest following the initial attack, along with a course of over-the-counter analgesics, sets most people on the road to recovery. If the pain is severe, you may want to ask your doctor about a prescription painkiller such as codeine or oxycodone (Percodan).

Keep On Moving

Once the I-can't-stand-it part of your pain is over, get yourself moving, says Leon Root, M.D., orthopedic surgeon at the Hospital for Special Surgery in New York City. You need to do exercises that increase circulation to the disk and strengthen the muscles of your abdomen and back to minimize the chances that a disk will act up again. One such exercise, as Dr. Root points out in his book *No More Aching Back*, involves lying on your back with your knees bent.

"Straighten your right knee, but keep your left knee bent," he suggests. "Stiffen your right thigh muscles so that your right knee is held rigid. Point your toes to the ceiling. Keeping your right knee stiff and your left knee bent, slowly raise your right leg off the floor. Lift it as high as you can without pain," Dr. Root says.

Hold for a count of five, then let the leg descend slowly to the floor. Hold the knee straight to achieve the maximum

Multipurpose Relief

For: **Muscle Strain, Disk Problems, Low Back Pain**

HEALING WITH TOUCH

When your back is hurting, does anything sound better than getting a massage from someone who has good understanding of your every muscle and ligament? Can't you just feel those strong, nimble fingers coaxing that nagging, throbbing pain right out of your back?

Well, what are you waiting for?

Many back centers offer deep muscle massage as a way to relieve back pain. After kneading and stroking you from neck to buttocks, the therapist gives you an all-over body stretch. If there are any sore places remaining, the therapist finishes them off by massaging ice over them.

In addition, after the initial pain of a back attack begins to recede, a massage from a shiatsu (acupressure) therapist is a wonderful way to send pain on an extended voyage, says Rudolph Ballentine, M.D., director of the combined therapy program at the Himalayan International Institute of Yoga Science and Philosophy in Honesdale, Pennsylvania.

Shiatsu is a Japanese form of massage that involves pressure on acupuncture points, says Dr. Ballentine. It relieves all sorts of back pain, including that from slipped or ruptured disks.

stretching effect upon the large hamstring muscles at the back of your thighs. Repeat using the other leg. (See "Basic Training for Your Back" on next page.)

Generally, try to avoid situations in which you have to do a lot of bending or twisting around, says Dr. White. Trying to be the disco-dancing star at your 30th college reunion is a good way to get attention all right—the attention of your former classmates as hospital attendants cart you and your disco disk away on a stretcher.

BASIC TRAINING FOR YOUR BACK

Most back problems are caused by letting your body get out of shape, says David Lehrman, M.D., director and founder of the Lehrman Back Center in Miami Beach, Florida. "As we get older we get more sedentary, lose a certain amount of flexibility, lose a certain amount of strength and endurance, and start developing back problems. We get tight, stiff, and inflexible," he says.

That's why exercise is frequently the key to preventing back pain, he says. If you can maintain the strength of your body, build endurance, and even increase flexibility, you can keep most back problems at bay.

But an important thing to remember is that regular exercise programs should be tailored to the individual, adds Edward A. Abraham, M.D., orthopedic surgeon at the University of California, Irvine. "We are all different ages and body builds, so exercise programs should vary," he says.

Such programs can be prepared by your doctor or by a physical therapist who consults with your doctor, says Dr. Abraham. Here's a sample of the exercises they're likely to recommend. Ask your doctor if these may be appropriate for you.

Pelvic tilt. Stand with your shoulders, back, and buttocks against a wall. Place your feet shoulder-width apart with your heels about 8 inches from the wall. Bend your knees slightly. Now tighten your buttocks and pull in your stomach. Try to make the small of your back touch the wall. Hold for a count of six. Relax, then repeat. Once you've got the hang of it, try flattening your back without the wall to help you.

Arm and leg raises. Lie face-down on a mat, with two pillows under your abdomen. Keep your arms at your sides. With your knee straight, lift one leg off the floor until it's even with the level of the pillows. Hold for 6 seconds. Lower that leg and repeat with the other leg. Next extend your left arm straight overhead and lift it. Simultaneously lift your right leg, keeping your knee straight, until it is level with the pillows. Hold for 6 seconds. Alternate arms and legs.

Curls. Lie on your back and bend both knees. Begin to

exhale slowly while lifting first your head, then your shoulders, off the floor. With your arms outstretched, hold this position for 6 seconds.

Side-to-side sit-ups. Lie on your back with your knees bent and your feet on the floor. Touch your chin to your chest, stretch your arms forward, and slowly curl up, reaching toward your right knee. Hold for 6 seconds, then reach for your left knee.

Cat pose. Get on your hands and knees, with your lower back relaxed. Drop your head, pull in your stomach muscles, and make your back as rounded and high as possible. Hold for 6 seconds.

Butt-tucks. Lie on your back with your knees bent and feet flat. Lift your buttocks off the floor while keeping your shoulders firm against the floor. Hold for 5 seconds, then slowly return to the floor.

Side-lying leg lifts. Lie on your right side, your bottom leg slightly bent, your top leg straight. Slowly lift your top leg up, keeping the kneecap facing forward and your body straight.

Know When to Stop

People who experience pain when they exercise should also remember to exercise their common sense, cautions Dr. Abraham. If you have a lot of pain when you exercise, you're probably not doing the exercise correctly. And doing it wrong can make the pain ten times worse than before. So when you have a lot of pain, stop, review the exercise with your doctor or physical therapist, and then try it again.

If you experience just a little discomfort and you feel otherwise okay, says Dr. Abraham, see if you can go ahead and finish the exercise.

If one part of an exercise program feels fine and one part hurts, don't drop the whole program or grit your teeth and do everything, says Dr. Abraham. Just drop the part that hurts. "Then try little bits at a time until you can work into a full program," he advises.

And don't forget to warm up.

When Surgery Is the Answer

For the few people who are not helped by bed rest, analgesics, and exercise, the only recourse may be surgery to remove the ruptured disk, says Dr. Wheeler.

But don't rush into anything. "There are a lot of people with back pain who have *not* gotten better following surgery," cautions Dr. Wheeler. "You don't want to be one of them."

Surgery should be performed only when the person shows evidence of neurological problems and signs of numbness or weakness, he explains. Those are the classic signs of a ruptured disk. If you don't have them, you don't have a ruptured disk, and surgery won't help.

If you are a candidate for surgery, your doctor will probably send you for either computer axial tomography (a CAT scan) or magnetic resonance imaging (MRI) before deciding whether an operation might help your disk problem. If you have any doubts, says Dr. Abraham, have a second or even a third doctor interpret those sophisticated computer pictures.

What's the point of a second opinion? Well, doctors once told actor/comedian Chevy Chase that surgery was the only way to fix his pratfall-tortured disks, says Dr. Root. Luckily, Chase didn't listen. Instead he got a second opinion—from Dr. Root, as a matter of fact—who realized that Chase's disk pain wouldn't respond to surgery. Dr. Root gave the comedian an exercise prescription that strengthened his back and relieved his pain. Today a new, stronger model Chevy continues to split his fans' sides— but not his disks.

LOW BACK PAIN

People with low back pain frequently blame a specific incident for their troubles. "If only I hadn't helped Mabel move," someone will grumble. "If only I hadn't danced that tango," someone else will say.

To a certain extent, they're right. Gravity dictates that more pressure is put on the lower spine than on the upper spine when you're active. The fact is, however, that the vast majority of low back problems are not caused by executing a single Latin-lover's dip on the dance floor. And you can stop blaming Mabel, too. The fact is, most low back pains, says Dr. White, are caused by arthritis. They simply result from the cumulative wear and tear of life. After age 30, people start losing water from the disks that separate their vertebrae, and the disk itself starts to wear away, says Dr. Abitbol.

Congenital defects in the spine, which may not have bothered you in the past, also can cause low back pain as you age, says Dr. Bassam. People can live with these defects for years without feeling pain, he explains. But if they gain weight, become physically unfit, or work in an occupation that puts stress on the back, pain may unexpectedly hit them one day.

Fortunately, adds Dr. White, most low back pain goes away sooner or later and does not become a major problem. Nonetheless, certain warning signs demand immediate medical attention. Pain accompanied by numbness or weakness in a leg, as well as pain that lasts more than a week or two, can indicate a significant problem, doctors say. If you do have any of these symptoms, see a physician without delay.

▶ INSTANT RELIEF

Low back pain can make sitting, standing, and walking so uncomfortable that you'd give your eyeteeth for a few moments of relief. Here are a few ways to keep your teeth and get the relief.

Seek heat. As long as your pain is not due to an injury, grab a heating pad and let the warmth radiate under your skin, says Dr. Abitbol.

Assume the position. If your back pain is a result of a particular joint that's acting up, getting into a position that takes the pressure off the joint will relieve the pain, says Dr. Root. In most cases, lying flat on the floor with your knees bent and your feet elevated on a chair will do the trick.

See also:

- Chapter 21, on hot and cold therapy.
- Chapter 26, on medications.
- "Rest Easy" on page 65.
- "Healing with Touch" on page 69.
- "Brace Yourself!" on page 81.

➡ PREVENTION PAIN-RELIEF PROGRAM

Most experts on low back pain say that one of the best ways to treat it and keep it from returning is to exercise, says Wendell P. Liemohn, Ph.D., professor of human performance and sports studies at the University of Tennessee in Knoxville. Exercise is not a panacea, says Dr. Liemohn, but it can often make you feel a lot better.

As the initial attack of pain begins to subside, ask your doctor for permission to perform the following simple exercises.

Stretch It

Here is a good beginning exercise for people who have suffered pain in the lower back, says Dr. Bassam. "Lie on your back with a pillow under your head and your arms at the side of your head," he says. "Slowly raise your knees to your chest ten times."

As the lower back improves, sit straight up in a chair,

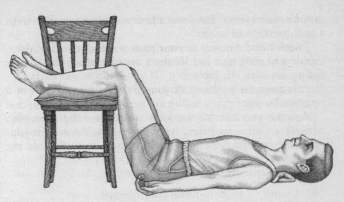

Lower back acting up? Try putting your legs instead of your bottom in the chair. Lie on the floor with your calves resting on the seat. You can put a rolled towel under your neck for support, if you like. Doctors say this position brings relief by helping to relax the muscles of the lower back.

says Dr. Bassam. "Now lower your head to your knees ten times." This exercise also aids flexibility, he says.

As your back gets stronger and pain retreats, try this exercise of Dr. Bassam's. "Stand with your back against the wall," he says. "Bend your knees and flex your hips. Slide down and get back up ten times."

Finally, when your back is its former self again, more activity can be permitted, says Dr. Bassam. "Lie on your back on a firm surface," he says. "Raise one leg as far as you can."

In this last exercise, Dr. Bassam recommends that each leg be lifted 10 to 20 times. Repeat the exercise with the other leg. Then do the exercise lifting both legs 10 to 20 times.

Walking is also excellent exercise for the lower back, says Dr. Liemohn, but it is important that you don't just shuffle along. Stand up straight and don't allow yourself to tilt forward. If you lean forward, what has to balance it out are the stressed-out muscles of the lower back.

Instead, walk softly "to cushion the joints" in the back,

says Dr. Liemohn. "But don't tiptoe—walk naturally with a heel-toe type of walk."

Joggers and runners must also beware of running flat-footed and making a lot of noise, because it jars the knees and spine, says Dr. Liemohn. "If you cushion as you land, there is going to be less strain placed on the spine when you run," he notes.

Another exercise that works particularly well for people who have gotten past the acute stage of back pain is yoga, provided that you're one of the fortunate few who live in an area where a yoga instructor works with one or more medical doctors, says Rudolph Ballentine, M.D., director

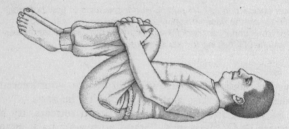

To stretch out the muscles in your lower back and improve hip mobility, here's an exercise recommended by Leon Root, M.D., author of No More Aching Back. Lie on the floor with your knees bent. Grasp your right knee with both hands and bring it up toward your right shoulder. Hold for a count of five. Now repeat, using your left knee. If you can, grasp one knee with each hand and raise both knees toward your shoulders and hold. Keep the back of your head relaxed against the floor throughout the exercise. Do not do this exercise if it causes you discomfort.

Here's another exercise from Dr. Root, designed to loosen up the lower back. (1) Lie on your back with your knees bent and your feet flat on the floor. Lace your fingers behind your head. Your elbows should be touching the floor. Cross your right leg over the left and (2) allow both legs to drop to the right. Don't force the stretch and don't allow your left elbow or shoulder to leave the floor. Hold for a count of five. Repeat five times. (3) Now cross your left leg over the right and (4) repeat the series to the left. These movements should provide a gentle, relaxing stretch and should feel good. Do not perform this exercise if it causes you discomfort.

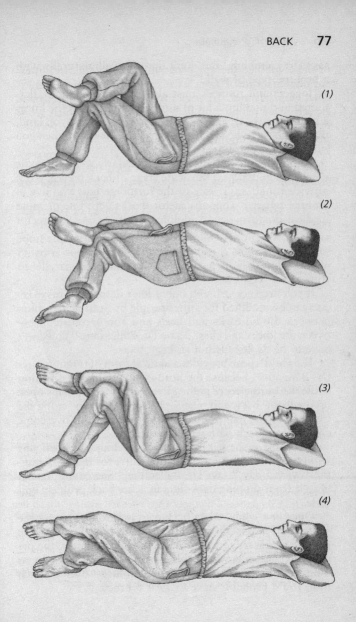

(1)

(2)

(3)

(4)

of the combined therapy program at the Himalayan International Institute of Yoga Science and Philosophy in Honesdale, Pennsylvania. "A yoga instructor individualizes back exercises for people and helps them discover which work best for them," he says. Always get your doctor's permission before attempting yoga.

One yoga exercise that works particularly well for people with chronic low back pain is called the child's pose (sometimes known as the folded leaf). "Most people can do it and derive benefit from it," says Dr. Ballentine.

"The posture involves sitting on the backs of your legs, resting on your heels, with your toes pointed backward," says Dr. Ballentine. "Slowly lower your head to the floor so that your chest is resting on your knees. Your arms go back so that they lie palms-up along your side, parallel to your lower legs."

If you are very stiff and tight, don't despair. "This exercise can be modified for stiffer people by putting a cushion between the buttocks and heels and another cushion between the knees and chest," says Dr. Ballentine. "You don't have to be as flexible but still can relax."

The child's pose provides a natural form of traction, says Dr. Ballentine, because the head is pulling in one direction while the buttocks are pulling in another. "That helps open up the lower back and relieve pressure," he says, citing the case of a nurse named Gabrielle who learned to overcome chronic low back pain with the exercise.

"As soon as she felt her back was feeling a little off, she would spend more time in that posture, for maybe 5 minutes twice a day," says Dr. Ballentine. "She could prevent herself from slipping back into an acute back problem episode."

Once in a while, when back pain is chronic because the spine itself is unstable, an operation to fuse the vertebrae may be necessary, says Dr. Bassam. Unfortunately, the period after the operation is quite painful, and it can take as long as 12 months for the vertebrae to fuse—during which time you'd probably have to wear a brace.

Luckily, the effectiveness of more conservative treatment such as using a back brace and pain-relief measures such as heat, exercise, and ibuprofen make the necessity for the operation rare.

SPINAL STENOSIS

As you pass age 50, a lifetime of wear and tear on your spine can culminate in enough bone spurs, swollen membranes, and ruptured disks in and around your spine to seriously narrow the space through which your spinal cord runs. And especially if you started off with a little less space at birth, the narrowing space—called a stenosis—can eventually squeeze the spinal cord until it screams in pain.

What's the first sign of stenosis? "The nerves in your back begin to complain," says Dr. White. They hurt when you walk—particularly downhill—and you may have a "pins and needles" sensation or even a loss of feeling in your legs. Eventually, standing, lifting, kneeling, coughing, and even going to the bathroom may cause or aggravate the pain.

▶ INSTANT RELIEF

What's available in the way of quick relief for spinal stenosis? "Not much," says Dr. White. However, he does offer a suggestion that may ease your discomfort. It probably won't do your wallet any good, however.

Go shopping. Many people report that leaning forward and pushing a shopping cart helps relieve their pain, says Dr. White. "It tends to open up the spinal cord a little bit," he says. The same effect can be achieved by squatting, lying on your side with your knees bent, or leaning forward while riding an exercise bike.

See also:

- Chapter 26, on medications.
- "Rest Easy" on page 65.
- "Brace Yourself!" on the opposite page.

▶ PREVENTION PAIN-RELIEF PROGRAM

You should not be trying to deal with the pain of spinal stenosis on your own. See your doctor.

Multipurpose Relief

For: Muscle Strain, Disk Problems, Low Back
        Pain, Spinal Stenosis

BRACE YOURSELF!

A brace is one way to support yourself through the initial stage of almost any back problem, doctors say.

"You don't want to use a back support to take over the natural function of your body," says Edward A. Abraham, M.D., orthopedic surgeon at the University of California, Irvine. In the long run, it's much better to strengthen your back and abdominal muscles. But in the short run, a brace can be helpful until you actually get those muscles strong enough to do their job.

Some individuals with lower back, disk, and spine problems are helped by back supports, notes David Lehrman, M.D., director and founder of the Lehrman Back Center in Miami Beach, Florida. You can find these supports at drugstores and orthopedic supply stores.

"They are aids that work for a percentage of people," he says. "They're designed to support the spine and to tilt the pelvis in a certain way to alter the posture and give relief."

Check with your doctor to see if one of these back supports might support you.

Any nerve that's being squeezed by its neighbors is going to kick up a pretty big fuss. That's why doctors prescribe strong painkillers—Percodan, for example—for this problem. They may also inject anesthesia near the spine, says David Lehrman, M.D., director and founder of the Lehrman Back Center in Miami Beach, Florida.

A back support can also relieve your pain, as can exercise.

"About 30 to 35 percent of patients with a spinal stenosis can be helped with exercise," says Dr. Lehrman, particularly walking.

But if exercise doesn't work, surgery to open up the

GETTING YOUR BACK BACK TO WORK

You've hurt your back. And although you'd like to spend another day or two in bed, you've got to get your body back to work. So how can you prevent yourself from aggravating your pain once you get there? How can you keep from reinjuring or restraining parts of your back?

No matter where you work, it's important to organize your workplace so that you don't routinely lift objects from the floor, says Augustus A. White III, M.D., professor of orthopedic surgery at Harvard Medical School. He suggests that those who perform manual labor rely on platforms to save their back, because the back is much more likely to forgive a load that's lifted from a height of 3 feet than one lifted from the ground.

Laws of Lifting

If your job is to pack ice cream pints into a cardboard box, for example, have the boxes stacked beside you on a platform. It doesn't have to be sophisticated—an old packing crate will do. Then, when the pint containers come off the production line, quickly load them into the box. When it's full, all you have to do is pick it up and swing it over to another platform.

Be careful to lift each load in a single smooth motion rather than jerking it, says Bassam A. Bassam, M.D., associate professor of neurology at the University of South Alabama College of Medicine in Mobile. "Always place your feet apart and keep the load close to your body, even for light weights," he says. Squatting or kneeling before lifting is also a good idea. "And don't bend or twist."

Another important strategy to stay pain-free is to frequently change positions while you're at work, says Edward A. Abraham, M.D., orthopedic surgeon at the University of California, Irvine.

Individuals who work at a computer terminal, for example, should condition themselves to stand every little while—say, every time the phone rings. And when you stand, lift one leg onto a book or two and shift your pelvis. Not only will this kind of periodic movement prevent back pain, it will also reduce any existing pain as well.

Strategy for Sitting

Don't forget to make sure that when you sit, you've put your bottom in the right chair to begin with, says David

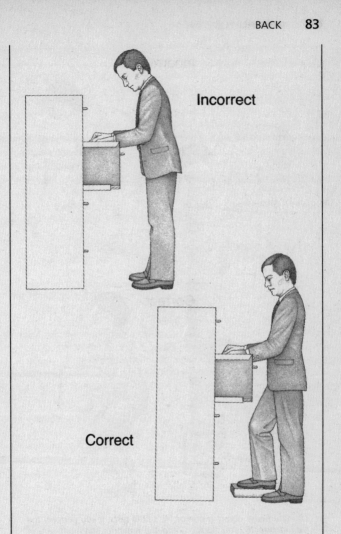

Incorrect

Correct

Keep your back happy on the job. If you must spend long hours standing, keep your back straight. Use a telephone book or some other object to elevate one foot a few inches off the ground. If you allow yourself to hunch over your work, your back muscles may go on strike.

Incorrect

Correct

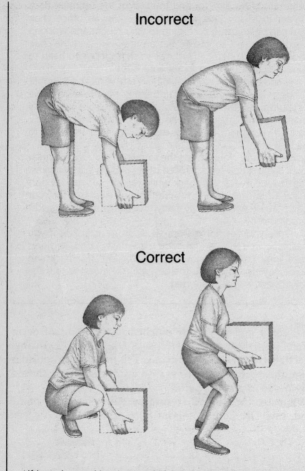

Lifting a heavy object is one of life's little tests. If you perform the task incorrectly, you flunk . . . and the reminder stays with you in the form of back pain. To lift a heavy object from the floor correctly, squat down, keeping your back straight. Keep the object close to your body and use the strong muscles in your legs to do the actual lifting. You're asking for trouble if you bend over and rely on the muscles of your lower back.

Lehrman, M.D., director and founder of the Lehrman Back Center in Miami Beach, Florida. Insist on an office chair that can be adjusted according to your height and working needs. Your feet should be flat on the floor, and the chair should be equipped with wheels so that when you need to turn, you turn the chair—not your body.

In addition, the chair should have arm rests and a lumbar support—a section of the chair that fits into the lower curve of your spine—that are adjustable. Suitable chairs are readily available from catalog sales houses and office supply stores, says Dr. Lehrman, but they cost anywhere from $500 to $2,000.

Fortunately, you can get the same benefit from a regular chair if you simply place a rolled towel or puffy pillow against the lower curve of your back while you sit, he says. Support pillows that are exactly the right shape and size for your back can be purchased at many drugstores and orthopedic supply stores.

Once you get home from work, sit in a recliner if you have one, and think about getting one if you don't. Recliners take some of the weight and pressure off your back and spine, says Dr. Lehrman. The best are contoured so that the lower back is well supported.

spinal canal and give your pinched nerves a bit of extra room is something to consider, says Dr. White. "I encourage active, elderly people who have this problem to consider having the operation," he says. "I don't think they should walk about in all that pain."

What are the odds that surgery will relieve the pain? Good, says Dr. White. "About 80 percent."

CHAPTER
3

CHEST

I t hurts. Right over the place where you pledged allegiance to the flag every day all those years ago in grammar school—it hurts. And every time you take a deep breath it hurts worse.

Are you having a heart attack? Ten to one you're not, says John Stone, M.D., a cardiologist at Emory University in Atlanta. The pain that signals a heart attack—or even the pain of angina—does not get worse when you take a breath. Nor does it get any better, for that matter. It generally maintains a constant pressure just behind your breastbone. The pain may radiate down to your stomach, up between your shoulder blades to your neck and lower jaw, or out to one or both of your arms. But wherever it goes, it doesn't get better or worse when you breathe.

Chest pain that gets worse when you breathe is more likely to be caused by pneumonia, says Dr. Stone. Or if you've been working out or mixing it up, the pain may indicate a strained muscle, broken rib, torn cartilage, or even a damaged vertebra. Chest pain that gets worse when you bend over, lie down, or stoop is more likely to be caused by heartburn or an inflammation of the sac that surrounds the heart.

On occasion, chest pain is also caused by weak spots in an arterial wall, leaky heart valves, anemia, shingles, arthritis, or even a ripped aorta.

PAIN-FINDER CHART FOR THE CHEST

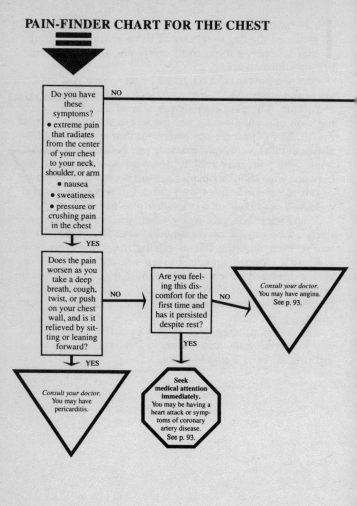

Do you have these symptoms?
- extreme pain that radiates from the center of your chest to your neck, shoulder, or arm
- nausea
- sweatiness
- pressure or crushing pain in the chest

NO

YES

Does the pain worsen as you take a deep breath, cough, twist, or push on your chest wall, and is it relieved by sitting or leaning forward?

NO

Are you feeling this discomfort for the first time and has it persisted despite rest?

NO

Consult your doctor. You may have angina. See p. 93.

YES

Consult your doctor. You may have pericarditis.

YES

Seek medical attention immediately. You may be having a heart attack or symptoms of coronary artery disease. See p. 93.

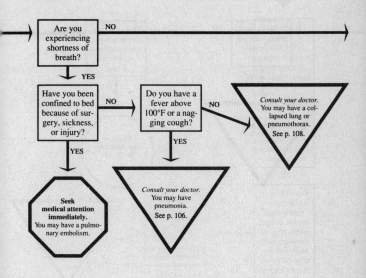

Are you experiencing shortness of breath?

NO

YES

Have you been confined to bed because of surgery, sickness, or injury?

NO

Do you have a fever above 100°F or a nagging cough?

NO

Consult your doctor. You may have a collapsed lung or pneumothorax. See p. 108.

YES

YES

Seek medical attention immediately. You may have a pulmonary embolism.

Consult your doctor. You may have pneumonia. See p. 106.

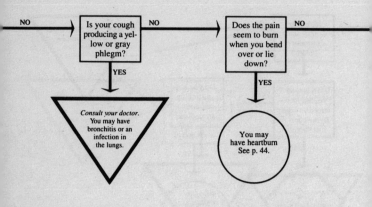

NO →

Is your cough producing a yellow or gray phlegm?

NO →

YES ↓

Consult your doctor. You may have bronchitis or an infection in the lungs.

Does the pain seem to burn when you bend over or lie down?

NO →

YES ↓

You may have heartburn See p. 44.

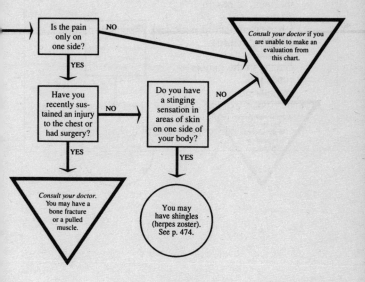

Is the pain only on one side?

NO →

Consult your doctor if you are unable to make an evaluation from this chart.

YES ↓

Have you recently sustained an injury to the chest or had surgery?

NO →

Do you have a stinging sensation in areas of skin on one side of your body?

NO →

YES ↓

YES ↓

Consult your doctor. You may have a bone fracture or a pulled muscle.

You may have shingles (herpes zoster). See p. 474.

GET PROFESSIONAL HELP IF:

- Your chest pain occurs with:
  shortness of breath
  dizziness
  radiation of pain to neck, jaw, shoulders, or arms
  sweating, nausea
  exertion
  tingling in the fingers
  inhalation
  irregular pulse
- Your pain is extreme and your chest is tender to the touch in the painful area
- There is bleeding from the area of a chest injury

HEART DISEASE

Chest pain that's caused by heart disease is usually your heart's desperate attempt to get your attention. Your heart can't very well leap out of your chest and grab you by the collar, so it does the next best thing: It sends a sharp message up the spinal nerves to your brain that's guaranteed to hit you in the head.

Why such desperate measures? Heart pain—whether it's the pain of angina or the pain of a heart attack—usually means your heart is not getting enough oxygen. And if it doesn't somehow manage to get more immediately—or to reduce its workload so that it doesn't need as much—then it and you are going to conk out.

Why would a hard-working heart ever have to deal with oxygen starvation? Over the years blood vessels in the heart become narrowed through a process called atherosclerosis. No one is exactly sure what starts it off, but something— a husband or co-worker's cigarette smoke, high blood pressure, too much cholesterol cruising your bloodstream, a viral invader—apparently slashes the inside wall of an artery and rips away a piece of the lining.

Then the body's repair squads arrive. Cells from inside the artery's walls try to patch the resulting hole by throwing themselves across it. Cells from your immune system arrive to shoot down any microbial invaders that might have slipped in, then hunker down in the artery wall to secrete growth factors that will help in the repairs. Any fats traveling by the building site are also drafted into service, weaving themselves in and among any tiny spaces the repair squads have overlooked.

Unfortunately, your body doesn't seem to know when to stop patching. Naturally occurring cholesterol from your liver, along with the extra cholesterol from last night's steak, stop to contribute their efforts as well. And platelets—tiny blood cells that are designed to adhere to uneven surfaces and form blood clots—also arrive at the scene and attach themselves to the patch, until eventually the patch bulges out into the artery.

Once the space inside the artery becomes so narrow that your blood—loaded with its precious oxygen cargo—can barely trickle through, you're likely to experience the pain of angina. It comes on whenever you increase your heart's need for oxygen by exerting yourself either physically or emotionally. If a piece of the patch breaks off and blocks the artery elsewhere, the blood can't get through at all and you're likely to experience the pain of a heart attack.

➤ INSTANT RELIEF

Although heart pain requires medical attention, once you know you have angina there are a number of things you can do to keep that pain at bay.

Sit. When angina pain grabs you, take a load off your feet and off your heart by sitting down immediately, doctors say.

Dynamite your arteries. If you've already been diagnosed with angina, use the nitroglycerin your doctor has prescribed when you need quick relief, says Joseph A. Gascho, M.D., a cardiologist at Pennsylvania State University's Milton S. Hershey Medical Center in Hershey. Squirt it on your tongue if you have the spray, or slip a pill under your tongue if you have the tablets. If you're still in pain 5 minutes later, take another dose. If you're still in pain after a second 5-minute interval, take a third dose. If you're still in pain 5 minutes after the third dose, get to the emergency room of your local hospital or call your local paramedics.

Do *not* go to your doctor's office, cautions Dr. Gascho. If the pain has lasted more than 15 minutes, chances are you're having a heart attack. And the high-tech medicine and equipment that can save your life are almost always available only at a hospital or paramedic unit.

➤ PREVENTION PAIN-RELIEF PROGRAM

Although angina is caused by the underlying atherosclerosis, it is actually triggered by a sudden disparity between the amount of oxygen your heart gets and the amount of oxygen it needs, says Dr. Gascho.

You run up a flight of stairs, pick up a bag of groceries, or jump up and down at a football game, and the pain signals that there's not enough oxygen for what you're doing. When this kind of angina—what doctors call "stable angina" or "exertional" angina—strikes, it's usually relieved within 3 to 5 minutes by a dose of nitroglycerin.

But a better way to handle the problem is to prevent it in the first place. That's why treatment is aimed at *preventing* a disparity between the amount of oxygen your heart gets and the amount of oxygen it needs, says Dr. Gascho. And that's done either by increasing the amount of oxygen available to your heart on a regular basis or by decreasing your heart's workload—as measured by your heart rate and blood pressure—so that it doesn't need as much oxygen to begin with.

Medications for Angina

Three different kinds of drugs form the antiangina lineup, explains Dr. Gascho. Beta-blockers such as propranolol help by decreasing your heart rate and blood pressure. Calcium channel blockers—nifedipine, verapamil, or diltiazem—help by decreasing blood pressure and dilating (opening) the arteries in your heart. Nitrates, prescribed for quick pain relief whenever you experience angina, are also used on a regular basis to lower blood pressure and cause the blood to pool in your legs. That may sound a bit alarming, says Dr. Gascho, but it's really not harmful. Its effect is to reduce the amount of physical pressure on your heart.

The timing of these drugs may also be important. The majority of heart attacks occur between 6:00 A.M. and noon. The problem, as researchers explain, is that the natural circadian rhythm of the body dictates a rise in both heart rate and blood pressure during that period of time, which increases the body's demand for oxygen. During the same period, your body produces naturally occurring chemicals that constrict blood vessels and reduce the flow of oxygen to your heart. So, in effect, you have the body working against itself.

On top of that, platelets—the tiny blood cells that clump together on arterial patches and make them bulge out into the arteries—seem to be superclumpable between 6:00 A.M. and noon. All this means that during these hours, your blood is at its thickest and moves more slowly than at other times of the day.

If you're beginning to think that your body is conspiring against you to trigger angina, you're really not far from the truth. But there is a way to outfox your body, reports Carl Pepine, M.D., a cardiologist at the University of Florida. And that's by timing the drugs your doctor prescribes to counter these natural rhythms.

Taking a long-acting beta-blocker at night before you go to bed, for example, can reduce your heart rate during the peak anginal period the next morning, he notes. It will also reduce your platelets' tendency to clump and redistribute oxygen to areas of the heart that may be in short supply. And taking a long-acting nitrate first thing in the morning, before you even get out of bed, can also dilate the arteries so that extra oxygen can get through during this peak anginal period.

Just remember that you need a break from nitrates at least once in every 24-hour period to keep their effect from weakening, cautions Dr. Pepine. Check with your doctor before you make any changes, but the best nitrate-free interval would probably be from about 10:00 P.M. until 8:00 A.M. while you're sleeping, he notes.

Exercise Until It (Almost) Hurts

Along with medications, your doctor will probably also prescribe exercise. There is some evidence that exercise may help increase the amount of oxygen available to your heart by conditioning other muscles in your body to use their oxygen more efficiently, says Dr. Gascho. The American Heart Association's (AHA) Committee on Exercise and

Cardiac Rehabilitation reports that regular exercise among people with heart disease lowers heart rate, lowers blood pressure, decreases the amount of oxygen your heart needs, and increases the amount of oxygen your heart has.

How much exercise does it take to achieve this miraculous effect? According to the AHA committee, if you already have heart disease or high blood pressure, you really need to ask your doctor. He'll probably put you on a treadmill, hook you up to a heart monitor, and tell you to start walking until you feel some pain. This test will allow him to judge how vigorously you should exercise. Then he'll write an exercise prescription that will let you get the exercise you need but stop short of where your pain starts. As you exercise over the weeks and months, of course, that threshold will change, and you'll gradually be able to exercise far more before the onset of pain than you did initially.

Generally speaking, your doctor is likely to suggest that you warm up slowly for 5 to 10 minutes, exercise the larger muscles in your body for 20 to 30 minutes (walking is a good choice), and then cool down for another 5 to 10 minutes. You'll probably be asked to do your workout three times a week, under direct medical supervision.

And don't be surprised if your doctor writes the prescription in terms of the calories you need to burn. Calories measure the amount of work being done by the body. Your doctor will be aware of studies that show fewer symptoms and decreased death rate from heart disease in people who exercise at a rate that burns off somewhere between 700 and 2,000 calories per week. Do *not* start an exercise program without checking with your doctor first.

Avoid Smoky Rooms

Another way to increase the amount of oxygen available to your heart is to avoid tobacco smoke. Smoke increases the amount of cholesterol that is deposited onto any of the patches bulging out from your artery walls, thus narrowing them even further, says Dr. Gascho. It also prevents red blood cells from releasing as much oxygen into your heart as they actually carry, and it increases the amount of oxygen your heart needs by increasing both your heart rate and your blood pressure, he says. And don't forget that scientists suspect smoking is one of the culprits—if not *the* culprit—that initiates injury to the artery wall to begin with.

The mind-boggling part is that you don't even have to be the person who's smoking to get hurt. Scientists from the University of California, San Francisco, who reviewed ten studies on environmental tobacco smoke and heart disease concluded that secondhand smoke from a spouse, a co-worker, or just one other person in the same room can reduce the amount of oxygen available to your heart. They also concluded that being exposed to other people's smoking can increase your risk of death from heart disease by 30 percent—even if you're perfectly healthy to begin with.

Can You Reverse Heart Disease?

Exercising and avoiding smoky rooms do more than provide your heart with more oxygen. There is at least some evidence that these things, when combined with a radically low-fat, low-cholesterol diet and a stress-management program, can actually reverse the underlying atherosclerosis that causes the angina to begin with.

In a multicenter study coordinated by researchers at the Preventive Medicine Research Institute and the University of California, San Francisco, 22 people with atherosclerosis were assigned to an experimental group that stopped smoking, started exercising, ate low-fat, low-cholesterol, high-fiber foods, and practiced a variety of stress-management techniques such as deep breathing, meditation, progressive relaxation, and guided imagery.

The diameter of their coronary arteries was measured before they started the program and again one year later. In between they ate fruits, vegetables, grains, legumes, and soybeans. No animal products were allowed, except for a cup of nonfat milk or yogurt once a day. Fats accounted for only about 10 percent of their total calories, and cholesterol was limited to 5 milligrams a day. Caffeine was eliminated, alcohol was limited, and a vitamin B_{12} supplement was given.

The participants also exercised—walking was the favored exercise—three times a week for a minimum of 30 minutes each time, not including warm-ups or cool-downs. And they meditated, relaxed, did visualization, or breathed deeply for an hour every day.

The result? These people lost weight, lowered their blood pressure, and dropped their cholesterol levels. And while the coronary arteries of another group in the study that made no lifestyle changes actually closed up another 3 percent, the group that had made such significant lifestyle changes found that the diameter of their arteries had actually *increased* by 2 percent.

That may not sound like much, but the effect it had on participants was nothing short of amazing. People in the group that made no lifestyle changes reported a 165 percent increase in frequency of angina, a 95 percent increase in duration of angina, and a 39 percent increase in severity of angina. But people in the group that made the changes reported a 91 percent *reduction* in the frequency, a 42 percent reduction in the duration, and a 28 percent reduction in the severity.

Cleaning Out the Arteries

If you're still having pain despite medication and lifestyle changes, however, your doctor may talk to you about some high-tech medical interventions that will improve the flow of blood and oxygen to your heart, says Dr. Gascho.

Percutaneous transluminal coronary angioplasty, for example, is the official mouthful that describes a procedure in which a tiny balloon is inserted into a coronary artery, inflated to smash the atherosclerotic patches back against the artery walls, and then withdrawn. Originally it was used only for those who had a single blockage in a single artery, but studies indicating its effectiveness in opening up arteries and relieving angina have encouraged doctors to use it in multivessel blockages as well. Thirty percent of the arteries that are opened by this procedure, however, become blocked again within six months.

A coronary artery bypass graft—frequently referred to simply as a "bypass"—is a procedure in which a surgeon takes part of an artery from somewhere else in the body and grafts it onto the heart to bypass a blocked artery. Twenty-five to 30 percent of the arteries opened by this procedure become blocked again with one year.

Why Operate?

"There are two reasons to perform either bypass surgery or angioplasty," explains Dr. Gascho. "One is to make someone feel better. And both of those procedures are very effective at doing that. So if someone has angina despite medicine and is very limited in what they can do, then these procedures are certainly indicated."

If someone's angina is well controlled by medication but their occupation demands that they exert themselves a lot, that's also an indication that one of these procedures is appropriate, he adds. A construction worker, for example, may have no angina at all when he's at home, but he does when he's hauling heavy pipes around on the job. "In this instance, a bypass or angioplasty will help the worker do what he has to do to earn a living. But the second reason for these procedures is to prolong life," says Dr. Gascho. "And that's where it really gets controversial."

Both procedures have their pluses and minuses, new techniques and technology are improving each procedure, and studies comparing the two are currently under way. The only study that has been completed to date—a comparison of people who had single-vessel disease and unstable angina—revealed that in limited instances, angioplasty and bypass surgery are equally effective in reducing angina, preventing a heart attack, and prolonging life.

So how do you know which procedure is best? Until more studies are completed, says Dr. Gascho, "the general rule is that if the left main coronary artery—which divides almost immediately into two other vessels—is significantly blocked, or if all three of these arteries are, then that's a definite indication for a bypass."

Electrify Your Pain

Of course not everyone is a good candidate for surgery. Some may have underlying problems—diabetes, for example—that make the procedures less likely to be successful. For these people, transcutaneous electrical nerve stimulation (TENS) may be the answer. A team of Swedish pain specialists did three studies showing that TENS may prevent at least some angina episodes.

In one study, for example, researchers divided a group of 21 people between the ages of 41 and 71 into two groups. Everyone in the experimental group was given a TENS unit and told to use it for 1 hour in the morning, at noon, and in the evening over a ten-week period. Everything else in their lives was to stay the same, including taking any medication for their angina. The other group conducted their lives as usual and did not use TENS.

Then, every other week, the researchers called everybody in and gave them an exercise test to see how much exertion they could take before their angina kicked in.

The result? People in the TENS group had increased their heart's ability to work by about 11 percent more than the non-TENS group. That meant that the number of angina attacks they experienced—and the amount of medicine they were required to take—were both significantly reduced. What really got the researchers excited, however, was the fact that fewer angina attacks occurred even *after* the study was over. In fact, an editorial in the *British Heart Journal* recently described the effect of TENS on angina as "impressive." (See chapter 32 for more information about TENS.)

Stopping a Heart Attack Before It Stops You

One thing that frightens people with angina is the possibility that the pain they're experiencing is actually from a heart attack. That's a real concern, says Dr. Gascho. That's why the rule for anyone with angina—or any kind of chest pain, for that matter—is that any pain that doesn't stop within 15 minutes should send you straight to the emergency room. You can call your doctor from there.

Heart cells start to die about 15 minutes into a heart attack, explains Dr. Gascho. So you don't have a lot of time to drive over to your doctor's office and find out he or she doesn't have the equipment or drugs to deal with a heart attack.

Nor do you have the time to fool around asking yourself, Is it or isn't it? As a general rule, it is probably *not* a heart attack if the pain comes and goes when you breathe, if it hits you "out of a clear blue sky," if it's sharp and jabbing, or if it's right smack in the center of your chest over your breastbone, says Dr. Gascho. It probably *is* a heart attack if you feel a burning pain or heaviness just to the left of your breastbone or if the pain is accompanied by nausea, sweating, or an intense feeling of dread.

Emotional Upset Triggers Trouble

Triggered by something as seemingly innocuous as the chemical effect of cigarette smoke, emotional upset, mental stress, or even moderate physical exertion on a vulnerable artery, heart attacks are usually caused by the rupture of an atherosclerotic patch on one of your coronary arteries.

In a study at Harvard Medical School, researchers found that emotional upset acted as a trigger in 18 percent of 412 men and women who had had heart attacks. Moderate physical exertion triggered another 14 percent, and a combination of factors—most commonly emotional upset and lack of sleep—triggered the heart attacks of another 4 percent.

When an atherosclerotic patch is ruptured, part of the patch—generally called a "clot" or "thrombus"—is thrown out into the artery, where it can partially or totally block the flow of blood, explains Dr. Gascho. If the blockage is partial, your doctor may say you have "unstable angina" or "pre-heart attack" angina. If it's total, he'll probably say you're having a heart attack. You don't want to hear him say either of those things.

Fighting Back

One thing can swing the balance in your favor, says Dr. Gascho. If you've made significant lifestyle changes in terms of diet, exercise, and stress reduction, you may have bought yourself enough time for collateral blood vessels to develop.

"There are frequently people who have totally blocked-off coronary arteries who do not develop a heart attack because these collaterals are present," says Dr. Gascho. Given enough time to develop, they can grow and expand until they can take over at least part of the job previously done by an artery that has become completely blocked.

They won't be big enough to give you enough blood and oxygen for a game of touch football, he adds. But they may be enough to prevent a heart attack.

Treating Heart Attacks

Fortunately, heart attacks are no longer the death sentences they used to be—as long as you get to the hospital emergency room *fast*, says Dr. Gascho.

Most of the deadly things that happen during a heart attack occur within the first couple of hours. Yet studies indicate that it takes most people between 2 and 4 hours of unremitting pain before they show up at an emergency room. They just don't want to believe they're having a heart attack.

Many people either die before reaching the hospital or are already past the most dangerous phase when they arrive at the emergency room entrance, says Dr. Gascho.

For people who get to the hospital quickly, however, doctors can administer a new generation of drugs that can actually dissolve the clot that's causing the attack. These drugs—generally either tissue plasminogen activator (tPA) or streptokinase—can dissolve the clot and restore the heart's blood and oxygen supply within 90 minutes. Once your heart is able to "breathe" again, the pain disappears.

There's also less damage done to your heart, adds Dr. Gascho. "If these drugs can be given within a half hour or even an hour, there will be a significant limitation in the size of the heart attack. If they're not given until 4 hours later, there will be no decrease in the size of the heart attack." That means chances of a second heart attack, post-heart attack angina, and an earlier death are all significantly increased.

A joint report by the American College of Cardiology and the AHA summarizes the statistics: "In patients whose treatment started within 3 to 6 hours, streptokinase resulted in a 17 percent reduction in mortality; in the 0-to-3-hour treatment group, it reduced mortality by 23 percent; and in those treated within 1 hour of symptoms, by 47 percent."

The difference in your chances is so significant, in fact, that doctors are now experimenting with allowing para-medic units to give tPA in the home or on the way to the hospital. A study at Tel Aviv University, for example, revealed that allowing paramedics to give tPA resulted in a 40-minute decrease in the time from symptom onset to treatment.

Preventing a Second Attack

Your doctor may also give you other drugs to help the clot-busters do their job, relieve pain, and reduce the possibility of a second heart attack. Heparin, aspirin, beta-blockers, and nitrates are the most likely while the attack is under way.

In one international study of over 17,000 patients, the simple addition of 160 milligrams of aspirin to the initial clot-busting treatment reduced the number of second heart attacks by *50 percent*. The aspirin was continued for one month after the initial heart attack and was so effective in preventing subsequent heart attacks that the researchers— drawn from 417 hospitals worldwide—suggested that it might well be appropriate for people who are having a heart attack to take aspirin at home—before they even go to the hospital. Moreover, aspirin is frequently the treatment of choice for one of the most common complications of a heart attack: pericarditis, an inflammation of the heart.

But drugs are not the only way to prevent a second heart attack, doctors emphasize. If you smoke, quitting will reduce your risk of heart disease by 37 percent within a matter of months. Reducing the amount of cholesterol in your diet by 10 percent can reduce your risk of another heart attack by 15 percent.

High-fiber/low-fat diets with plenty of fish—two or three servings a week of mackerel, tuna, herring, or salmon—can also reduce your risks, and scientists are beginning to suspect that adequate amounts of magnesium and vitamin E are important as well.

Exercise has a significant effect on delivering more oxygen to your heart, teaching it to use less and slowing the underlying progression of atherosclerosis that can set you up for another heart attack. It may also increase the small amounts of tPA that—believe it or not—naturally occur in your body. For these reasons, the AHA's Committee on Exercise and Cardiac Rehabilitation suggests that people who have had a heart attack participate in a cardiac exercise program under medical supervision.

Keeping the lid on stress is also important. In a study at Briar Cliff College in Sioux City, Iowa, researchers found that the stresses people were most likely to encounter after a heart attack included worrying about their jobs and when they could return to work (44 percent), worrying about their health (36 percent), worrying about activities they enjoyed but could not immediately do (29 percent), and feeling guilty about not doing things they thought they should (21 percent).

A second study, this one conducted in a coronary care unit in Washington, D.C., revealed that both relaxation techniques and music therapy are effective ways of reducing stress in people who have just had a heart attack. (See chapter 22.)

PNEUMONIA

You're over the flu.

But now, just when you thought you were getting well, you're starting to cough. Your fever's gone up, your chest hurts, you can't breathe, and you never knew the human body could produce so much mucus.

No, it's not the flu, part 2. It's pneumonia, an inflammation of the lungs that can be caused by the flu or by an invasion of a variety of other viral and bacterial characters.

Particularly among the elderly, pneumonia may be caused by accidentally inhaling the contents of the stomach or by coughing up lung secretions following surgery.

▶ INSTANT RELIEF

There really is no quick relief for pneumonia. It requires medical attention. However, there is one thing you can do for yourself.

Reach for the aspirin. Nonsteroidal anti-inflammatory drugs such as aspirin relieve mild to moderate pain, doctors say.

▶ PREVENTION PAIN-RELIEF PROGRAM

Pneumonia is nothing to fool around with. It kills 40,000 to 60,000 people every year. In 1990, Muppeteer Jim Henson, the much-loved creator of Kermit the Frog, Miss Piggy, Big Bird, and Oscar the Grouch, succumbed. As Henson would probably say, "Anything that can get Kermit must sit in a pret-ty tough pond."

Most cases of pneumonia can be treated with antibiotics, says Frederick Ruben, M.D., a professor of medicine at the University of Pittsburgh. A mild case often responds to oral medication, while a tougher case needs the heavy-duty kind administered intravenously. Just a couple of days' worth will usually do the trick, he adds; then your immune system mops up the field of battle.

An annual flu shot will prevent a lot of cases, as will a one-time shot of pneumonia vaccine. Both are highly recommended for older folks, according to Dr. Ruben, since 25 percent of those over age 65 do not survive a battle with the germs that cause pneumonia.

PNEUMOTHORAX

When a balloon gets a leak, it deflates. When a tire gets a leak, it deflates. Not surprisingly, when a human lung gets a leak, it deflates, too.

While a balloon or tire usually gets deflated by a sharp object, the lung is deflated by a pneumothorax—literally a tiny bubble of air that has leaked out of the lung into the sac that surrounds it, explains Norman H. Edelman, M.D., consultant on scientific affairs to the American Lung Association. Pneumothorax may be caused by an infection or an injury. That injury can be as seemingly insignificant as a tiny blisterlike formation at the top of a lung, says Dr. Edelman.

▶ INSTANT RELIEF

There is no quick relief for pneumothorax, and the pain—sudden and localized in one lung—is such that you won't have to ask yourself whether or not you need to get yourself to the doctor.

▶ PREVENTION PAIN-RELIEF PROGRAM

Your lung may have sealed itself by the time you see the doctor. So if the pneumothorax is minor, your doctor will probably do nothing more than give you a little oxygen and watch to see how you do, says Dr. Edelman. If your pain continues, he or she may give you a nonsteroidal anti-inflammatory drug such as aspirin, and may add a narcotic if it's severe.

The pain may disappear within 2 or 3 hours. If it doesn't, adds Dr. Edelman, your doctor may admit you to the hospital and insert a tube into the sac surrounding the lung to extract the bubble of trapped air.

CHAPTER
4

EARS

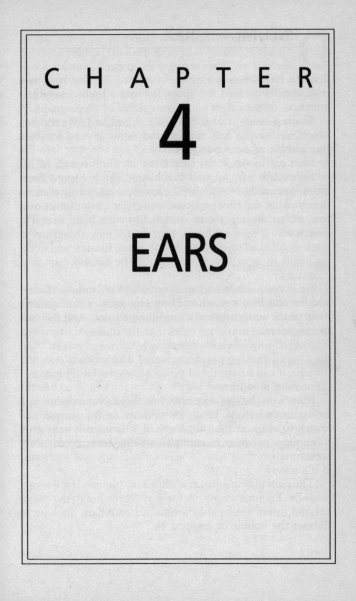

D octors seem to delight in coming up with new names for ear problems—leprechaun's ear, cauliflower ear, surfer's ear. Patients may get a quick chuckle when they discover their condition is named for the fairy tale character, vegetable, or sport it most closely resembles. Patients, on the other hand, may think of their condition as firecracker ear, water balloon ear, or hand grenade ear. Their ear may be hot, tender, and itchy. It may feel full, pounding, and near bursting.

Pain can come from infections in the outer canal or in the middle ear, located just behind the eardrum; from blockages inside or outside the ear that create an air vacuum that pulls at the eardrum; and sometimes from infections, tumors, or abnormalities elsewhere in the head or neck. That's why if your ear hurts, your doctor may also examine your mouth and teeth, jaw, throat, nose, sinuses, and neck. Problems in any of these areas could be sending pain into your ears.

As anyone who's had an earache can tell you—it hurts! The ear canal is a narrow, bony passageway that doesn't have room to accommodate swelling tissues. And the eardrum normally moves no more than the diameter of a single hydrogen atom when it's vibrating from sound waves. With the kind of vacuum pressure created with altitude changes, though, it can be stretched up to $1\frac{1}{2}$ excruciating millimeters before it ruptures.

It's not just babies who cry when they have ear blockages on an airplane, says James Donaldson, M.D., professor of otolaryngology at the University of Washington in Seattle. "That kind of pain is enough to bring tears to anyone's eyes."

GET PROFESSIONAL HELP IF:

- You have hearing loss not caused by a cold, allergy, or wax buildup
- You have suffered any trauma or injury to your ear (inner or outer)
- You have a yellowish, bloody discharge
- You feel dizzy or have trouble balancing
- You have itching, pain, or redness that lasts more than five days

PAIN-FINDER CHART FOR THE EARS

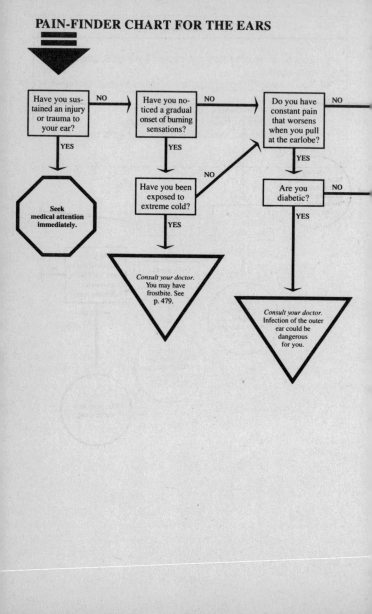

Have you sustained an injury or trauma to your ear? — NO →

Have you noticed a gradual onset of burning sensations? — NO →

Do you have constant pain that worsens when you pull at the earlobe? — NO →

YES ↓

Seek medical attention immediately.

YES ↓

Have you been exposed to extreme cold? — NO →

YES ↓

YES ↓

Are you diabetic? — NO →

YES ↓

Consult your doctor. You may have frostbite. See p. 479.

Consult your doctor. Infection of the outer ear could be dangerous for you.

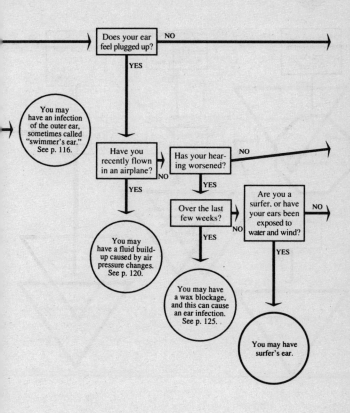

Does your ear feel plugged up? → NO →

YES ↓

You may have an infection of the outer ear, sometimes called "swimmer's ear." See p. 116.

Have you recently flown in an airplane?

YES ↓

You may have a fluid build-up caused by air pressure changes. See p. 120.

NO →

Has your hearing worsened? → NO →

YES ↓

Over the last few weeks?

YES ↓

You may have a wax blockage, and this can cause an ear infection. See p. 125.

NO →

Are you a surfer, or have your ears been exposed to water and wind? → NO →

YES ↓

You may have surfer's ear.

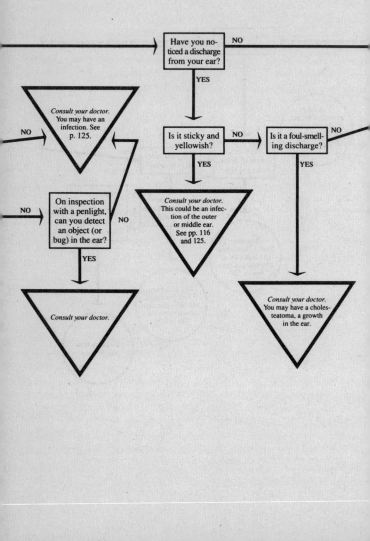

Have you noticed a discharge from your ear?

NO

YES

Consult your doctor. You may have an infection. See p. 125.

NO

Is it sticky and yellowish?

NO

Is it a foul-smelling discharge?

NO

YES

YES

On inspection with a penlight, can you detect an object (or bug) in the ear?

NO

Consult your doctor. This could be an infection of the outer or middle ear. See pp. 116 and 125.

YES

Consult your doctor.

Consult your doctor. You may have a cholesteatoma, a growth in the ear.

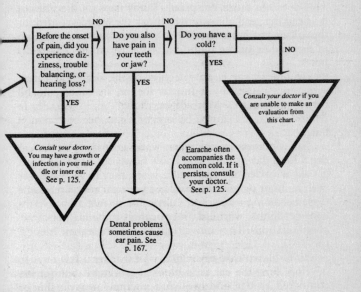

Before the onset of pain, did you experience dizziness, trouble balancing, or hearing loss?

NO → Do you also have pain in your teeth or jaw?

NO → Do you have a cold?

NO →

YES ↓

Consult your doctor. You may have a growth or infection in your middle or inner ear. See p. 125.

YES ↓

Dental problems sometimes cause ear pain. See p. 167.

YES ↓

Earache often accompanies the common cold. If it persists, consult your doctor. See p. 125.

Consult your doctor if you are unable to make an evaluation from this chart.

SWIMMER'S EAR

Your kid's been in the water so long you wouldn't be surprised if he grew gills. Instead, he develops swimmer's ear. This does not mean he sprouts funny flaps on the sides of his head that will allow him to break the world's record for the 100-meter butterfly. It does mean he will wake you up in the middle of the night and say, "Mom, my ear *really* hurts."

Swimmer's ear is an infection of the outer ear canal, sometimes caused by a fungus (hence, its other colorful name—*jungle ear*). More often, though, and especially in painful cases, it's caused by one of a number of common bacteria.

The condition begins when water gets stuck in the ear canal for a day or two. You know how your hands and feet get all wrinkled up and white when they're in water for even an hour or so? The inside of your ear reacts the same way, becoming soggy and vulnerable to infection. Germs consider moist, warm, dark ear canals to be high-class accommodations. They move right in and invite their friends, too.

A full-blown case of swimmer's ear takes a few days to develop. First the ear feels blocked and itchy. Soon it becomes red, tender, and swollen. Sometimes it swells shut or starts draining a milky liquid. It is also very sensitive to touch, especially on the triangular bit of cartilage in front of the ear canal, called the tragus.

➤ INSTANT RELIEF

When the infection reaches the painful stage, a doctor is usually a welcome sight. What can you do in the meantime?

Eat ice cream and watch cartoons. If your child says he feels better doing fun things, don't think he's faking his symptoms as a way to indulge. Enjoyable activities can distract young and old alike from their pain.

Multipurpose Relief

For: Swimmer's Ear, Middle Ear Infection

WARM IT UP

People's ears jut out from their heads for a reason—to catch every passing sound. Unfortunately, they also catch every passing breeze. And for anyone with an earache, cold drafts can mean more pain.

Just as cold can make people cringe with ear pain, warmth makes those ears feel comfortable. Even cupping your hands over your ears can provide soothing relief. So can snuggling your ear up to a heating pad or hot water bottle.

Some doctors suggest using a blow dryer to warm up that aching ear. Forget the blow dryer if you have a perforated eardrum, however. It can blow dust and other particles into your ear.

Remember to keep your ears covered when you venture outdoors. Earmuffs may make you feel like a polar bear, but without them you'll feel like growling—in pain.

See also:

- "Warm It Up" above.
- "Analgesics for Auditory Aches" on page 127.

▶ PREVENTION PAIN-RELIEF PROGRAM

Swimmer's ear usually clears up readily with antibiotic eardrops, which your doctor can prescribe. If the ear is too swollen to allow the drops to penetrate, the doctor can place a wick in the ear canal, which will draw the solution into the ear. The wick may fall out in a day or two as swelling subsides. An expanding spongy wick, however, will have to be removed by the doctor. Antibiotic drops are used for three to five days; during that time it's important to keep your ears dry, says Robert Schindler, M.D., professor and chairman of the Department of Otolaryngology—Head and Neck Surgery at the University of California, San Francisco.

Staying Dry

Since swimmer's ear has a nasty habit of revisiting the previously afflicted, doctors suggest a preventive measure that, used faithfully, should prevent further recurrences.

Within an hour after you've gone swimming, put four or five drops of isopropyl (rubbing) alcohol in each ear. To do this, turn the ear skyward, put the drops in, and wiggle the ear by grasping the outside and gently tugging to work the drops all the way in. Then turn your head and let the fluid drain out. "You might also twist the corner of a tissue into a little point and use it to wick water out of your ear," suggests Jack Pulec, M.D., a Los Angeles ear, nose, and throat specialist.

Isopropyl alcohol works two ways. Because it has a lower surface tension than water, it breaks up water molecules and makes it easier for trapped water to find its way out of a long and winding ear canal. And the tiny amount of alcohol/water mixture remaining in your ear evaporates quickly, leaving your ear canal too inhospitably dry for any microbes that might be looking for a home. Inexpensive commercial eardrops such as Auro-dri contain mostly isopropyl alcohol. Others, such as Star-Otic, contain boric acid. Those that contain boric acid or acetic acid (white vinegar) kill potential infecting organisms by making the ear canal slightly acidic. (You can make up your own mix of alcohol and vinegar.)

If water is frequently trapped in your ears, you may have a dam of wax retaining water. If so, use a commercial earwax remover, such as Debrox, or see your doctor. You may do well to have your ears cleaned out by a doctor before swimming season starts, says Dr. Schindler.

People whose ears are frequently exposed to cold water—northern California surfers, professional lifeguards, or members of the Polar Bear Club—may develop growths under the skin in their ear canals. These bony bumps, which take years to develop, are the ear's attempt to protect itself from the cold, but they can also trap water in the ear. The bumps can be planed away just as a plastic surgeon would remove a bump on the nose, in an outpatient surgical procedure, says Dr. Pulec.

Get the Wet Out

Just about all ear specialists say earplugs designed to keep water out of the ears don't work. "I'd rather have my patients expose their ears to the water and then use alcohol to dry them out," Dr. Pulec says. If they insist, he will make customized earplugs from plastic molds of a patient's ears.

A swimming pool can cause an epidemic of swimmer's ear if its water is not being properly disinfected. Warm, stagnant water is more likely to cause ear canal infections than fast-moving water, because it contains many more microorganisms, says Dr. Donaldson. So if your canoe tips over while you're out on the bayou, dousing your ears in alcohol would be a wise preventive move.

ALTITUDE/FLIGHT-RELATED EAR PAIN

"We'll be landing in mumble mumble blah blah blah in approximately 20 minutes. We hope you've had a pleasant time flying with mumble mumble blah blah blah airlines and that you will mumble mumble blah blah blah with us again."

You're not listening. You feel like your ears are going to explode. You automatically start gulping down air, hoping the pain will stop.

What's going on here? Chances are that a cold or allergy has blocked your eustachian tubes—the tiny passageways that lead from your throat to your middle ears, supplying them with the air they need to function properly.

A blocked eustachian tube means that the air pressure inside your ear is lower than the air pressure outside your ear. Air pressure drops as altitude increases. In this case, what goes down must come up, and as the plane descends, the pressure gradually increases again. The cabins of most commercial planes are pressurized at 5,000 to 8,000 feet, but there is still a fairly rapid pressure change to which your ears must adjust. This can be a real problem on the way down, as pressure builds rapidly on the outside of the eardrum. It creates a vacuum inside your ear that pulls at your eardrum. That's what causes the pain.

▶ INSTANT RELIEF

If you can get air through the eustachian tube and to your ear, the pain and pressure will be relieved.

Clear your ears. Pinch your nostrils shut, take a mouthful of air, close your lips tightly, and try to blow out firmly against your closed nose and mouth. Increase the pressure gradually until you hear a pop, which signals that you have forced a bubble of air through the eustachian tube, equalizing the pressure inside and outside your ear, advises

Dr. Donaldson. Continue to clear your ears in this manner every few minutes during the entire descent.

Experts warn, though, that once pain has set in, it becomes harder and harder to clear your ears. That's because the same air vacuum that tugs at your eardrums also sucks the eustachian tubes closed, collapsing them. It may take more air pressure than you can muster up to force air into the tubes. So start clearing your ears the minute the plane begins its first descent.

"On a flight from Los Angeles to Philadelphia, you'd want to start clearing your ears over Ohio," Dr. Pulec says. If you're not sure when the plane will start its descent, ask a flight attendant.

▶ **PREVENTION PAIN-RELIEF PROGRAM**

If you want to ensure a pain-free trip, you must do a little homework before you leave.

If you have either a head cold or allergies and you must fly, use a nasal spray or oral decongestant. (Check with your doctor first, though, if you have high blood pressure, heart disease, diabetes, thyroid disease, or are pregnant.)

Most doctors recommend a long-lasting nasal spray containing oxymetazoline hydrochloride, such as Afrin. "I tell my patients to take one spray of Afrin on each side of their nose about 1 hour before their first descent, then a second spray in each side of their nose 10 minutes later," Dr. Donaldson says.

As far as relieving ear pain is concerned, it's the second spray that does the job. "The first spray just opens the nose; the second one shoots way back and shrinks down all the mucous membranes," Dr. Donaldson says. When you spray your nose, be sure to inhale deeply.

Some doctors recommend taking decongestant tablets containing phenylpropanolamine hydrochloride, such as Comtrex. "I tell people to take an amount equivalent to 50 milligrams of phenylpropanolamine at least an hour before their first descent," says Dr. Pulec. "That amount is going to make them a little shaky and nervous, but it will definitely keep their ears open." Other doctors say nasal sprays work just as well, with fewer unpleasant side effects.

Gulp and Chew

Before and during the descent, swallow frequently. That makes your eustachian tubes open briefly. Chewing gum also helps. And do make sure you're not in dreamland when the plane makes its descent. (Ask your neighbor or a flight attendant to wake you up if necessary.)

If you're using earplugs, remember to remove them during both ascent and descent. "They can create another sealed air space, which only adds to your problem," warns Dr. Pulec. He also suggests you drink plenty of plain water, but avoid alcohol while you're flying.

Delaying Action

If you've gotten psyched up over that special trip, the last thing you want to do is put it off. But your ears are too precious to endanger for the sake of a brief fling in vacationland.

Consider postponing your flight or taking a train if you have a really bad cold or sinus infection, experts agree. The back of your throat is probably coated with virus or bacteria-laden mucus, and an air pressure-induced vacuum could draw germs into the middle ear, Dr. Donaldson says. "They might have gone there anyway, but when you fly with an upper respiratory infection, you're actively promoting the problem."

If you're about to embark on the vacation of your lifetime and have no intention of canceling your flight plans because of a stuffy head, or if you fly for a living and can't afford to take days off for earaches, it may be possible to have ventilating (tympanostomy) tubes inserted through your eardrums, Dr. Pulec says.

Because they provide a constant source of air to the middle ear, these tubes equalize air pressure on both sides of the eardrum. The tubes are inserted in a doctor's office in a procedure that takes just a few minutes and has little risk of infection as long as the ears are kept dry. The tubes can be removed when you return from your vacation or will fall out on their own in about a year.

If your ears refuse to clear during your plane's descent, you may have head-splitting pain when you touch down. But your pain shouldn't get any worse once you've landed, Dr. Donaldson says, and if you tough it out, the pain will slowly resolve over a few days.

However, you will be left with fluid in your middle ear, which will muffle your hearing for some time before it's reabsorbed into the body. If you see an ear, nose, and throat specialist, he or she may make tiny slits in your eardrums to relieve pressure and vacuum the fluid out. Always see a doctor if your pain persists or if you're dizzy, Dr. Donaldson warns. It may mean you've damaged your middle ear or even your inner ear.

Air Babies

If you're planning to take a child or infant on a trip, you should take special precautions to protect their sensitive ears.

Ear infections and earaches are the bane of many children's young lives. If your child has frequent earaches, ask your pediatrician about using a decongestant or nasal spray during the flight.

"If the nasal lining is so swollen that it's closing off the tube, a decongestant may help," explains Allan DeJong, M.D., clinical professor of pediatrics at Thomas Jefferson Medical College in Philadelphia.

A parent who has to fly with a congested infant or small child "should use good judgment based on the child's age and experience," Dr. DeJong says. "If it's a very young infant who has not had decongestants before, you're better off not using a decongestant for the first time on an airplane. (They can cause irritability and agitation.) If it's an older child who's taken antihistamines or decongestants with no ill effects, they may be helpful and are probably not going to hurt."

Don't rely on drugs alone to solve your child's ear problem, Dr. DeJong cautions. Breastfeed or bottle-feed an infant during the descent to encourage frequent swallowing. And keep the baby upright, at a level at least 20 degrees above the horizon. This allows the eustachian tubes to function better. Give older children gum to chew or hard candies to suck. Or give them a balloon or other inflatable toy; be sure to tell them to hold their nose while blowing up the balloon or toy.

MIDDLE EAR INFECTION

It's hard to believe such a tiny portion of the anatomy can cause so much agony—especially in children.

Right behind the eardrum lies the middle ear, a small air space sheltering the delicate bridge of bones that transfers sound vibrations from the eardrum to the inner ear. The middle ear can become infected when bacteria or viruses move in from the throat and establish squatter's rights. (The middle ear can also become inflamed—tender and swollen—without an infection.)

Middle ear problems are fairly common in children age ten or younger. In adults, they are much less frequent and are usually associated with a bad cold or allergies, says Dr. Schindler.

In adults, a middle ear infection may set in three to five days after the onset of a cold. Warning signals are fatigue, fever, swollen glands, and ear pain—which may be constant or intermittent, mild to excruciating, and accompanied by drainage, hearing loss, dizziness, and ringing.

In an adult, chronic middle ear problems could be linked to a structural abnormality in the ear that may require surgery, says Dr. Schindler.

A hole in the eardrum, for example, makes a person more vulnerable to middle ear infections because it is easier for germs to enter the ear from the eustachian tube or ear canal. "We may recommend repair in some instances, but if someone's had a hole in their eardrum for a long time with no problems, usually there's no need to repair it," says Dr. Schindler.

▶ INSTANT RELIEF

Earaches are usually worse at night. The eustachian tubes are less active, which means air pressure can build up in the middle ear.

Get an angle on it. Try sleeping with your head propped up on an additional pillow to allow the eustachian tubes to function, says Dr. Donaldson. But don't try to prop up a baby with pillows.

Breastfeeding or bottle-feeding a baby while it's lying flat on its back has been associated with an increase in middle ear infections. This feeding position may wash liquid and germs into the middle ear as the child sucks and swallows. So always keep a baby at least semi-upright to feed, suggests Dr. DeJong.

See also:

- "Warm it Up" on page 117.
- "Analgesics for Auditory Aches" on the opposite page.

➡ PREVENTION PAIN-RELIEF PROGRAM

There's no doubt: Middle ear infections require a doctor's prompt treatment. Before World War II, bad ear infections often were fatal. These days, thanks to prompt treatment with antibiotics, few people die from ear infections.

Once you've seen your doctor, the next part of your program to banish middle ear infections should involve a few household adjustments.

The same kinds of lifestyle tactics that reduce the number and relieve the severity of head colds and allergies can help reduce ear infections.

Avoiding cigarette smoke tops the list of every otolaryngologist. "And that includes passive smoking," Dr. Donaldson says. "Kids whose parents smoke are much more likely to have upper respiratory infections that can lead to ear problems." Doctors suggest that parents not smoke in the house.

Allergies to airborne substances, such as pollen, dust, or animal dander, can swell shut a child's eustachian tubes, causing ear blockage. (Constant congestion without a fever, along with itchy, watering eyes, is the tip-off of allergy.) Minimizing contact with these allergy-causing substances, using an antihistamine, or getting desensitizing shots may help prevent allergy-related ear problems, says Dr. DeJong.

Most pediatricians believe allergies to airborne substances rather than to food are most likely to be involved in ear problems, says Dr. DeJong. Still, some doctors believe it's helpful to try eliminating certain foods from an infant's or child's diet to see if ear problems improve. Tops on their scratch-it list is dairy products. They also sometimes suggest eliminating eggs, peanuts, soy, wheat, or fish.

Whether the person suffering from a middle ear infection is a child or an adult, it pays to keep the house moderately humidified, to about 50 or 60 percent. Make sure you drink lots of fluids to keep mucus thin and running when you have a cold. Blow your nose gently: Blasts that summon the troops can also push germ-laden mucus into your ears, some experts say.

Multipurpose Relief

For: Swimmer's Ear, Middle Ear Infection

ANALGESICS FOR AUDITORY ACHES

It's the middle of the night and your child is crying with an earache. You feel like crying, too. The pediatrician is likely to prescribe antibiotics to treat the infection and a painkiller such as codeine to provide relief until the antibiotics kick in and blast out those microbes. Once you *see* the pediatrician, that is.

But what do you do *now*, while you're holding your child and watching the luminous dial on the clock creeping oh so slowly toward the hour of your appointment?

Over-the-counter drugs such as aspirin or ibuprofen can relieve many kinds of aches, including those of the ear variety. These analgesics are fine for adults. But pediatricians warn that children should be given acetaminophen, not aspirin. Aspirin has been linked with a potentially deadly childhood disease, Reye's syndrome. (See chapter 26).

C H A P T E R
5

EYES

Your eyes are a delicate, vital, irreplaceable part of your body. That's why nature protects them.

A protective barrier of bones encircles most of the eye. The eyelid forms an additional line of defense, snapping shut in response to an intense flash of light or the glimpse of an incoming object. Like a tiny windshield wiper, the lid sweeps fluid across the eye, moistening and cleaning it.

The cornea forms a structure much like a watch crystal that sits on top of your eye, protecting the iris and pupil. (The white part of your eye is relatively insensitive to pain, but the iris—the colored portion—contains receptors that can scream with pain.) Inside the cornea is a chamber filled with a clear, watery liquid that nourishes and maintains pressure in the eye.

Still, even with all this protection, there are things that can make your eyes hurt: an errant champagne cork, a full day spent staring at a computer screen, or a bout with "pinkeye" or some other eye disease.

Oddly, most major diseases that can cause blindness—such as cataracts and most forms of glaucoma—do *not* cause pain.

However, eye pain is a signal that something is seriously wrong, says Paul Vinger, M.D., a Lexington, Massachusetts, ophthalmologist. Your doctor won't simply give you anesthetic drops and send you on your way. He or she will make every effort to find what's wrong.

PAIN-FINDER CHART FOR THE EYES

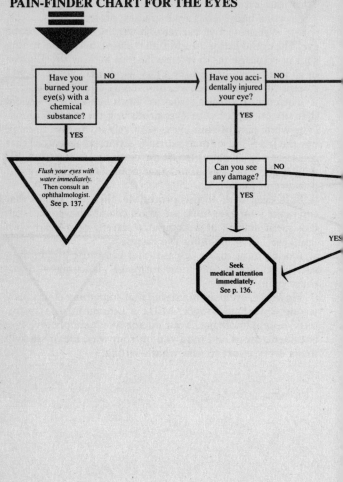

Have you burned your eye(s) with a chemical substance?

NO

Have you accidentally injured your eye?

NO

YES

Flush your eyes with water immediately. Then consult an ophthalmologist. See p. 137.

YES

Can you see any damage?

NO

YES

Seek medical attention immediately. See p. 136.

YES

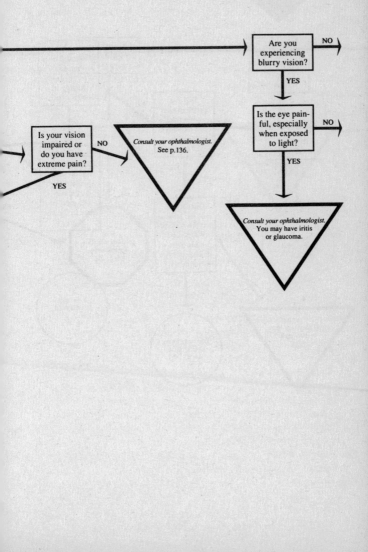

Are you experiencing blurry vision?

NO →

YES ↓

Is the eye painful, especially when exposed to light?

NO →

YES ↓

Consult your ophthalmologist. You may have iritis or glaucoma.

Is your vision impaired or do you have extreme pain?

NO →

Consult your ophthalmologist. See p.136.

YES

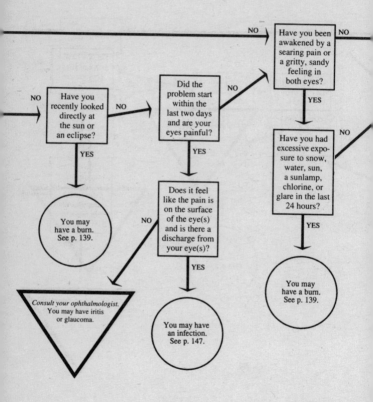

NO →

Have you been awakened by a searing pain or a gritty, sandy feeling in both eyes?

NO →

NO →

Have you recently looked directly at the sun or an eclipse?

NO →

Did the problem start within the last two days and are your eyes painful?

NO →

YES ↓

YES ↓

YES ↓

Have you had excessive exposure to snow, water, sun, a sunlamp, chlorine, or glare in the last 24 hours?

NO →

You may have a burn. See p. 139.

Does it feel like the pain is on the surface of the eye(s) and is there a discharge from your eye(s)?

NO

YES ↓

Consult your ophthalmologist. You may have iritis or glaucoma.

You may have an infection. See p. 147.

You may have a burn. See p. 139.

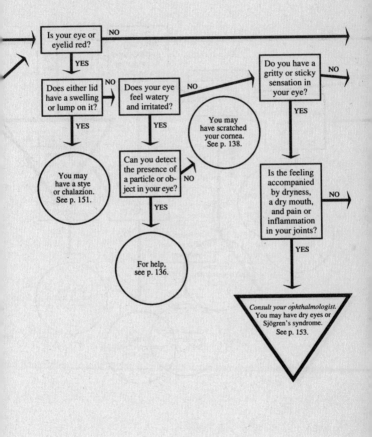

Is your eye or eyelid red?

NO →

YES ↓

Does either lid have a swelling or lump on it?

NO →

YES ↓

You may have a stye or chalazion. See p. 151.

Does your eye feel watery and irritated?

NO →

YES ↓

Can you detect the presence of a particle or object in your eye?

NO →

YES ↓

For help, see p. 136.

You may have scratched your cornea. See p. 138.

Do you have a gritty or sticky sensation in your eye?

NO →

YES ↓

Is the feeling accompanied by dryness, a dry mouth, and pain or inflammation in your joints?

NO →

YES ↓

Consult your ophthalmologist. You may have dry eyes or Sjögren's syndrome. See p. 153.

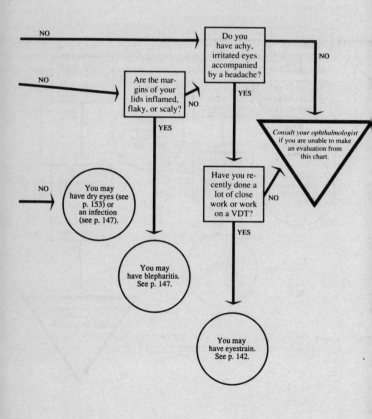

GET PROFESSIONAL HELP IF:

- You have an eye injury
- You have blurred or impaired vision
- You have double vision or loss of a portion of the visual field
- You have pain behind the eye, with a severe headache, sensitivity to bright light, drowsiness, confusion, or pain when you bend your head forward
- You have persistent redness of the eye
- There is blood in the eye
- There is an unmovable or embedded object or particle in your eye
- Your pupil is an irregular shape

INJURIES

Every once in a while you get a sharp reminder that your eyes can indeed feel pain. It may come in the form of a grain of sand that lands in your eye, a splash of household chemical, even an out-of-bounds tennis ball that socks you in the face. Or you may spend too long in the sun and sunburn your eyes. (The right kind of sunglasses do more than enhance your beach image.)

▶ INSTANT RELIEF

The techniques you use to banish pain will, of course, depend on the type of injury to the eye.

A speck in your eye no bigger than the period at the end of this sentence can feel like a creature with claws. This is one instance in which pain is sending you a helpful message—left in your eye, that speck could scratch the cornea.

If you can see a foreign body on the white of your eye, you may be able to remove it yourself. If it's on the colored part, however, you probably need to get your doctor to remove it, says Dr. Vinger. Be careful, he warns. If you can't wash or wipe the speck away, don't reach into your eye and yank—even if the speck seems to be sticking up. See a doctor instead. That "speck" could be a part of your eye.

"You must be positive that what you see is something on your eye and not a cut in your eye," Dr. Vinger says. "When in doubt, leave it alone."

Winken and blinken. If it's simply a speck of dust or an eyelash, a few sharp blinks may push the foreign body off your cornea into the white part of your eye, where it is more easily removed.

Wipe it out. Use a clean cotton swab or the tip of a moistened, clean handkerchief to gently wipe the speck toward the corner of your eye.

Push-me pull-me. If blinking and wiping don't work,

gently pull your upper lid down over your lower lashes, causing your eye to tear. Those tears may wash the object out. Or the lower lashes may wipe the undersurface of the lid and push the object out.

Flush it. If your eye has been hit with a splash of a chemical—such as drain cleaner or toilet bowl cleaner—flush the eyes with water immediately. Hold your head over the sink and use your fingers to pry your eye open, says ophthalmologist C. Douglas Witherspoon, M.D., a member of the American Academy of Ophthalmology's Eye Safety and Sports Ophthalmology Committee and co-director of the Eye Injury Registry of Alabama. Because of the pain, you may need to enlist someone else to hold your eyes open under the water, he says.

Multipurpose Relief

For: Infection, Stye, Chalazion

WASH THAT EYE!

Under the right set of conditions, bacteria can grow in your eye as fast as they can in egg salad on a warm summer's day.

If you are particularly prone to eye infections, styes, or chalazions, your doctor may advise washing your eyes, says Paul Vinger, M.D., a Lexington, Massachusetts, ophthalmologist. If you feel the irritation that sometimes precedes these conditions, a splash in time can do wonders.

Here's how.

Mix a soapy solution of half water and half baby shampoo, or get an eye preparation like I-Scrub or OCuSoft. With clean fingers, pull one eyelid at a time away from your eye. Dip a cotton swab into the mixture, then gently massage it along the edge of your eyelid. Use another swab dipped in clear water to rinse. Do this with each of your eyelids.

Whatever it takes, "your eye *must* be rinsed immediately and copiously," says Oliver D. Schein, M.D., ophthalmologist at the Wilmer Institute at Johns Hopkins University School of Medicine. "You don't have to have any special equipment. No eye cups or special eye washes. Shower water or tap water will do. Some of the chemicals that are damaging to the eyes do their damage within seconds, so you want to wash them out as quickly as possible."

Keep flushing your eyes with water until someone can drive you to the emergency room, or for at least 10 minutes, Dr. Witherspoon says. Flushing quickly may save your eyesight.

Cup it. If you can't remove the foreign body or if you have chemicals in your eyes, close them while someone takes you to the doctor. Keep both eyes closed to minimize your eye movement and cut down on the pain, says Dr. Vinger.

Chill out. If you get socked in the eye with a ball or some other object, apply a clean, cold compress. The cold will help anesthetize your eye and face while keeping swelling to a minimum.

"Swelling could make the eye hard to evaluate," Dr. Witherspoon says. "Use very little pressure against the eye in case it is ruptured or there has been a cut from the blunt force."

See also:

- "Wash that Eye!" on page 137.

▶ PREVENTION PAIN-RELIEF PROGRAM

If you successfully remove a foreign object from your eye and pain lingers to remind you of the unpleasant experience, you should probably see your ophthalmologist. For that matter, you should make an appointment for any painful injury to your eye.

The ABCs of Abrasions

What looks like a harmless speck might leave behind a corneal abrasion—a scratch on the surface of the cornea.

Small pieces of metal can rust in your eye and cause damage. You also can get an abrasion from scratching yourself with a fingernail while inserting contact lenses. Or if you fall asleep with your contacts in your eyes, you could wake up with a scratch.

If you have an abrasion, it will feel like there's something still in your eye. Your eye will hurt, appear red, and probably tear. Your vision may be distorted.

If your ophthalmologist detects an abrasion, he or she will prescribe a course of antibiotics. And you'll get an eyepatch to wear for 24 to 48 hours to allow your eye to rest and to ease the pain.

If the injury resulted from activity that you're likely to repeat in the near future—a job-related task, for example—your doctor will undoubtedly advise investing in a pair of safety goggles or glasses. (See "Put Up a Good Front" on page 140.)

Here's Fire in Your Eyes

If you've spent the weekend skiing, that eye pain could come from an injury that slipped up on you. Just like the rest of your body, your eyes can sunburn, but you probably won't think of burning when you're romping in the snow.

Your eyes can also get burned from a suntan lamp or from looking at the flash from welding equipment without protection. It takes about 12 to 24 hours from the time you burn your eyes until you feel the effects. That means you may go to sleep and wake in the middle of the night or the next morning with searing pain and the feeling of sand in your eyes.

"We see burns in skiers who aren't properly protected," says Ivan Schwab, M.D., associate professor of ophthalmology at the University of California, Davis. "Ultraviolet light burns happen when the sun is reflected off sand or snow. It burns the surface of the eye, the epithelium. That surface is injured or sick, or it dies. Then it drops off, leaving an abrasion on the cornea. That's painful."

Sunglasses with ultraviolet-protective lenses can prevent

the burn, he says. Look for a label that gives light transmission factors, telling you what percentage of the light gets through the lenses. For protection from the sun, look for a light transmission factor of 30 percent or less. To protect against the glare from sand, water, or snow, 15 to 10 percent is best. Polarized or mirrored glasses can also protect against glare. Choose gray, brown, or green lenses.

PUT UP A GOOD FRONT

Don crouched like a cat ready to spring, every muscle tensed. His eyes followed the little blue rubber ball as it bounced off the wall of the racquetball court.

Thock.

The ball leapt back toward Don. And he caught it . . . right in the face.

Thock.

Don crumpled to the floor. His opponent rushed to his side.

Don looked up, smiling. He peeled off his wraparound safety goggles. No harm done.

Most eye injuries are just as fast, just as unexpected, and just as easily prevented.

Forty-eight percent of all eye injuries happen at work. In a machine shop, for instance, a tiny piece of metal flies up from a metal grinder and lands in an eye. Twenty-seven percent happen at home: Steam and chemicals can spew up with violent force when a drain cleaner hits a clog. Even spraying your roses can prove hazardous if the wind shifts at the wrong time.

With a little forethought, avoiding eye injury is a piece of cake. Before you undertake any project that might put your eyes in jeopardy, put on a pair of good-quality safety glasses or goggles made with polycarbonate lenses, says Oliver D. Schein, M.D., ophthalmologist at the Wilmer Institute at Johns Hopkins University School of Medicine. The National Society to Prevent Blindness estimates that 90 percent of all eye injuries could be prevented by wearing a pair of safety glasses.

"Regular glasses will stand up to some impact, but they may crack," says C. Douglas Witherspoon, M.D., ophthalmologist and member of the American Academy of Ophthalmology's Eye Safety and Sports Ophthalmology Committee. "If you're in a machine shop, a metal projectile could fly up from the side and could go under the glasses or through the side."

Goggles or glasses should bear the code ANSI Z87 to show they meet the requirements set by the American National Standard Institute Practice for Occupational and Educational Eye and Face Protection. For sports use, be sure the package around the glasses or goggles says "polycarbonate lenses" or "lexan," not just "impact resistant."

You'll find goggles or safety glasses with side shields at your optician's office, in some hardware stores, and in some sporting goods shops. They cost about $15 to $40. It is also possible to have the lenses in your safety glasses made to fit with your eyeglasses prescription. Ask your optician about this option.

If you want to test your glasses, put them on and look in the mirror. You shouldn't be able to see your eyes, says Dr. Schwab.

For swimming, consider buying a pair of watertight, $5 goggles for use in the pool. Chlorine can mildly burn your cornea and make your eyes feel dry and scratchy.

EYESTRAIN

It's a myth, Mom. Reading in poor light, going without your glasses, or working on one project too long will *not* injure your eyes.

However, all these things *may* make your eyes feel tired and sore. The condition is called eyestrain, and it means you've overused your eyes or misused your eyes, says Dr. Vinger. It may also mean you need a new pair of glasses or a new prescription.

➤ INSTANT RELIEF

If you look up from your work and your eyeballs feel like they've been fried, take a pause that refreshes. Here are a number of techniques often recommended by medical experts.

Stare off into space. Rest your eyes every half hour. Gaze off into the distance. Let your eyes unfocus for a few minutes occasionally when you're doing close work such as sewing or reading.

Wet your eyes. Over-the-counter eyedrops won't cure eyestrain, but they will soothe eyes irritated by overwork, dust, smoke, pollution, or dryness.

Get cheeky. Acupressure points on your face can relieve the pain of eyestrain. (Used before eyestrain sets in, they can also help prevent it.) For their correct locations, see the drawings on pages 143 and 144. Press each of the points lightly for 1 minute.

➤ PREVENTION PAIN-RELIEF PROGRAM

Headache, fatigue, and eye pain can follow a demanding task that requires close concentration. These symptoms can mean you've overdone it and strained your eyes. They can also mean it's time to get a new prescription for your glasses. If you are bothered by repeated bouts of eyestrain,

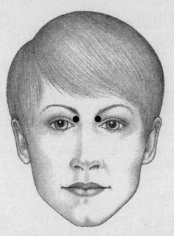

Press your thumbs up under the ridge of bone at the inside edge of your eyebrows.

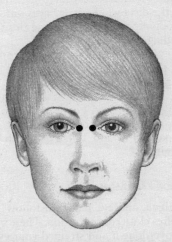

Use your forefingers to press either side of the bridge of your nose. Many people naturally massage this area when their eyes are tired.

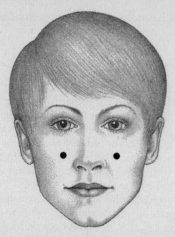

To find the correct point on the cheeks, put your middle and index fingers on either side of your nose. Now lift your middle finger and press with your index finger.

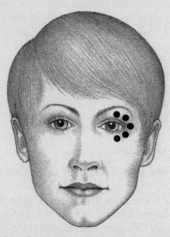

There are a number of points along the bony ridge that surrounds your eye. After you've finished pressing the other points, massage the outer edges of the ridge above and below your eyes.

see your ophthalmologist for an evaluation, says Dr. Vinger.

Focus on Fit

If your glasses don't feel right, take a lesson from Goldilocks. She didn't want to eat the porridge that was too hot, sit in a rocking chair that was too big, or sleep in a bed that was too soft. She wanted everything "just right."

That's the way you should feel about your glasses, says Dr. Vinger. Sometimes, when glasses don't fit exactly right, they can cause those eyestrain symptoms that you complain about at the end of the day.

"Look at eyeglasses the way you choose your sneakers," Dr. Vinger says. "If you're working in them all day, they have to fit right. That means you have to look through the whole lens."

When you look through your glasses, you should see equally well with both eyes. The center of each lens should go directly over the center of each eye. That means if you've chosen frames too large, you'll end up looking through the top part of the frames and you won't see the way your doctor meant you to when he or she wrote your prescription. Your eyes will have to work harder, and that will make them tired and cranky.

"If your eyes aren't centered, you'll get a lot of peripheral distortion, especially if you wear progressive [line-free] bifocals," Dr. Vinger says.

Beating VDT Blahs

Glasses aren't the only thing that can cause that burned-out feeling.

People who stare at a computer screen all day often complain of blurred vision, headaches, eye irritation, and eyestrain, says Dr. Vinger. These symptoms are caused by holding the eye muscles rigidly and focusing on one particular distance instead of a variety of distances. That's why it helps to shift your focus from time to time.

Arranging your workspace will give your eyes a better working environment, too. "Imagine if you were trying to read a book that had been glued down," Dr. Vinger says. "You'd have to adjust yourself around it. The same is true in your workplace. You have to adjust yourself to fit the fixed computer."

He suggests you find a comfortable reading distance and place your computer screen at that distance. An intermediate viewing distance ranges from 22 to 26 inches. The proper height for your terminal is just below eye level.

Glare from the computer screen can also contribute to eye fatigue, says Dr. Vinger. Turn your screen so it won't reflect light from the windows or ceiling, he advises. If that's not possible—and in many offices you aren't allowed to rearrange the furniture—there are other things that you can do.

You can ask your eye care specialist to add an antireflective coating to your glasses or get a special antiglare screen to place over your computer screen. Or wear a hat with a brim or an old-fashioned green eyeshade to block the glare, says Dr. Vinger.

Check the lighting on your screen, he advises. Some people are especially sensitive to it. If you are used to working on a screen with a light background and dark letters, try to swap it for a screen with a dark background with light letters, advises Dr. Vinger.

If you can't switch screens, try changing the contrast. Most people work better with great visual contrast between the screen and the letters, says Dr. Vinger. Adjust the print on the screen so that it is five to ten times brighter than the background. And adjust the screen's brightness so that it is three or four times brighter than the room lighting. (It may help to dim the room lights somewhat.)

Finally, if you've done all these things and your eyes still feel dry and gritty at the end of the day, check the ventilation around your computer to be sure it isn't blowing air into your eyes. You can redirect that air with a piece of cardboard taped to your computer.

INFECTIONS

Red eyes? And you didn't even paint the town last night? It could be an eye infection.

Red eyes are one of the most common reasons people see their eye doctor, says Dr. Vinger. The problem could be something as simple as too much partying and not enough sleep. Then again, it might mean disease. When your eyes are red *and* painful, that's a signal to see your doctor, says Dr. Vinger.

Red, gritty, painful eyes could mean a bacterial or viral infection, says Dr. Vinger. The redness could also be a symptom of uveitis—an inflammation caused by allergy.

Redness of the eyelids, rather than of the eyes themselves, could be blepharitis—an infection that features greasy scales, itching, and the feeling that there's something in your eye.

▶ Instant Relief

While you're waiting for that doctor's appointment to roll around, try some of these pain-relieving tips.

Cool it off. If you have a viral infection, cold is better than warmth. A viral infection makes your eyes red like a bacterial infection, but the discharge is watery, not puslike, and there is very little debris on your eyelashes, says Dr. Schwab. One eye may look worse than the other. A viral infection is generally not as severe as a bacterial infection, but it can be uncomfortable. A cold compress, "as cold as you can get it," applied to the eyelid will decrease the blood flow to your eyes and lids and give some relief, says Dr. Schwab.

Drop in on them. If your eyes are especially irritated from a viral infection, try artificial tears without preservatives. They'll put a soothing film over your red eyes. Preservatives, Dr. Schwab warns, may make your eyes even more sore. You can purchase artificial tears at your local pharmacy.

Go incognito. Some infections can make your eyes sensitive to light, especially bright light. Put on a pair of dark glasses and you'll spare your eyes discomfort. Sensitivity to light can be a sign of more severe eye problems. If it persists, see your doctor.

Rest a little. If you give your eyes a break, they'll have less pain. Try closing your eyes for a nap or simply sitting in the dark for a while.

See also:

- "Wet and Warm" on page 150.

▶ PREVENTION PAIN-RELIEF PROGRAM

Once your doctor diagnoses your eye problem, he or she will be able to prescribe the appropriate medications to clear it up. If you want to avoid a return visit with the same problem, a little prevention is in order, says Dr. Vinger. Preventing an eye infection can be as simple as washing your hands and taking extra care with makeup and contact lenses, he says.

Don't Give Bacteria a Toehold

Suppose you use the same makeup day after day. Then you get an eye infection and continue to use the same mascara. The wand that touches your eyelashes and the bacteria growing on them goes back into the tube, where it sits until you color your eyelashes again.

You might get rid of the infection, but you'll daub it back on again every time you do your lashes.

If you have had an infection, start over with fresh, germ-free makeup, Dr. Vinger says, because "makeup gives bacteria a scaffold on which to grow."

To help prevent the infection from recurring, Dr. Vinger suggests a nightly eyelid wash. (See "Wash That Eye!" on page 137.)

Other ways to avoid bacterial and viral infections include washing your hands frequently, changing your towel and washcloth daily, changing your pillowcase each night, and not sharing towels, washcloths, or makeup with other people. Sharing personal items spreads infection.

Watch What Comes in Contact

Contact lenses can also become a source of recurring infection.

Sometimes people accidentally scratch their corneas while inserting the lenses, leaving their iris open for bacteria. And you're just asking for an infection if you don't disinfect your lenses properly. If you're going to wear contacts, you can't take shortcuts, says Dr. Vinger.

"Anytime you put something onto or into your eye, you risk infection," he cautions.

Steps for preventing infection include a regular schedule of daily and weekly lens cleaning. Here is the recommended procedure for the care of your contact lenses.

- Wash your hands before inserting or removing lenses.
- Insert contacts before putting on makeup and remove them before you remove your makeup.
- While wearing your lenses, leave your lens case upside down on a paper towel to dry.
- Daily, clean your lenses with a thimerosol-free solution. (Thimerosol has been implicated in an irritating eye condition known as keratoconjunctivitis.)
- Weekly, use an enzymatic cleaner, which removes protein deposits from your lenses.
- Use commercially prepared cleaning solutions. Doctors say homemade solutions of salt and distilled water may contain bacteria or the one-celled organism acanthamoeba. This organism can infect your cornea and cause an ulcer. It is hard to get rid of medically or surgically and may cause blindness.
- Do not wear lenses while you swim. They can absorb chemicals from the water.
- Do not use hairspray or other aerosol sprays when wearing your lenses. (Use them before inserting the lenses.)

- Do not moisten or clean contacts in your mouth.
- If you wear a MedicAlert bracelet, add the fact that you wear contact lenses to the information on your bracelet. If you are in an accident, the contacts should be removed by a doctor before they can cause damage.

Multipurpose Relief

For: Infection, Stye, Chalazion

WET AND WARM

After a hard day of physical labor, there's nothing quite like a warm shower. Giving your eyes a little warmth—in the form of a soothing compress—can make them feel good, too.

To take advantage of this feel-good remedy, fill a bowl with warm water. Test the water on the inside of your wrist to be sure it won't be too hot for your eyelids. Then immerse several clean washcloths in the water. Pull one cloth at a time from the bowl, wring it, and place it against your closed eye. Use one washcloth per eye. Don't put the used compresses back into your bowl of clean water.

Hold the compresses in place until they cool. Then replace them with new, clean compresses. Use warm compresses for 15 minutes each session.

Dispose of or launder your compresses separately from your family laundry to avoid sharing your infection.

You can also make a warm compress from a first aid gel pack, says Elaine Harris, president and founder of the Sjögren's Syndrome Foundation. Heat the gel packs, she says. (Don't forget to test them on your wrist before you put them against your eyes!) Wrap them in two thick, clean washcloths. Lie down and apply the packs to your eyes. Relax and listen to music while you wait for your 10- to 20-minute treatment to end.

STYE AND CHALAZION

If the eyes really are the windows of your soul, as the saying goes, you probably don't want a frog sitting in your window. That's what a stye or a chalazion—a bump on your eyelid—looks like.

Most people have experienced a stye or a chalazion on one of their eyelids at some point in their life. Besides being not particularly attractive, they hurt.

Styes and chalazions are two types of bumps that grow along the eyelid's edge. Although similar in appearance, they are caused by two different problems, doctors say.

A chalazion is a swollen meibomian gland. Meibomian glands, which secrete oil, ring the upper and lower eyelids. If a gland swells—usually due to a plugged duct—it can create a hard little bump that presses against the eyeball, possibly causing astigmatism, a vision problem.

A stye is a type of infection in the eyelid's edge. An eyelash follicle gets infected and forms a bump that may include a head of pus.

▶ INSTANT RELIEF

Here's something that may help ease the discomfort of either type of eyelid bump.

Warm it up. Doctors recommend using a warm compress for either a chalazion or a stye. Apply the compress for 10 to 15 minutes, four times a day, for three to four days. The warmth will relieve the pain in both cases. With a stye, the warmth may help the bump burst, allowing the pus to drain. If you have a chalazion, heat may help open the gland, allowing it to drain naturally.

▶ PREVENTION PAIN-RELIEF PROGRAM

Whatever you do, don't be tempted to squeeze a stye or chalazion to speed draining. Squeezing can spread infection and may cause other eye problems.

Both styes and chalazions can recur. So once you've had one, experts say, you should be on the alert and use a warm compress as soon as your lids appear to be irritated. This treatment increases the blood supply to your eyelids and helps keep natural drainage systems open. If you get chalazions or styes frequently, your doctor may also recommend a daily eyelid wash. (See "Wash That Eye!" on page 137.)

Your doctor may recommend surgery to remove a chalazion, especially if the bump is painful and affects your vision. Surgery takes only a few minutes and is done under local anesthesia.

Afterward, the doctor will probably have you wear a pressure eyepatch for 8 to 24 hours to control bleeding and swelling. Following surgery, doctors recommend using an antimicrobial ointment to reduce the chance of getting another infection.

DRY EYES

For more than a year, Elaine Harris's eyes felt dry and gritty. She also felt exhausted and run down. During that time, she visited 13 different doctors. Dozens of preliminary tests showed nothing wrong. One of the doctors told her that her eye pain was psychosomatic. No matter what she did, her eyes remained so dry that they caused her continual discomfort.

Dry eyes may not sound like a problem worthy of 13 doctors, a battery of tests, and a year-long search for relief. However, for Harris and more than nine million other people who have chronic dry eyes, that dryness is enough to make them cry . . . if only they could.

If dry eyes aren't treated, the chronic dryness can damage the cornea and possibly lead to a loss of sight. Drafts, reading, fumes, smoke, bright lights, air conditioning, and sleeping with your eyes partly open can lead to a dry-eye problem.

In Harris's case, doctors finally discovered that her dry eyes were caused by an autoimmune disease called Sjögren's (SHOW-grins) syndrome. As a result of her experience she founded the Sjögren's Syndrome Foundation and wrote *The Sjögren's Handbook*.

If your eyes feel gritty, as if you have sand, gravel, soap, or shampoo in them, see your ophthalmologist.

▶ INSTANT RELIEF

For people such as Elaine Harris, there is no cure, although science has a lot of ways to treat the symptoms of Sjögren's. Treatment for dry eyes caused by other things usually is simple and inexpensive.

Cool down. You can cool your dry, irritated eyes with a slice of a cucumber. Close your eyes and place a slice on each lid for a few minutes. A cool, wet washcloth will also do.

Make yourself cry. Try an artificial tears preparation, available without a prescription at your pharmacy. They are good for rewetting dry, gritty eyes, says Daniel Nelson, M.D., chief of ophthalmology at Ramsey Clinic and St. Paul–Ramsey Medical Center and associate professor of ophthalmology at the University of Minnesota. You can use them four to five times a day.

Watch the weather. Air conditioning in the summer and heat in the winter are eye-drying hazards. If you keep the humidity in your home and office high, you'll do your eyes a favor.

Put your eyes on the blink. Computer terminals and televisions can cause dry eyes—but not because of any weird radiation coming from them. When you read or stare at a screen, you blink less. Blinking restores the tear film over your eyes. So when you're working on something that takes close concentration, give your eyes a break and look away every half hour. And remember to blink.

Enclose your eyes. If you enclose a hot tub in a plastic bubble, the water won't evaporate, says Dr. Nelson. You can do the same for your eyes by wearing ski goggles, swim goggles, or special moisture-chamber glasses.

Harris uses moisture-chamber glasses and says they are excellent for keeping eyes damp. Her glasses have a clear vinyl cone between each lens and her eyes, so they form a relatively airtight chamber. As her tears evaporate, the chamber becomes more humid. That keeps more tears from evaporating and leaves her eyes in a comfortable, moist atmosphere.

Protect yourself. When you go outside, if you don't have a pair of special glasses, pull on a pair of wraparound sunglasses or glasses with nonprescription lenses. They will help protect your eyes from the drying effects of the wind.

Read your prescription. Many common prescription and nonprescription drugs can cause eye dryness, says Dr. Nelson. Some of the drug categories include antihistamines, beta-blockers, decongestants, diuretics, oral contraceptives, sleeping medications, tranquilizers, and tricyclic antidepressants. Talk to your doctor or pharmacist if you think your dry eyes are caused by medication.

➡️ PREVENTION PAIN-RELIEF PROGRAM

Doctors compare the eyes to a sink, says Dr. Nelson. "Think about a kitchen sink. Water comes into the sink through the spigot. It stays in the sink. It goes out of the sink through the drain," he says.

To treat dry eyes, you can pour in water using artificial tears or plug the drain through surgery. There are no approved drugs, Dr. Nelson says, that turn the faucet back on.

Get Tears in Your Eyes

If you have a mild case of dry eyes, you'll use over-the-counter artificial tears, says Vincent P. deLuise, M.D., director of the cornea unit at Opticare Eye Health Center, Waterbury, Connecticut. These are the mainstay for most people with dry eyes. There are about 30 brands on the market, and most of them are a mixture of saline solution and a film-forming substance, such as polyvinyl alcohol or synthetic cellulose.

Apply artificial tears one drop at a time, four or five times a day, advises Dr. deLuise. This should be done whether your eyes feel dry or not, because prevention is important in chronic dry-eye problems, he says. (See "Drop In on Your Eyes" on page 159.)

Either the preserved or nonpreserved artificial tears are all right to use if you have mild dry-eye symptoms, Dr. deLuise says. However, steer clear of any preparations containing thimerosol or benzylkonium chloride, which are irritating ingredients. Doctors say you should try several brands of tears to see which work best in your eyes.

If you have mild eye dryness, don't use preservative-containing drops more than five times a day. If you overuse these eyedrops, the preservatives can build up to a toxic concentration and start killing cells on the surface of your eye. Possibly the least irritating preservative currently in use is sorbic acid.

People with a moderate dry-eye problem have very little natural tear film, so they probably have some dry spots on their corneas, says Dr. deLuise. They need artificial tears *without* preservatives, he says. Some must use these drops once an hour and others may need them as often as every 15 minutes.

Even when your eyes are closed, they need to be moisturized. Dr. deLuise recommends using a moisturizing ointment, such as Lacri-Lube, Refresh PM, or Duratears Naturale, at night. Ointments usually contain petrolatum, mineral oil, and other ingredients. They keep eyes damp for a much longer period of time than an application of drops just before sleeping.

One preservative-free tear-replacement product comes in a solid form. Lacrisert is an oblong pellet made of cellulose and tear-replacer. Every morning, you place a pellet under your lower eyelid. The pellet slowly dissolves during the day, making your tear film thicker. Lacrisert is available by prescription only.

"You might think of it as a slow-release sponge," says Dr. Nelson. "If you don't have enough tears to dissolve the pellet, it can be like a little rock. It's the diameter of a pencil lead. If you have too many tears, it can make your eyes mucousy and blur your vision. It's hard to use, and we've had our best success with women in their thirties or forties. We've found you either have great success with it or no success at all."

If you soak Lacrisert pellets for 10 to 15 minutes in a nonpreserved artificial tears solution before you insert them, they'll be more comfortable to use, notes Harris.

Plugging the Drain

If you have severe dry-eye problems, you have no tear film at all to cover your cornea, says Dr. deLuise. Your cornea will lack luster and the top layer of cornea will look almost dead.

"For that, we need aggressive therapy. We use oily drops and ointments that stay in the eye," he says. "Eyelids are taped shut at night. Sometimes we close up tear ducts with silicone plastic plugs so that tears don't drain from the eyes. These plugs have the advantage of being reversible."

The Driest: Sjögren's Syndrome

Some people with dry eyes also have a dry mouth, feel a general malaise, and may have swelling in their joints. These people have Sjögren's syndrome, a disease that affects about one million people in the United States.

Sjögren's is an autoimmune disease, like rheumatoid arthritis, says Dr. deLuise. Many people who have Sjögren's also have an arthritic disease, he says.

An autoimmune disease is caused by a glitch in the body's natural defenses, the immune system. Immune system cells usually protect the body by killing foreign organisms, such as viruses and bacteria. In an autoimmune disease, these defenses turn and attack the body's own cells. In Sjögren's syndrome, the immune system attacks and kills the lacrimal (tear) and other moisture-making glands, says Dr. deLuise.

More women than men have Sjögren's, by about nine to one.

"We aren't sure why," Dr. deLuise says. "We know there are hormonal differences between men and women, and some people feel it's those hormonal differences that influence dry eyes."

Unfortunately, your doctor can't just prescribe the hormones or kill the virus and cure Sjögren's. Instead, you need to control the symptoms.

The Future Looks Wetter

Scientists and doctors are investigating a variety of products that may offer hope to people with dry eyes.

Some doctors, such as Dr. deLuise, are using a certain type of eyedrops to protect the cornea. Healon is the brand name of hyaluronic acid, a liquid derived from the collagen in rooster combs. Usually, it's injected into the eye during cataract surgery to maintain the shape of and protect the cornea.

Healon diluted with saline has proven to be a good preservative-free artificial tear formula, says Dr. deLuise. Some ophthalmologists will make it on request, although it's expensive: $50 to $75 per bottle.

"Many of our patients think it's more soothing than commercial drops," Dr. deLuise says.

Doctors are also studying the malaria drug Plaquenil, an anti-inflammatory, at Scripps Clinic and Research Foundation in La Jolla, California.

In the early stages of Sjögren's, an anti-inflammatory drug may help save the lacrimal glands, according to Mitchell H. Friedlaender, M.D., an ophthalmologist at Scripps. As part of a study, ten Sjögren's patients who took 200 milligrams of Plaquenil every day for a year were compared to ten Sjögren's patients who had no treatment. Those who took Plaquenil had significantly reduced autoimmune response. Further study is under way.

DROP IN ON YOUR EYES

You tip your head up, poise the dropper over your eye, and squeeze. It's time for the eyedrops your doctor prescribed.

Ouch. The first drop hits your cornea, so you blink. Oops. Another splashes, then rolls down your cheek. You wonder how much medication your eye actually received.

Ointment isn't any easier to use. You dab the ointment at your eye, and instead of the medication going where it counts, it gums up your lashes.

So how do you get your medication where it's supposed to go?

Follow a few simple steps and you'll get eyedrops where they belong and get maximum absorption, says William L. White, M.D., chief of the ophthalmology service at Ireland Army Community Hospital in Fort Knox, Kentucky.

Begin with a thorough hand-washing. Whenever your fingers are going to touch your eyes, you want them to be clean, he says. Also, don't touch the bottle to your eye— you don't want to pick up bacteria that could be inserted into your eye with your next dose.

Also, make sure you close the top tightly on all medications. Drops are usually considered safe for four weeks and ointments for three months after they have been opened.

Applying Drops

1. You can lie on your back when putting drops in your eyes.

2. Don't plop the drop in the middle of your eye, says Dr. White. The drop can irritate the cornea, causing blinking and tears, which washes the medication out of your eye. Instead, using gentle pressure, pull your lower eyelid down toward your cheek. You'll create a small pocket between the lid and the eye. That's where your medication should go.

3. Place a single drop of medicine into the pocket. If your doctor prescribes more than one drop at a time in your eye, plan to wait 15 minutes before you apply the second drop. You will dilute the medicine if you try to insert the drops more quickly.

4. If your other eye needs a dose, apply it immediately after your first dose. Be quick. You don't want to blink either eye.

5. Then gently close both eyes for 2 minutes (even if you only medicate one eye). Keeping your eyes closed for a full 2 minutes enhances the absorption of the medication and reduces the chance of side effects, says Dr. White.

Each time you blink, Dr. White says, you flush the eye, possibly washing away medication before the eye can absorb it.

As part of a study, Dr. White gave 12 volunteers eyedrops containing a radioactive tracer. Using a special camera, he measured how long the drops stayed in the volunteers' eyes when they were allowed to blink normally. Then he measured how long drops stayed in their eyes when they kept them closed after the eyedrops were applied.

Eyedrops stayed on the volunteers' eyes ten times longer with the eyes closed than when they were open and blinking normally.

Keeping the eyes closed for 2 minutes seems to be the optimum time, says Dr. White. "We didn't find any statistically significant improvement by keeping the eyes closed longer than 2 minutes," he notes.

6. As an added measure, it helps to use a fingertip to apply gentle pressure to the inside corner of the eye at the base of the nose. The pressure will help slow drainage of the medication from your eye. Keep the pressure up for 2 to 5 minutes after the drops are in your eyes.

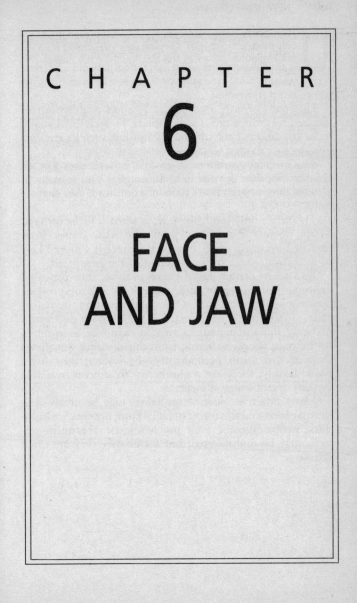

CHAPTER
6

FACE
AND JAW

Unless you're wearing a mask, it's hard to hide the truth when your face hurts. Whether it's sinus pain, a throbbing tooth, or tense, tender jaw muscles, that scrunched-up, why-me expression can betray even the most poker-faced individual.

Face pain is most often traced to sinus problems or to infected teeth or gums. (See chapters 11 and 13.) Usually these conditions have obvious symptoms such as gumline abscesses or nasal drainage.

Any medical condition or sensitivity that causes a headache can localize in your face, although it's most likely to also produce pain in other parts of your head. (See chapter 8.)

The face's only joint, the jaw, is often a focus of pain. Many doctors these days think the pain comes from clenched muscles; some, however, believe it's more likely to be a disturbance of the function of the joint itself.

And when certain facial nerves misfire, they can send lightning bolts of pain into a cheek or jaw or produce continuous, burning pain. One such condition, tic doloreaux, or trigeminal neuralgia, has the dubious distinction of being the worst pain known to man—or to woman. In the past, people suffering from this disorder sometimes stopped their pain permanently—by ending their lives. Now, luckily, there are a number of treatments available for this excruciating ailment.

Many different medical specialists may be involved in the diagnosis and treatment of facial pain: dentists, neurologists, neurosurgeons, even psychologists. Treatment options may be multifaceted, but fortunately they are often effective.

GET PROFESSIONAL HELP IF:

- You have severe pain radiating from one bloodshot eye
- You have continuous, throbbing pain on one side of your face that is worse at night or when you chew
- You have sudden pain in both temples and you feel generally ill or your scalp is suddenly sensitive to touch
- You have weakness, numbness, or paralysis in the face

PAIN-FINDER CHART FOR THE FACE AND JAW

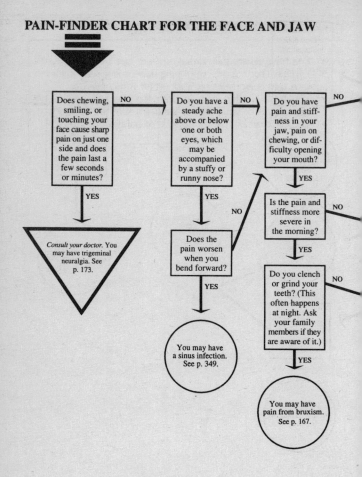

Does chewing, smiling, or touching your face cause sharp pain on just one side and does the pain last a few seconds or minutes?

NO →

Do you have a steady ache above or below one or both eyes, which may be accompanied by a stuffy or runny nose?

NO →

Do you have pain and stiffness in your jaw, pain on chewing, or difficulty opening your mouth?

NO →

YES ↓

Consult your doctor. You may have trigeminal neuralgia. See p. 173.

YES ↓

Does the pain worsen when you bend forward?

NO

YES ↓

You may have a sinus infection. See p. 349.

YES ↓

Is the pain and stiffness more severe in the morning?

NO →

YES ↓

Do you clench or grind your teeth? (This often happens at night. Ask your family members if they are aware of it.)

NO →

YES ↓

You may have pain from bruxism. See p. 167.

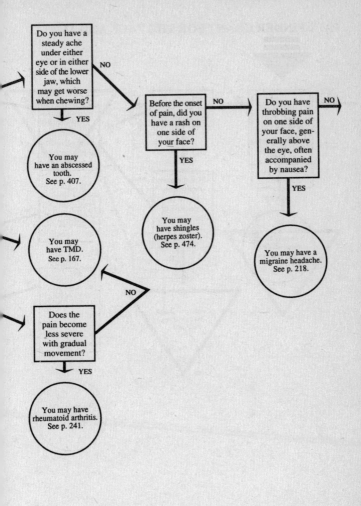

Do you have a steady ache under either eye or in either side of the lower jaw, which may get worse when chewing?

NO →

YES ↓

You may have an abscessed tooth. See p. 407.

You may have TMD. See p. 167.

Does the pain become less severe with gradual movement?

YES ↓

You may have rheumatoid arthritis. See p. 241.

NO →

Before the onset of pain, did you have a rash on one side of your face?

NO →

YES ↓

You may have shingles (herpes zoster). See p. 474.

Do you have throbbing pain on one side of your face, generally above the eye, often accompanied by nausea?

NO →

YES ↓

You may have a migraine headache. See p. 218.

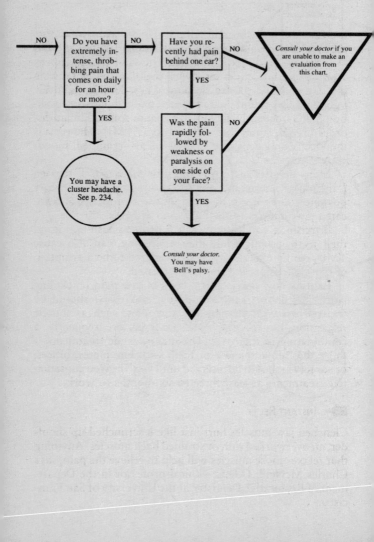

NO →

Do you have extremely intense, throbbing pain that comes on daily for an hour or more?

NO →

Have you recently had pain behind one ear?

NO →

Consult your doctor if you are unable to make an evaluation from this chart.

↓ YES

You may have a cluster headache. See p. 234.

↓ YES

Was the pain rapidly followed by weakness or paralysis on one side of your face?

NO →

↓ YES

Consult your doctor. You may have Bell's palsy.

TMD: TEMPOROMANDIBULAR DISORDER

Imagine walking around all day long with your fists clenched. Your hands would be stiff and aching by the end of the day—no doubt about that. The same thing happens when people unconsciously clench their jaw muscles during the day or while they're sleeping. They develop painfully tight muscles around their jaw, ears, and temples—a condition that's frequently diagnosed as temporomandibular disorder (TMD, sometimes referred to as TMJ). The pain is the facial equivalent of a charley horse—cramped, blood-starved muscles.

Many dentists and physicians now think muscle tension is the most common cause of TMD. Among the many other possible causes: teeth that do not meet properly, a dislocated jaw, injuries to the joint, and arthritis.

Bruxism, a condition in which people gnash and grind their teeth, usually while they're sleeping, can also cause TMD, dental experts say. It's considered to be a symptom of muscle tension and should be treated.

Experts now agree: Most cases of jaw pain (excluding pain caused by fractures, tumors, and cysts) should be treated first with simple, safe therapies, such as muscle relaxation, hot or cold packs, massage, or, frequently, a combination of therapies. The major-league treatments—those that move the jaw or teeth with bite plates, braces, or surgery—should be reserved until you've given conservative treatments at least three to six months to work.

▶ INSTANT RELIEF

Clenched jaw muscles hurt just like a scrunched-up shoulder, an overworked calf, or strained back muscles. Anything that relaxes those muscles will help to relieve the pain, says Charles McNeill, D.D.S., clinical professor in the Department of Restorative Dentistry at the University of San Francisco.

Follow fire with ice. Relax for 15 or 20 minutes with a steaming hot towel draped around your jaw. Chase it with either 2 to 3 minutes of ice massage on the muscles around your jaw joints or an ice pack, followed by another 5 minutes of heat, Dr. McNeill suggests. This treatment reduces pain by increasing blood circulation to muscles.

Try aspirin. Over-the-counter analgesics such as aspirin and ibuprofen may help to relieve an occasional acute attack. And they can be particularly helpful when your jaw pain is due to arthritis. But if you find yourself relying on drugs for long-term relief from TMD, you should discuss nondrug forms of therapy with your doctor or dentist, says Dr. McNeill.

Press where it hurts. Use your fingertips to probe for tender spots that may be radiating pain, suggests David Nickel, a doctor of Oriental medicine and a licensed acupuncturist. Press the spot and slowly increase pressure. Or press on and off a few seconds at a time. Like acupuncture, acupressure is thought to ease an ache by stimulating the release of the body's own pain-relieving chemicals.

Rub circles around the pain. Massage the muscles of your jaw joint just as you would an aching calf or tense shoulders, suggests Jocelyn Granger, a registered massage therapist and spokesperson for the American Massage Therapy Association. Beginning with light pressure, use your fingertips to make small circles in front of your ears.

Massage helps to relax muscles and thus reduces pain. It may also help to improve tissue elasticity and so make your jaw easier to open. (See chapter 24 for more on massage.)

Imagine your jaw as a screen door, hanging limply on a lazy summer day. Researchers at the University of Washington's School of Dentistry use mental images to treat TMD pain. Under their guidance, people with TMD do deep abdominal breathing, progressive relaxation, and guided imagery to learn to relax their whole body, and especially their shoulders, neck, and jaw. (See chapter 34 for more on this technique.)

A mental scene that people find particularly soothing,

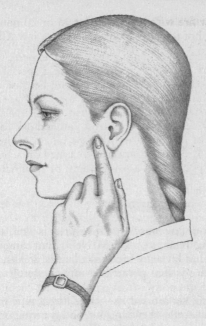

To relieve jaw pain, use your fingertips to massage the bony area directly in front of your ears.

for example, takes you to a sunlit meadow. There, at the edge of the woods, is a summer cabin, complete with a front porch and—you guessed it—a screen door. That screen door is your jaw, hanging loosely on its hinges, perfectly inert, not giving a hoot if a fly or two find their way into the cabin.

"By putting themselves into this sort of scene, teeth apart, lips barely touching, breathing deeply, face smooth and peaceful, drained of all energy, people can experience the feeling of letting the tension melt out of their muscles," says Leanne Wilson, Ph.D., a clinical psychologist who works with TMD patients.

➡ **PREVENTION PAIN-RELIEF PROGRAM**

Regular use of instant pain-relief techniques may be all you need to keep TMD pain at bay, some experts say. If relief eludes you, however, you should see a specialist. Finding the right one is particularly important because many orthodontic and surgical treatments for TMD are considered controversial. Your best bet: Visit or call the dean of the university dental school nearest you and ask for a referral to a dentist in your area who specializes in the treatment of TMD. A dentist connected to a medical school can call in other specialists—a psychologist or rheumatologist, for example.

Lay Off the Hard Stuff

Getting your jaw muscles to take a rest is likely to be a part of your treatment, says Dr. McNeill. That can be as easy as replacing hard, chewy foods like bagels, steaks, and carrot sticks with mashed potatoes, soups, casseroles, and meat loaf.

Breaking certain habits—clenching a pipe or cigar between your teeth, chewing gum, and gnawing on pencils or fingernails—may also help relieve your jaw pain.

Alternately, coaching by a biofeedback therapist or physical therapist might help you tune in on tension and consciously relax those jaw muscles, even when habit would have you champing at the bit, Dr. McNeill says.

Your dentist may recommend a bite plate (also called an occlusal splint or oral appliance)—an acrylic mold that fits over some or all of your teeth and holds your jaw in a relaxed position, says John Dodes, D.D.S., a Woodhaven, New York, dentist and chapter president of the National Council Against Health Fraud. A dentist is likely to suggest a bite plate if you grind your teeth at night, he says.

Bite plates help some people with TMD, and for some, wearing a bite plate at night is all that's needed to relieve jaw pain, says Dr. Dodes. Most people see improvement in about a month, but some develop additional problems by using an inappropriately prescribed dental appliance, he says.

Make sure you know what a bite plate is designed to do. You should probably not wear an oral appliance for more than 18 hours a day, says Dr. Dodes. "In certain cases, people have been wearing plastic TMD appliances 24 hours a day for years," he says. "This can lead to excessive tooth migration."

"Certain people need to wear an appliance 24 hours a day at first, but the appliance must cover all the teeth," Dr. McNeill says.

Relaxation of a different sort may also be a part of your program to relieve TMD pain: Some TMD specialists say stress management is a crucial element in treatment. "It's considered good medicine in general to get counseling to improve your coping skills if stress is contributing to a health problem," Dr. McNeill says.

Some people benefit from trigger-point injections to the painful areas around their jaw, followed by exercises that stretch and relax the jaw muscles, says Andrew Fischer, M.D., Ph.D., chief of the Department of Rehabilitation Medicine at the Bronx Veterans Affairs Medical Center. (See chapter 33.) The exercises involve slowly opening and closing your mouth against resistance provided by placing your fist under your jaw. Similarly, moving your jaw to the left and right against your fist relaxes additional muscles, says Dr. Fischer.

Surgery: Unlikely

Rarely, you may have a joint problem that is best corrected by surgery, says Dr. McNeill. Most doctors prefer *not* to operate on dislocated jaw disks. "The trend is not to do surgery just because a disk is out of position or a jaw is clicking," he says. "That's because we've found out that we can't seem to reposition that disk anyway, and recent research suggests that we just need to get the disk moving, not reposition it."

Surgery is recommended and useful only in cases of extreme, unrelenting pain not reversible by any other medical treatment, severe degeneration of the jaw joint, tumors, or displaced fractures, says Dr. McNeill. "Probably fewer than 5 percent of people with jaw pain require surgery," says Dr. Dodes.

Don't let a dentist or orthodontist treat your jaw in an attempt to correct such far-removed physical ailments as scoliosis (curvature of the spine) or menstrual problems, warns Dr. Dodes. Such treatments have been offered and are pure quackery, he says.

TRIGEMINAL NEURALGIA

Pain carried by the nerves of the face can present a baffling array of symptoms—brief, intense pain; constant, burning pain; dull aching that lasts all day long.

Perhaps the best known of these conditions, trigeminal neuralgia, produces bolts of electrifying pain on only one side of the face, following the pathways of the trigeminal nerve, says Seymour Solomon, M.D., professor of neurology at Albert Einstein Medical College in New York City and director of the Headache Unit at Montefiore Medical Center. Chewing, swallowing, shaving, or even exposure to a strong, cold wind can trigger an attack. Simply touching the upper lip or face is often enough to trigger pain. Between attacks, most people have no pain at all, he says.

Other neuralgias ("nerve pains") can cause similar sudden, severe, and fortunately brief pain in your throat or ear. (Neuralgia must be distinguished from neuritis—inflamed nerves that cause continuous, burning pain in areas of the face, tongue, or mouth. Neuritis develops most frequently in people with diabetes. It's treated by bringing the diabetes under control and with anti-inflammatory drugs.)

Neuralgias are not uncommon. The trigeminal nerve seems to be more prone to neuralgias than other parts of the body, Dr. Solomon says.

With trigeminal neuralgia, pain attacks tend to become longer or more frequent with time. Episodes that earlier lasted only a few seconds may persist for many minutes and occur up to 50 times each day. Trigeminal neuralgia becomes more common as we get older, and it seems to strike more women than men. Doctors who are stumped by a facial pain may attempt to label it psychosomatic. Most experts, however, agree with Dr. Solomon, who says, "Very few cases are psychological in nature."

▶ INSTANT RELIEF

Most forms of facial nerve pain don't respond to home care. In a few cases they do.

Try hot-pepper cream. For lingering, burning pain from a herpes zoster (shingles) infection of the face, try capsaicin cream (marketed as Zostrix or Axsain), made from hot peppers. (See page 474 for more about shingles.) "It can provide good relief for people with postherpetic neuralgia," says Raymond Maciewicz, M.D., Ph.D., director of the Spaulding Rehabilitation Hospital Pain Program in Boston. "You have to be careful, though; it is extremely irritating to the eyes. If you rub it into your forehead, you have to be careful sweat doesn't bring it into your eyes."

Take an anti-inflammatory pain reliever. Some kinds of facial pain are caused by inflamed nerves. If you've been diagnosed as having neuritis, aspirin or ibuprofen may help ease the ache, Dr. Solomon says.

Put it on ice. Shingles or neuritis may respond to gentle ice massage. Neuralgia, though—especially trigeminal neuralgia—is unlikely to be relieved and may even worsen with exposure to cold.

▶ PREVENTION PAIN-RELIEF PROGRAM

Trigeminal nerve pain can strike suddenly and is usually disturbing enough that people see a doctor without delay. That's good, because a doctor can provide valuable help.

Drugs are usually the first line of defense for trigeminal nerve pain, says Dr. Solomon. Anticonvulsant medication prevents the recurrent pain of neuralgia. Analgesics or anti-inflammatory drugs can ease the pain and inflammation of neuritis. Steroids may be used during severe attacks.

Nerve-Calming Drugs

An anticonvulsant, carbamazepine (Tegretol), helps calm the irritated misfiring of nerves, says Dr. Maciewicz. Doctors also often prescribe other anticonvulsants or muscle-relaxing drugs like baclofen (Lioresal). "All these drugs inhibit the flow of sharp, lightninglike sensations through the nervous system and may work on the abnormal discharges of the injured nerves," Dr. Maciewicz says.

For trigeminal neuralgia, certain antidepressant drugs are sometimes prescribed in addition to an anticonvulsant, says Dr. Maciewicz. Antidepressants may be used alone for postherpetic neuralgia. And they are sometimes tried for trigeminal nerve pain that defies diagnosis (sometimes called "atypical facial pain"). These drugs have pain-relieving properties independent of their mood-lifting effects. (See chapter 26.)

Needling Nerve Pain

At the Kriser Oro-facial Pain Center at New York University College of Dentistry in New York City, acupuncture is frequently used as a treatment for trigeminal neuralgia and for atypical facial pain, says director William Greenfield, D.D.S. "We have found acupuncture to be of significant help, particularly for trigeminal neuralgia, in quite a few of our patients." Other experts in the field say more work needs to be done before acupuncture can be recommended as a treatment for any kind of trigeminal nerve pain. Consult a dentist or physician familiar with acupuncture to see whether this treatment may be appropriate for you. (And see chapter 16 for more on acupuncture.)

In most cases of trigeminal neuralgia, if drugs fail to control symptoms, surgery is tried next, says Dr. Maciewicz.

"There is a long history of different kinds of surgery for trigeminal neuralgia," he says. "It's now clear that a large number of people who continue to have pain despite the appropriate use of drugs will be able to get pain relief following a surgical procedure to the trigeminal nerve."

Two of the procedures involve a permanent nerve block to the root of the nerve, at the base of the skull. Both are equally effective, Dr. Maciewicz says. (See chapter 27.)

Surgery that corrects the probable cause of trigeminal

neuralgia is also available. Many doctors believe the nerve irritation is caused by a convoluted or sagging artery in the base of the brain that is throbbing against the nerve. The surgery repositions the artery and nerve, and sometimes a sterile protective pad is positioned to cushion the nerve.

The operation is effective, but it is major surgery, says Dr. Maciewicz. "The advantage is that you are not injuring the nerve at all in this procedure," he says. Younger, healthy adults are the best candidates for this surgery, he says. "Someone with significant medical problems would be better suited to the nerve block, which takes only a needle and is done in 30 minutes."

Nerve blocks are seldom done for other kinds of facial nerve pain.

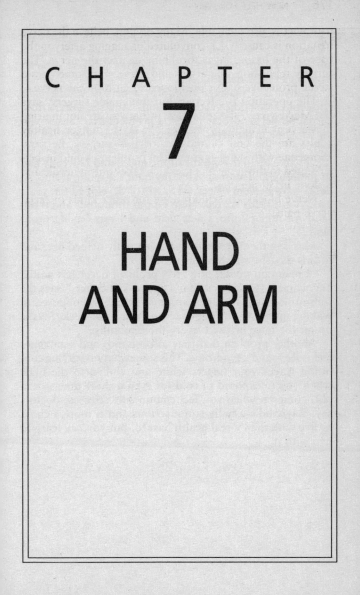

CHAPTER
7

HAND
AND ARM

Jan Benlein has a problem with her job. Like a pilot with vertigo or an interior designer with color blindness, she has a health problem that makes her job very difficult to manage on a daily basis.

Benlein is a massage therapist, a person who kneads tense and sore bodies with her hands. And she suffers from carpal tunnel syndrome (CTS), a problem that causes pain and tingling in the arms, wrists, and fingers. Herein lies the rub.

"I woke up in the middle of the night, and I literally had to jump up and start shaking my hands around, it hurt so bad," says Benlein of her CTS, which developed ten years ago. "I got really scared. Here I'd put thousands and thousands of dollars into a new field and I was having problems."

Massage therapy treatments eventually helped her, and to this day she still receives them.

"I maintain myself now. My problem never has gotten any worse. I don't know if it's gotten any better," says the California-based therapist and instructor. "As opposed to waking up five nights out of seven during the week, I wake up maybe once or twice every three months."

Another problem that may affect hands and sometimes feet is Raynaud's syndrome. This somewhat mystifying condition leaves your fingers white and chilled to the bone when you're exposed to cold for even a short time. It can also come on when you feel emotionally stressed, doctors say. Raynaud's usually is not serious and is more a chore to live with than a real health hazard. But you *can* learn to live with it.

GET PROFESSIONAL HELP IF:

- The pain immediately follows an injury and the area looks misshapen
- The pain extends down your left arm, begins during exercise, and disappears with rest

PAIN-FINDER CHART FOR THE HANDS AND ARMS

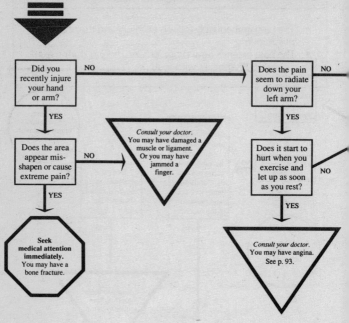

Did you recently injure your hand or arm?

NO →

Does the pain seem to radiate down your left arm?

NO →

YES ↓

YES ↓

Does the area appear mis-shapen or cause extreme pain?

NO →

Consult your doctor. You may have damaged a muscle or ligament. Or you may have jammed a finger.

Does it start to hurt when you exercise and let up as soon as you rest?

NO →

YES ↓

YES ↓

Seek medical attention immediately. You may have a bone fracture.

Consult your doctor. You may have angina. See p. 93.

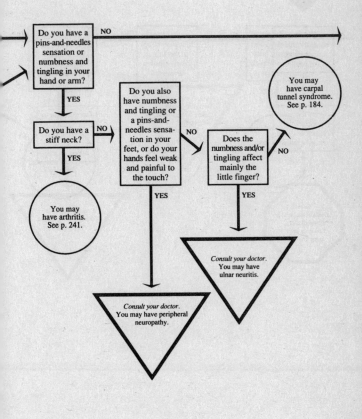

Do you have a pins-and-needles sensation or numbness and tingling in your hand or arm?

NO →

YES ↓

Do you have a stiff neck?

YES ↓

You may have arthritis. See p. 241.

NO →

Do you also have numbness and tingling or a pins-and-needles sensation in your feet, or do your hands feel weak and painful to the touch?

YES ↓

Consult your doctor. You may have peripheral neuropathy.

NO →

Does the numbness and/or tingling affect mainly the little finger?

YES ↓

Consult your doctor. You may have ulnar neuritis.

NO →

You may have carpal tunnel syndrome. See p. 184.

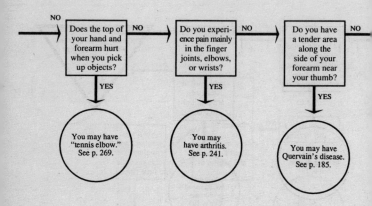

NO →

Does the top of your hand and forearm hurt when you pick up objects?

NO →

YES ↓

You may have "tennis elbow." See p. 269.

Do you experience pain mainly in the finger joints, elbows, or wrists?

NO →

YES ↓

You may have arthritis. See p. 241.

Do you have a tender area along the side of your forearm near your thumb?

NO →

YES ↓

You may have Quervain's disease. See p. 185.

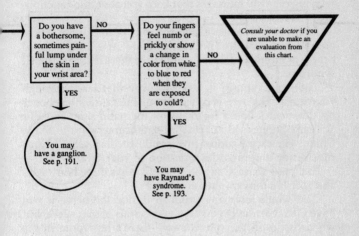

Do you have a bothersome, sometimes painful lump under the skin in your wrist area?

NO →

Do your fingers feel numb or prickly or show a change in color from white to blue to red when they are exposed to cold?

NO →

Consult your doctor if you are unable to make an evaluation from this chart.

YES ↓

You may have a ganglion. See p. 191.

YES ↓

You may have Raynaud's syndrome. See p. 193.

CARPAL TUNNEL SYNDROME

Nerves run to and fro—the body's own telegraph wires relaying the vital messages that keep you alive and functioning.

Interfere with a nerve, and you may be in trouble. There are pinched nerves in necks, the agony of sciatica, frayed nerves in moms and dads . . . and then there is carpal tunnel syndrome.

The carpal tunnel is a passageway that leads through your wrist. The area is called a tunnel because it has bones on three sides and a ligament on the palm side, explains William Cooney, M.D., chief of hand surgery at the Mayo Clinic. The carpal tunnel protects the median nerve, which runs inside and provides sensation to your fingers.

Feel your wrist. Can you feel that it has three bony sides and soft tendons on the underside?

You won't have any problem feeling the nerve if you have CTS. Normally you aren't conscious of that nerve, but when tissues in the tunnel swell, there's less room in the area and the median nerve becomes irritated, Dr. Cooney explains. Most people with CTS experience numbness, tingling, and pain in the fingers, wrist, and even the arm.

"It's commonly described as fingers going to sleep, as when you've rested on a part of your body for a long time, then you wake up and that part of your body is asleep. It is also described as a pins-and-needles tingling. It can be quite uncomfortable for some people," says H. Jay Boulas, M.D., assistant professor of hand and upper extremity surgery in the Department of Orthopedics at the University of Texas Southwestern Medical Center in Dallas.

What causes the problem? Sometimes the motions a person performs repeatedly with the wrist and fingers—such as pinching or gripping—cause swelling of the tissues in the canal, which puts pressure on the median nerve, doctors say. Repetitive motions and/or certain wrist positions that can lead to CTS range from typing all day at a computer to biking or golfing for a few hours on a regular basis, especially if you have any problems with technique that add strain to your wrist.

Swelling and pressure—and CTS—also can be caused by conditions such as low levels of thyroid hormone, arthritis, diabetes, pregnancy, hormonal changes associated with menopause, and broken or dislocated bones in the wrist, says Dr. Cooney.

Some doctors think it's also possible to irritate the median nerve by sleeping on your stomach with your wrists in a somewhat stressed position under your body.

In all, there are many reasons why people develop CTS, one member of a group of arm and hand pain problems that doctors call "cumulative trauma disorders," Dr. Boulas explains.

Two other common hand conditions related to CTS are Quervain's disease and trigger finger, which are also cumulative trauma disorders, Dr. Cooney says. These two conditions are the most common forms of tenosynovitis—the inflammation of a tendon and its sheath (the layer of tissue that houses the tendon and through which the tendon moves). Quervain's involves inflammation of the tendons that extend and bring the thumb away from the hand, explains Chris McGrew, M.D., assistant professor in the Division of Sports Medicine at the University of New Mexico Medical School in Albuquerque. Trigger finger, a disorder of tendons and pulleys in the hand, can cause pain when you flex your fingers.

Remember: If you have CTS, you have swelling. Since Quervain's and trigger finger involve swollen tendons often associated with repetitive movements, you may have these problems in addition to CTS.

"It may not be causal, but often we do see them together," says neurologist Peter Barbour, M.D., chief of the Division of Neurology, Lehigh Valley Hospital Center, Allentown, Pennsylvania. "Any time you have any inflammation, there's just so much room in the area. The blood vessels don't get compromised, but the nerve does."

If you notice changes in your penmanship or have trouble combing your hair or holding a telephone or driving, you may have CTS. You may notice the symptoms more at night or in the morning, although doctors aren't sure why.

➡ **INSTANT RELIEF**

Most doctors agree that if you have CTS symptoms for a week or so, you should seek professional help. But don't despair. Treatments are in hand for your pain.

Hands off activity. Maybe the carpentry project you started last week or all those loaves of bread you made over the weekend irritated your wrist. Take some time off until you feel better. Don't work through the pain, Dr. Cooney says, because you'll aggravate the problem.

Ice may be right. Massage therapy treatments usually begin and end with ice, in the form of a soft, pliable ice wrap, says Benlein. You can use the soft ice bags that are made for eyes by attaching them to wrists with Velcro, she says. Strapping them on for 10 to 20 minutes can cool the inflammation.

"Soaking the wrists in an ice water bath might help out some," says Dr. McGrew.

See also:

• Chapter 26, on medications.

➡ **PREVENTION PAIN-RELIEF PROGRAM**

Take this job and . . . change it.

Change the way you work or play, that is.

You may be placing extra strain on your wrists by the way you hold them during certain activities—typing, playing the piano, holding a woodworking chisel, using a staple gun, kneading bread, wringing wet laundry, or gripping bicycle handlebars or golf clubs. All of these activities and others may cause pain or tingling in the wrists and hands, doctors agree.

Remember: Anything that causes you to bend your wrist continually or work in an awkward posture may contribute to CTS, says Marvin Dainoff, Ph.D., director of the Center for Ergonomic Research at Miami University in Oxford, Ohio. Dr. Dainoff's work involves ergonomics, which he defines as the physical and psychological fit between people and their work environment.

Computer Maneuvers

If you and your job are as compatible as sunshine and snowballs, you may find yourself saying hello to CTS.

Let's take the computer keyboard as an example. A standard keyboard guarantees that your wrists are in their least optimal working position.

What's the best position?

"If you ask someone to let their arms fall naturally to their side, then raise them and bend the arms 90 degrees, you're going to be in what would be an optimal keying position," Dr. Dainoff explains. "If you do that, you find that your hand is positioned sort of like you're holding a melon."

Every time you move your hands up or down from that position, you have to bend or angle your hands or arms, pulling the tendons from the optimum position, he explains. And if you work all day every day in the wrong position, you may be heading for CTS.

So look around you. Try to alleviate any awkward postures where your wrists or arms are bent, Dr. Dainoff says.

"If you have to bend forward at the waist, if you have to angle your upper arm forward and bend your wrist, if you have to stay in these postures, that's where trouble is going to arise," he explains.

When sitting at the keyboard, make sure your hands are at elbow level or slightly below elbow level to prevent excess bending or stretching in the wrist, says physical therapist Denise Wise of Isernhagen and Associates, a physical therapy consulting firm in Duluth, Minnesota. A physical therapist may be able to provide a wrist rest, a foam pad placed at the end of the keyboard for extra support, Wise says.

Take a break every hour or so, or whenever you feel tired, to change your posture. Lean back and take your hands off the keys, she suggests. Open and close your fists a few times.

"Although many people try sometimes to associate movement with the problem, CTS can also be caused when people are in a static position for so long that it causes compression on the nerve," Wise says. "And so, if you can get out of that position and release the compression, then that's going to improve the situation."

The same advice holds true for people who ride bikes or play tennis, or for anyone who continually bends the wrist or absorbs vibrations in the hands and arms during activity. You should wear properly padded biking gloves and change positions during a long ride or during breaks in competition. Or take a few days off if you have a flare-up. Make sure you're properly fitted for your bicycle before you begin riding. And take tennis or golf lessons to learn the proper grip and avoid developing possible injuries, advises Dr. McGrew.

Let's Get Digital

Long hours spent sitting at a typewriter or computer keyboard can produce awkward or prolonged pressure on your wrists. Here are a few exercises Wise says may help you loosen up.

Try finger winging. This simple exercise involves spreading your fingers apart and bringing them back together.

Now take a second to bend your wrists the opposite way from the position they normally maintain, Wise explains. Also, stretch your fingers and shoulders, moving them around naturally, to get them out of a fixed position.

To stretch your wrists, try this. Place the palms of your hands together in prayer position and try to push the heels of your hands down. Now try again, only use your fingertips so the heels of your hands aren't touching, Wise says. Now try turning your hands—palm up, palm down—in a slow, controlled manner, she explains.

These exercises provide a nice break from typing's tedium. "They basically just break up the compression on the wrist, if there is compression from chronic posturing. They will also help improve blood flow. And if there is any swelling, that type of muscle action will help pump that out," Wise explains.

If you've got rubber bands handy, you've got a convenient exerciser that can help, Benlein says. Take a thick rubber band and place it around the tips of your fingers, including your thumb. Now open and close your fingers like a flower petal.

"I keep rubber bands in the pocket of my lab coat and I walk around the office working my hands," Benlein says.

Instead of taking breaks from work by squeezing a tennis ball, which is sometimes recommended for stretching muscles and ligaments, try a sports dough Benlein recommends called "Power Putty." This material, available at sporting goods stores, is softer than a ball and easier on your hands than a metal handgrip. Available in four degrees of softness, the dough should be squeezed several times a day. Start with the softest form and work from there, Benlein advises.

Finally, here's an exercise Dr. Dainoff recommends that's designed to ease muscle tension by keeping you from pounding the keys while typing: The first time you sit down to type during the day, deliberately type so softly that you hit only half of the keys. Then gradually increase the force until you're hitting all of them. (Just make sure you're not typing the boss's memo when you do your warm-ups.)

"The point at which you're just comfortable that you're hitting all of the keys is the force you should be using," Dr. Dainoff says.

Even just paying attention to your body's position may help you head off CTS, Dr. Dainoff notes. In one study, which Dr. Dainoff helped complete in the early 1980s at the National Institute for Occupational Safety and Health, workplace changes relieved some pain symptoms in one week. Many people in the study experienced less shoulder and back pains, while their productivity increased. Making such simple changes as improving your posture would probably have an impact on CTS pain, Dr. Dainoff says.

"It's pretty dramatic," he says of the study results. "These were just complaints of pain. But on the other hand, physicians call complaints 'symptoms.' So yes, you can see rather immediate reductions in these things."

Dial a Doc

Your doctor can offer pain-relief remedies if your carpal tunnel symptoms seem too much to bear. If making changes in the way you work or play doesn't seem to help, your doctor may suggest that you wear a splint "to hold the wrist in an upward position," Dr. Cooney says.

The splint, which Dr. Cooney calls "the first line of treatment," allows your fingers freedom but keeps the wrist immobilized in the neutral position. This position is important, Dr. Boulas says, because it allows the nerve the room it needs.

Some doctors advise wearing the splint round-the-clock, while others advise wearing it only at night or only during the day. In some cases, a splint can relieve pain in a day or so. But you may have to wear it for several weeks, Dr. Boulas says, depending on how long you've had symptoms.

You may be referred to an occupational or physical therapist for a custom-made splint. These therapists may also advise you about additional exercises, posture, and adapting your tools at work, Wise says. (Massage therapists also see people with CTS and may treat with ice, a paraffin or hot wax bath, and compression, which is done by carefully squeezing and manipulating the wrist and fingers, Benlein says.)

Medications That Help

Your doctor most likely will prescribe nonsteroidal anti-inflammatories along with the splint and will tell you to rest and stay away from work for a few days, or to go on light duty until you feel better, Dr. Cooney says.

If you're not feeling better after a few weeks, the next line of treatment probably will be a cortisone injection, he says. The purpose of the cortisone is to decrease swelling around the tendons. "It's like putting the aspirin or Motrin [ibuprofen] right in the wrist," he explains.

THINGS THAT GO BUMP ON YOUR WRIST

What the heck is that? you ask, as your doctor presses on the bump on your wrist.

That's a ganglion.

A ganglion is a cyst that may pop up on either side of your wrist. Ganglions tend to come and go, says Chris McGrew, M.D., a sports medicine specialist at the University of New Mexico Medical Center in Albuquerque. Sometimes they're here, sometimes they aren't. Sometimes they hurt, sometimes they don't.

"I had a patient once who, when he did handstands, they'd pop up. When he didn't do handstands, they wouldn't pop up," Dr. McGrew says.

Ganglions occur when a jellylike substance leaks from a joint or a tendon sheath.

They are fairly harmless, says Dr. McGrew. But have a doctor look at yours if it's really painful, limits your activities, or worries you, he advises.

Treatments range from draining and rest to cortisone injections to surgical removal, says William Cooney, M.D., chief of hand surgery at the Mayo Clinic.

Myths and legends surround at-home treatments, Dr. McGrew says, citing a classic example: Bible bashing. "Because the Bible was the biggest book in a person's house, they'd use it to slam and smash the ganglion," he says. "I've had patients tell me they did that and wound up fracturing their hand. I wouldn't advise doing it."

Instead, try rest, patience, and perhaps your doctor's care.

Cortisone injections frequently are used for these problems, but almost all doctors agree cortisone should not be used frequently because it may cause tendons to degenerate. Some studies have shown a high success rate with the drug, although the relapse rates are high. Ask your doctor about cortisone.

"Some people, after an injection, will get better and never see you again. Some will get better and come back a year later. Some people get relief for one day, then it's back," Dr. Boulas says.

B Stands for Better

Some doctors espouse vitamin B_6 supplements as a CTS treatment. A B_6 deficiency can bring on CTS symptoms, says John M. Ellis, M.D., a surgeon and family practitioner in Mount Pleasant, Texas, who has done extensive research on the vitamin.

Yet other studies have shown no convincing evidence of the effectiveness of B_6 supplements. "There's no good evidence that it works," says Dr. Cooney. "We have occasionally used it for patients who have blood tests showing they are anemic. We have given people vitamin B_6 or all of the B vitamins."

Not only that, but taking large doses of the vitamin may cause nerve damage. Your best bet is to check with your doctor before adding supplements.

The Surgical Solution

Once you've tried all of the conservative treatments, surgery is the last option, says Dr. Cooney. The procedure, called a "release," involves cutting the ligament forming the roof of the carpal tunnel to relieve pressure on the median nerve. The operation, usually done on an outpatient basis, is fairly routine and successful in most cases, Dr. Cooney says.

Before you consider surgery, make sure you've tried the other options—changes in the workplace and seeing a physical or occupational therapist to learn new ways to work or play. Surgery may not be able to undo muscle or nerve problems brought on by years of strain.

"If the CTS was brought about by the workplace, then I suggest a change at work, even if surgery is performed," Dr. Boulas says. "I'll always ask them, even after surgery, if they can't change their work a bit. I think that's better, because I can't guarantee that CTS symptoms won't come back."

RAYNAUD'S SYNDROME

Take a Texan and drop her in Alaska.

After shaking a fist at the fleeing prop plane, she looks around. All is white. All is hushed . . . and it's d-a-a-a-a-a-ng cold.

Suddenly she realizes her hands and feet are fast losing feeling. Her fashionable cotton gloves are no protection from the wind. She has no matches, and they don't teach you to build snowcaves in the Lone Star State. She wishes for home. She wishes for warmth.

And she almost wishes this scenario were true.

Why? Because her hands and feet feel ice cold, and she's dressed normally, sitting in the kitchen of her home on a cool autumn morning. She's stuck inside, daydreaming, hoping the periodic attacks of cold, numbing pain, the kind that turn her hands white, won't come today. She has Raynaud's syndrome, and she might as well be tiptoeing through the tundra. The attacks come anyway.

Raynaud's is a problem involving small blood vessels that feed the skin. During a Raynaud's attack, these arteries contract, limiting blood flow. Lack of blood flow turns the fingertips white, then blue. Fingers turn pink or red when blood flow returns, explains Carolyn Bowles, M.D., assistant professor of medicine and consultant in rheumatology at the Mayo Clinic in Rochester, Minnesota.

Classic Raynaud's involves white/blue/red color changes, says James Edwards, M.D., assistant professor of vascular surgery at Oregon Health Sciences University. Some people experience only white or only blue or only red, he says, but the numbness, tingling, and sometimes pain are always there.

Of course, it's normal for your hands to turn pale and feel cold when you walk outside on a cold day or dig in the freezer for a pint of ice cream. When are the pain and color changes a sign of Raynaud's?

"In Raynaud's there is a well-demarcated line above

which it's just pure white," Dr. Bowles says. "This is really dramatic. It's like a white page in a book."

So if you see this white line, it's a sign to see your doctor. Don't be surprised, though, if your doctor can't give you a clear-cut explanation of what's causing your condition.

Doctors aren't sure what causes Raynaud's, only that attacks seem to be related to exposure to cold and to emotional stress, says Dr. Edwards. Women between the ages of 15 and 50 most commonly have Raynaud's.

▶ INSTANT RELIEF

There are several things you can do to help yourself if you have Raynaud's symptoms.

Protect yourself from the cold. Try to avoid exposure to cold weather or refrigerated air, Dr. Bowles says.

Put on gloves and warm socks. Wear mittens or gloves, even while you're inside. Or hold your hands next to your chest to warm them, Dr. Edwards says.

Burrow down in an electric blanket. Keeping your body warm may help alleviate blood vessel contractions in your fingers and toes.

Do the windmill. You can force your hands to warm up by performing this procedure, developed by Donald McIntyre, M.D., of Rutland, Vermont. Swing your arm downward behind your body, then upward in front of you at about 80 twirls per minute. (Don't worry, it's not as fast as it sounds.) The windmill effect, based on a skiers' warm-up exercise, forces blood to the fingers through gravitational and centrifugal forces. In one case, the exercise reversed a Raynaud's attack in 90 seconds.

▶ PREVENTION PAIN-RELIEF PROGRAM

If you have Raynaud's symptoms, be aware that it may be a sign of another problem such as scleroderma, systemic lupus, or rheumatoid arthritis. That's a good reason to see your doctor if you notice Raynaud's symptoms on a regular basis.

A key portion of your program consists of keeping your circulation healthy. A rich supply of blood helps keep your hands and feet nice and pink and warm. And what tops the list when it comes to healthy circulation?

"One of the most important things to do is stop smoking," says Dr. Bowles. "It's a very critical thing."

"Smoking causes your arteries to constrict," Dr. Edwards says, "so if you have an exaggerated response to cold and you smoke, or if you have a slightly exaggerated response and you smoke, you can get a very exaggerated response."

Even other people's smoke may cause a problem if you have Raynaud's. (For more information on quitting smoking, see chapter 23.)

You may also want to watch your caffeine intake because it may cause the blood vessels to contract. Some doctors believe you should avoid the stimulating substance because it causes blood vessel spasms. Others aren't sure it has any effect on Raynaud's. Ask your doctor, or alter your intake and see if it makes any difference.

Here's something else to ask a doctor about: taking fish-oil capsules. Preliminary evidence from a study at Albany Medical College of Union University in New York suggests that fish oil may ease blood vessel spasms. Researchers found that Raynaud's symptoms stopped completely in 5 out of 11 people taking fish-oil capsules daily for 12 weeks. The other 6 people extended the length of time they could keep their hands submerged in cold water from 31 to 46 minutes before blood flow to their fingers shut down.

And keep this in mind: Certain medications may make Raynaud's symptoms worse, Dr. Edwards says. Beta-blockers—frequently prescribed as blood pressure medication—and ergotamines—used for treatment of migraine headaches—can bring on Raynaud's symptoms. Tell your doctor if you're currently taking these medications and notice any symptoms.

Dress for the Occasion

What you take for your insides is important, but so is what goes on the outside.

Make sure you're properly equipped for any occasion when you may experience cold. Don't go outside without a scarf, gloves, or a hat during cold weather. Wear warm socks and boots and keep your feet dry. When inside, keep your hands and feet warm. Keep a pair of gloves or potholders handy for reaching into the refrigerator or freezer.

"It's really important to keep your extremities warm," Dr. Bowles says. "And keep your body warm. Keep a hat on your head." Much heat is lost through an uncovered head—heat that your body needs.

Training Your Blood Vessels

One of the most frustrating aspects of Raynaud's is the nuisance factor. But you may be able to sidestep it, with a little training.

This technique, developed by Murray P. Hamlet, D.V.M., director of the Research Program and Operations Division at the U.S. Army Research Institute of Environmental Medicine in Natick, Massachusetts, involves teaching or "conditioning" the hands to warm up when temperatures turn cold.

Here's how it works: Fill two containers, each large enough for both hands, with warm water. Place one container in a warm room and the other in a cold room or outdoors. Dress lightly, as you would for indoors, and place your hands in the indoor container for 2 to 5 minutes. Now go outside or to the cold room and dip your hands again, for 10 minutes. Come back inside and dip your hands again for 2 to 5 minutes. Repeat the procedure three to six times a day, every other day, about 50 times—or less if you get relief sooner.

The point? Normally the chilly environment constricts blood vessels, leaving your hands cold and numb. But the sensation of warm water keeps them open. Repeatedly training the blood vessels to open despite the cold enables you to counter the constriction reflex *without* the warm water.

In army experiments, this procedure was repeated every other day, three to six times, on 150 people. After 54 treatments, their hands were 7 degrees warmer in the cold than before, Dr. Hamlet reports.

It just may be worth a try.

Another procedure that may work is biofeedback, Dr. Edwards says. This involves learning to stop or prevent attacks by using biofeedback machines—training yourself to think your fingers or toes are warm. Since Raynaud's symptoms may be brought on by emotional stress, biofeedback may help you learn to relax muscles and prevent attacks, Dr. Bowles says. (See chapter 17.)

Medications May Help

If such training seems inappropriate for you, there are drug therapies that work, Dr. Edwards says. Doctors commonly prescribe nifedipine—a calcium channel blocker—which works in about 75 percent of cases. Side effects of headaches and ankle swelling keep some people away from it, but these are not considered serious drawbacks, Dr. Edwards adds. Plus, most people take such medication only during the winter, or when they're going skiing, or when they know they'll be exposed to cold weather, he says.

The last choice is a surgical procedure known as a sympathectomy, which involves cutting the nerves that control the blood vessels. The operation is very meticulous and tedious, Dr. Boulas says, and is done only in rare cases for unrelenting pain or potential loss of a finger.

WATCH FOR THE KNUCKLEBALL

You're at second base, ready to pivot and throw to first to complete a double play. Suddenly your vision is obscured by a large man wearing the other team's uniform. His head looms in your view, then disappears as his feet slide heavily into the bag you're standing on. Then everything goes upside down.

Your head hits the dirt, your arms and hands crunch underneath you in a dusty pile.

You stand and shake yourself off. But there's one thing you won't shake. Your jammed finger.

From major league to Little League, from volleyball to family horseplay in the rec room, jammed fingers are commonplace.

When a jam occurs near the finger's last joint, it's known as mallet finger. It hurts because the tendon that connects the muscles at the end of the finger is forcibly separated from the bone. Jams also may occur in the middle knuckle of your finger, says Chris McGrew, M.D., a sports medicine specialist at the University of New Mexico Medical Center in Albuquerque.

But what do you do about them? Your finger has been hit, it's swollen, and it hurts. How do you know if it's broken? Should you keep playing or should you call time out?

First, check the movement. If you can bend your finger and you're not in too much pain, you can tape it to the finger next to it and keep playing, Dr. McGrew says.

"But most people are pretty uncomfortable and not willing to go through that. So what we tell people is: Put ice on it initially and tape it to the adjoining finger," he says.

Apply ice to your finger and soak it in an ice bath for a few days, he advises. Take anti-inflammatories to control pain and swelling. "If it's still really hurting a few days later or if you can't straighten or bend it completely so that it looks like the other fingers, that's a good time to see a doctor," he says.

And remember, whenever you're engaged in sports, it's a good idea to remove your rings, says Dr. McGrew. If you do jam a finger while wearing a ring, try to remove the ring as quickly as possible. Soap your finger to help it slip off. If you can't get it off, "you're going to be heading to the hospital to get that ring cut off," he says.

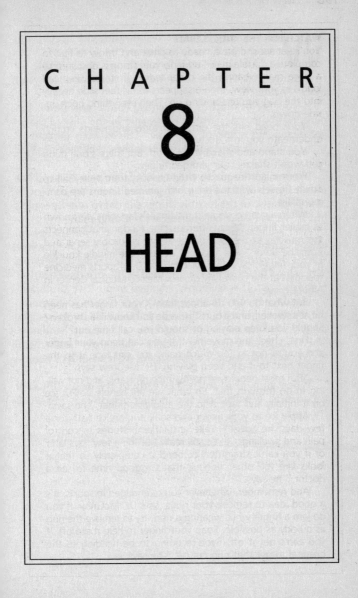

C H A P T E R

8

HEAD

What do sex, Chinese restaurants, the beach, and ice cream have in common?

All these wonderful things are capable of triggering a not-quite-so-wonderful sensation in your body—headache.

If you get headaches frequently, you're not alone. Experts estimate that 50 million people in the United States get headaches some of the time. Thirty-seven percent of that number are so plagued by headaches, they seek medical help.

No one is immune to chronic headache pain. Legend has it that Queen Mary Tudor, who was also known as Bloody Mary because of the terrible things she did to *other* people's heads, went to her coronation with a migraine.

And some experts think that Lewis Carroll's fictional use of flamingo heads as mallets is evidence that he wrote *Alice's Adventures in Wonderland* while having a migraine. When his Queen of Hearts shouted "Off with their heads!" perhaps Carroll was simply engaged in positive thinking.

Headaches come in a few basic types. The most common, the tension headache, is thought to be caused by stress. The most talked-about is the migraine, a vascular headache. The vascular category also includes the cluster headache, a severe pain that usually concentrates itself around or behind one eye.

When your head hurts, be ready to try many different treatments. What works for another person may not work for you.

GET PROFESSIONAL HELP IF:

- Your headache is accompanied by fever and a stiff neck
- Your headache has persisted for more than 24 hours
- You're experiencing visual difficulties
- You have injured your head
- You're experiencing mental or speech changes or general loss of coordination
- Your headache is worse in the mornings

PAIN-FINDER CHART FOR THE HEAD

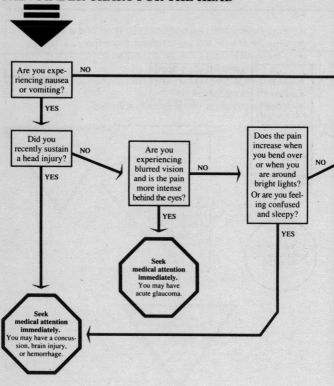

Are you experiencing nausea or vomiting?

NO

YES

Did you recently sustain a head injury?

NO

YES

Are you experiencing blurred vision and is the pain more intense behind the eyes?

NO

YES

Does the pain increase when you bend over or when you are around bright lights? Or are you feeling confused and sleepy?

NO

YES

Seek medical attention immediately. You may have acute glaucoma.

Seek medical attention immediately. You may have a concussion, brain injury, or hemorrhage.

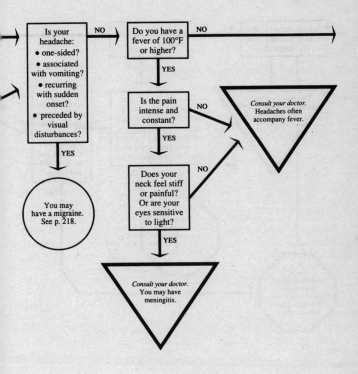

Is your headache:
- one-sided?
- associated with vomiting?
- recurring with sudden onset?
- preceded by visual disturbances?

NO →

Do you have a fever of 100°F or higher?

NO →

YES ↓

Is the pain intense and constant?

NO →

YES ↓

You may have a migraine. See p. 218.

Does your neck feel stiff or painful? Or are your eyes sensitive to light?

NO →

Consult your doctor. Headaches often accompany fever.

YES ↓

Consult your doctor. You may have meningitis.

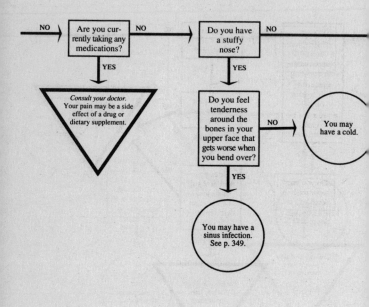

NO → Are you currently taking any medications?

NO → Do you have a stuffy nose?

NO →

YES ↓

Consult your doctor. Your pain may be a side effect of a drug or dietary supplement.

YES ↓

Do you feel tenderness around the bones in your upper face that gets worse when you bend over?

NO → You may have a cold.

YES ↓

You may have a sinus infection. See p. 349.

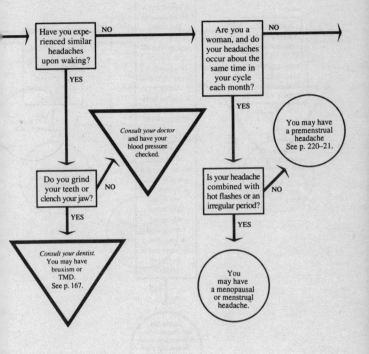

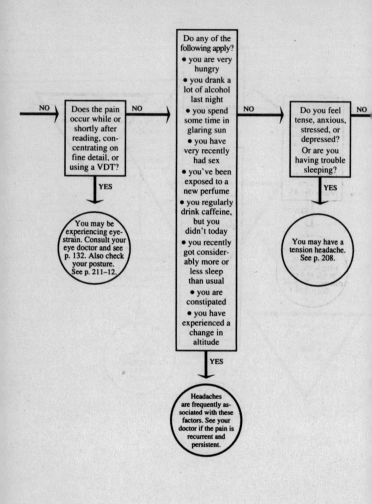

NO → Does the pain occur while or shortly after reading, concentrating on fine detail, or using a VDT? → **NO**

YES ↓

You may be experiencing eye-strain. Consult your eye doctor and see p. 132. Also check your posture. See p. 211–12.

Do any of the following apply?
- you are very hungry
- you drank a lot of alcohol last night
- you spend some time in glaring sun
- you have very recently had sex
- you've been exposed to a new perfume
- you regularly drink caffeine, but you didn't today
- you recently got considerably more or less sleep than usual
- you are constipated
- you have experienced a change in altitude

→ **NO**

YES ↓

Headaches are frequently associated with these factors. See your doctor if the pain is recurrent and persistent.

Do you feel tense, anxious, stressed, or depressed? Or are you having trouble sleeping? → **NO**

YES ↓

You may have a tension headache. See p. 208.

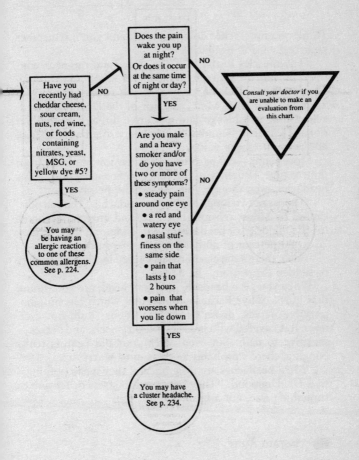

Have you recently had cheddar cheese, sour cream, nuts, red wine, or foods containing nitrates, yeast, MSG, or yellow dye #5?

NO →

Does the pain wake you up at night? Or does it occur at the same time of night or day?

NO →

Consult your doctor if you are unable to make an evaluation from this chart.

↓ YES

You may be having an allergic reaction to one of these common allergens. See p. 224.

↓ YES

Are you male and a heavy smoker and/or do you have two or more of these symptoms?

• steady pain around one eye
• a red and watery eye
• nasal stuffiness on the same side
• pain that lasts $\frac{1}{2}$ to 2 hours
• pain that worsens when you lie down

NO →

↓ YES

You may have a cluster headache. See p. 234.

TENSION HEADACHES

Think of a nutcracker doing its work and you'll remember your last tension headache.

"The muscles in the face, the scalp, and the neck contract, putting the squeeze on the blood supply to the brain. The result is a lack of oxygen, which causes pain," says Seymour Diamond, M.D., director of the Diamond Headache Clinic in Chicago and executive director of the National Headache Foundation. He has written a number of books on headache pain.

Most people—90 percent—get a tension headache from time to time. Usually you can function normally during this headache, even though you are in pain, he says.

"There are two kinds of tension headaches. The episodic, caused by stress, tension, hostility, and anxiety, accounts for the majority of headaches," Dr. Diamond says. In fact, 75 to 80 percent of all headaches are episodic.

"Also, there's the chronic type caused by chronic anxiety or hidden depression," he adds.

When you get a headache, it's your head, not your brain, that hurts. Why? Because your brain, which has no pain-sensitive nerves, doesn't feel pain. Your skull, however, does. It is covered with muscles, blood vessels, and nerves—sensitive to pain. But even when your old bean is really banging, there's probably no reason to worry.

"Most headaches are insignificant, they mean nothing," says Dr. Diamond. "They're related to stress or tension or something else, not a brain tumor."

▶ INSTANT RELIEF

Finding relief from tension headaches is usually fairly simple. Here are some strategies.

Sleep it off. Some people find a short nap sends a tension headache packing. If you can sneak off for a short snooze, it's certainly worth a try.

Take a deep breath, then yawn. When your head feels as if it is expanding while your hatband is shrinking, take a deep breath. Then begin a type of relaxation that experts say may stop your headache short.

Clench your fists and breathe in deeply. Hold that breath. Now breathe out slowly and let your body go limp, like a rag doll. Now yawn (and don't be surprised if others around you yawn and begin relaxing, too).

Take a hike. Try a brisk walk around the block the next time you get a mild tension headache. Some experts think that walking may ease your pain by releasing the body's own natural painkillers, the endorphins. Others think walking may help because it drains the tension from your body.

Give exercise a try, says Dr. Diamond. It's successful for one out of two people who try it. Beware, however, that some people find exercise worsens their head pain. If that's true for you, skip walking.

Good vibrations. Electric massage—vibration—used with moderate pressure on a specific spot on the head can relieve some or all of the pain of a tension headache, according to Margo McCaffery, R.N., a specialist in nursing people who are in pain. Vibration for 25 minutes may offer pain relief for several hours. To try this, find the area at the back of your head just below the bony bump at your hairline. Press a small, hand-held vibrator against this area. (For an alternate point, see the illustration on page 210.)

For chronic pain, lengthen each treatment to 30 to 45 minutes, twice a day. Do not use this technique to treat a migraine headache.

Brush the pain off. You'll find another massage tool on your bureau. Use your hairbrush to give your scalp a massage. Brushing improves the poor blood circulation that may cause a headache. Start at the right temple, just above the eyebrow. While keeping the bristles against your scalp, move the brush in small circles, gradually working toward the back of your head. Repeat on the other side. Move to the top of your head, just left of center. Brush in small circles again, moving toward the crown and then down the back of your head. Repeat on the right side.

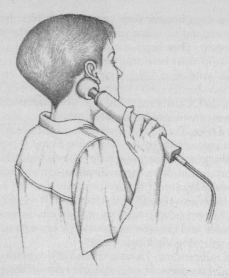

Try z-z-z-z-z-zapping a tension headache. Place the tip of a hand-held vibrator against the bony area just behind the ear at the hairline. A 25-minute session may relieve pain for up to several hours.

See also:

- "Take 2, Not 4 or 8" on page 212.
- "Take the Pressure Off" on page 214.
- "Hot News about Heat and Cold" on page 219.
- "Guiding Yourself Free" on page 228.

➡ PREVENTION PAIN-RELIEF PROGRAM

Few people turn to their doctor for help with a tension headache. They take a couple of aspirin or take a nap. Once the headache is gone, it's forgotten.

However, if that tension headache seems to creep up on you day after day, you probably should be looking into ways to banish that pain from your life. First, see your doctor to be sure there's no serious underlying cause for your pain. At the same time, you can take action on your own by learning to deal with the tension that is provoking your chronic pain.

Mirror Your Emotions

One way to spot the tension in your body before it turns into a full-blown tension headache is to see it and relax before it starts. Here's how to do a tension checkup several times a day, according to Fred Sheftell, M.D., and Alan Rapoport, M.D., directors of the New England Center for Headache in Stamford, Connecticut, and authors of *Headache Relief*.

Take a minute to stop and look in the mirror. Can you feel pain or tightness in your lower back? Are your shoulders straight or hunched? How do you feel when you consciously relax your shoulders? Do you look like a ruffled bird with your shoulders tight in a protective position? Check the back of your neck . . . is it feeling loose or tight? Now examine your face. Are you frowning? Do you look serious? Are you forcing a smile? Are you clenching your jaw or grinding your teeth?

If you do a physical tension check several times a day, you'll begin to understand how your emotions translate into the muscle contractions that tighten your body and give you a headache.

As you become aware of your emotions and your physical response to them, you may be able to stop tension before it turns to hurt.

Sit Pretty

Being physically aware can help in other ways, too. Take Margaret, who spends most of her workday sitting in one place. She types. She answers the phone. She adds data to a computer disk. When she leaves at 5:00 P.M., she carries her work home with her in the form of a headache.

Yet on weekends, she's headache-free.

What makes the difference?

In addition to the psychological tension caused by Margaret's desire to do a good job, she puts *physical* tension on her body by sitting in a fixed position for hours and hours. And because Margaret tends to hunch over her work, her posture adds even more stress and strain to an already burdened body.

Headache experts Dr. Rapoport and Dr. Sheftell sent Margaret to a physical therapist. The therapist taught her better posture, suggested a chair with a lumbar support, and encouraged Margaret to change her position every 20 minutes to get her blood circulating freely again. Margaret's headaches were gone within six weeks. Perhaps you should check your posture if your headaches seem to come at the end of your workday and vanish on weekends.

TAKE 2, NOT 4 OR 8

For quite a number of people, relief is spelled P-A-I-N-K-I-L-L-E-R. For others, painkiller spells T-R-O-U-B-L-E.

For best results, follow the directions on the bottle, says Fred Sheftell, M.D., a director of the New England Center for Headache in Stamford, Connecticut. Take the recommended dosage. More can *give* you a headache, he warns.

Experts have discovered that overuse of certain analgesics can *cause* the headaches they were meant to cure. The headache that bounces back at you because of what you did to slap it out of the way is known as the rebound migraine. All painkilling drugs are potential problems when overused: aspirin, ibuprofen, and acetaminophen, as well as prescription painkillers and the ergotamine drugs, which are specifically prescribed for migraines.

"People begin to medicate at the earliest sign of minor head pain to prevent having a migraine that sidelines their life," says Dr. Sheftell. "Then, when they think they can't afford to have a headache tomorrow, they take a couple of aspirin tonight. Their headaches become more chronic because they overuse their medications. We have some people who have taken up to 50 tablets per day, although 6 to 8 is the average," he says.

Dosing a mild headache with prescription medication designed for a severe one can lead to a rebound headache, according to Joel R. Saper, M.D., clinical associate professor of neurology at Michigan State University and director of the Michigan Headache and Neurological Institute in Ann Arbor.

If you need an over-the-counter painkiller more than three times a week or more than twice a day, or if you feel as if you can't leave home without a bottle of something in your purse or briefcase, you need to get help with your headaches, Dr. Sheftell advises.

Your best bet is to take painkillers two days in a row if necessary, then give your body five medication-free days in between. If you need more medication, you probably need preventive therapy.

Here are some clues that your headaches might be medication-related.

- You feel pain more often than you used to and it occurs more than one or two days a week.
- You use painkillers more frequently.
- You get a headache within several hours or a day after your last dose of medication.
- You can feel a rhythm of pain/medication/pain/medication.

To break this cycle, Dr. Sheftell says, a person must check into a hospital, where the medications are gradually "washed out" of the body. During the hospital stay a person breaking this cycle would get the minimum amount of medication until the body no longer needs the drugs to function.

Once the person's body has readjusted, the doctor helps them learn how to deal with headache pain without such heavy reliance on medication.

Get Moving

Regular aerobic exercise such as walking, running, bicycling, or swimming can make a big difference in how you feel, too, Dr. Sheftell says. Exercise improves blood circulation, providing your tissues with more oxygen and speeding up the removal of waste products. And when you work out, your body manufactures natural morphinelike chemicals

Multipurpose Relief

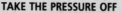

For: Tension Headache, Migraine

TAKE THE PRESSURE OFF

In ancient times, the Chinese discovered that pressing certain points on the body could relieve headache pain. You can use those same ancient techniques today to relieve your headache pain.

Sit comfortably and press one or two of these points to relieve your headaches.

- Find the ropy muscles on the back of your neck below the base of your skull and ½ inch from your spine. Curve your fingers against the muscles as you press. Breathe deeply and press for a minute.
- Find the depression on either side of the back of your neck, just below your skull. Place your hands behind your head, with your thumbs tucked into each hollow. Now your thumbs will be about 2 to 3 inches apart. Close your eyes and tilt your head back slightly. Press in firmly on these points until you can feel your pulse. Then hold that position lightly.
- Locate a point in the webbing between your thumb and index finger where the muscle mounds when you bring these bones together. Angle the pressure toward the bone in the hand. Press the point on each hand for about a minute. These points will relieve pain in the front of your head.
- Locate a sensitive point, in the indentation between the big toe and the second toe, on each foot. Slide your index fingers about 2 inches toward your leg, between the bones on the top of your feet. Press at an angle toward the bone of the second toe or rub briskly for 30 seconds.

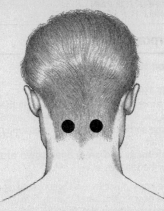

You can find two pain-relief points ½ inch below the base of your skull. Each is about ½ inch out from the middle of the neck. Press into these sensitive areas with your thumbs for about a minute. Tilt your head back as you do so.

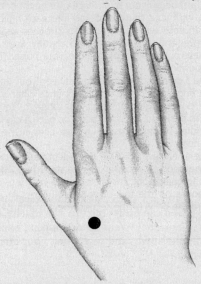

If you press your thumb and index finger together, the muscle bulges out. The point is right at the top of that bulge. Find the point, spread your thumb and finger apart, and press in toward the bone of the hand for 1 minute. Make sure you do both hands.

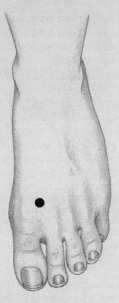

Next time you want to get rid of a headache, try slipping off your shoes. Place your index fingers on each foot between the big toe and second toe. Slide the fingers up 2 inches along the groove between the bones. Now press firmly in toward the bone that attaches to the second toe. You can also rub this point briskly for about 30 seconds.

called endorphins, which raise your pain threshold and give you a sense of well-being.

However, if you are unaccustomed to exercising, sudden strenuous exertion can push you into a headache, especially on cold days. You may want to develop an exercise program—beginning slowly and increasing your effort as you become fitter.

Food, Air, and Water

Sometimes the cause of a headache is as basic as, well, the basics. Let's take a look at the link between food and head pain. Think back to the last time you skipped lunch. Did you have a headache about midafternoon? Lack of food does more than make your stomach growl. Hunger can result in low blood sugar, which causes a headache. You can beat that feeling simply by eating small meals and frequent snacks, according to Dr. Diamond.

Lack of air, too, can cause problems—and you don't have to be choking. Just pull the blankets over your head at night and you'll awaken with alarm—the headache alarm—because you're not getting enough oxygen. Of course the cure is both simple and obvious.

If too little food and air are problems, so is too much sun. Those burning rays deplete the fluid around your brain and spinal column, resulting in a headache. To help prevent headaches, avoid the sun between 11:00 A.M. and 2:00 P.M., wear a hat, and drink plenty of fluids.

Rx: Prescription Analgesics

For chronic headaches, your doctor may prescribe one of several pain relievers. (See chapter 26.) Low doses of antidepressants, for instance, have been shown to be effective in controlling headaches. Commonly prescribed are amitriptyline HCL, doxepin HCL, imipramine HCL, or desipramine HCL.

Muscle relaxants, too, can work to ease head pain. This type of medication includes drugs such as cyclobenzaprine, orphenadrine citrate, and carisoprodol. Nonsteroidal anti-inflammatory drugs (NSAIDs), such as ketoprofen, naproxen, and ibuprofen, also can be effective.

Short-Circuit Your Headache

When the tension settles in your shoulders and telegraphs pain to your head, there's another way to ease the pain. Transcutaneous electrical nerve stimulation (TENS) may short-circuit that headache by using electrical current to relax muscle spasms, according to a California study. (See chapter 32 for more on this pain-relief technique.)

MIGRAINE

There's probably little comfort in knowing that people have been getting migraines for more than 4,000 years. One of the first doctors to recognize these head-pounders was Aretaeus of Cappadocia, who called them *hemicrania*. Meaning "half a head," the term accurately reflects the fact that migraines usually do occur on only one side of your head.

People who suffer from migraines usually experience the first one between the ages of 20 and 35. And twice as many women as men get migraines. Some 50 percent to 70 percent of migraine suffers have a family history of the problem.

The *classic* migraine begins with a warning called an aura. During this time you might have blurred or cloudy vision. You may see shimmering heat waves, zig-zag lines, or bright lights. You may feel numbness in your face or you might feel dizzy.

When the headache itself arrives some 30 minutes later, it is a dull ache that eventually turns into a throbbing pain. It may feel worse behind an eye or ear. The pain may be accompanied by nausea and vomiting. You may have diarrhea, sweating, chills, or cold hands. Also, you may find that light or noise intensifies your pain.

The *common* migraine arrives without the warning aura, and the pain is usually more severe.

Usually, migraine pain remains on one side of the head, but it can shift from side to side. Most migraines can last anywhere from an hour to two days, although the average pounding lasts about 6 hours.

Doctors know that the initial migraine symptoms are caused by the narrowing of the blood vessels in the brain— a process called vasoconstriction—which causes the brain to have a low supply of blood. This narrowing happens during the aura stage and may explain why you feel tingling or numbness or have visual disturbances.

This vasoconstriction is then followed by the rapid dilation of the blood vessels in the brain and scalp. The throbbing pain that follows comes from pressure on nerves in the blood vessels.

A migraine attack can be triggered by stress, fatigue, low blood sugar, and hormonal changes, as well as environmental factors such as a change of weather or altitude, extremes of heat or sound, certain smells, carbon monoxide, and even looking at bright lights, according to Dr. Diamond.

Multipurpose Relief

For: Tension Headache, Migraine

HOT NEWS ABOUT HEAT AND COLD

Emily remembers the last time she nipped a migraine before it nipped her.

"I could feel my head starting to hurt. I remembered reading somewhere that cold helped, so I held ice against my face. It went away," she says, still a little amazed by the speedy recovery.

If you want easy relief, use heat to prevent a headache and ice to relieve it, according to Fred Sheftell, M.D., and Alan Rapoport, M.D., directors of the New England Center for Headache in Stamford, Connecticut.

Heat, the doctors say, will increase the blood flow to your head and neck muscles. And these muscles will relax. This is especially important with tension headaches.

Cold will reduce circulation by constricting the capillaries and arteries, which is especially helpful in a migraine, where blood vessels swell. Cold also reduces nerve sensitivity, especially those in the back of your head and in your neck. Cold blocks pain messages to the brain because it uses those same nerve pathways.

Some people prefer one sensation over the other—hot or cold—and it's all right to choose the one that feels more comfortable, the doctors say.

A hot compress is one way to use heat. Fold cotton towels into rectangles measuring 4 or 5 by 19 inches. Soak them in hot water and wring them out. They should be as warm as you can stand, but not hot enough to cause discomfort.

Lie down with a pillow under your knees and a rolled-up

towel or small cushion under your neck so that your neck muscles don't have to work. Apply one compress behind your neck, another across your forehead, and two over your collarbone so that your shoulders are covered. When your compresses cool—in about 5 minutes—reheat them and reapply until you've had 20 minutes of treatment. Top this off with a hot compress over your face for 10 minutes, with only your nostrils free.

Here's an easy way to get rid of a headache: Apply cold directly to the places you feel the headache pain. Here are some other places that pain-relief experts recommend putting that ice pack.

- On the forehead, halfway between your eyebrows and hairline, for a tension headache
- Squarely in the center of the top of your head for an ache inside
- In a curving area that begins at the tip of your eyebrow and extends like a rainbow halfway between your ear and the back of your head for a tension headache
- Against the bony area between the top of the eye and the brow
- About two-thirds of the way between the ear and the crown of the head
- On the occipital bone—the bone that sticks out causing a little bump on the back of your head

A Headache by Any Other Name

Migraine, the most common vascular headache, also can be caused by something you eat. Many migraines have been named for their food triggers—the Chinese Restaurant headache, the hot dog headache, and the ice cream headache.

Other "named" migraines include the altitude headache, the constipation headache, and the PMS headache.

The "altitude headache" actually isn't caused by altitude at all, but by physical stress, emotional stress, and the higher ozone level in a plane. Fear of flying, combined with the airplane's dry air and your resulting dehydration, cramped quarters, and even the noise of preflight preparation, can trigger the biological mechanisms that cause migraines, according to a study by Dr. Diamond.

The "constipation headache" is a dull, throbbing migraine that sometimes accompanies this condition. The distention from a full urinary bladder or bowel causes a nervous reflex that is believed to trigger the headache.

The "PMS headache" is the migraine that many women get about a week before their menstrual period. It is triggered by hormones, says Dr. Diamond. This kind of migraine usually will disappear with menopause, unless you get postmenopausal hormone therapy. If you have a history of PMS migraines, mention it to your doctor if you are considering hormone replacement therapy.

▶ INSTANT RELIEF

No matter what the underlying cause of the migraine, there are several strategies for quick relief.

Be in the dark. People who are sensitive to light and sound get their best relief by lying down in a darkened room.

Think hot thoughts. Researchers have found that if you imagine that your hands are growing warmer, it may help relieve migraine. The technique works by directing blood flow out of the head and into the hands. If you'd like to try it, picture your hands in a bucket of hot water or on a hot radiator. You might also imagine holding your hands in front of a hot fire or cupping a warm bowl of soup. Researchers have measured actual temperature changes in the hands in response to these imaginary warming methods.

No one knows why or how raising the temperature of your hands can stop a migraine, but it's a very effective tool, Dr. Diamond says. Curiously, only the heat generated by your mind will do the trick. Placing your hands in hot water at the beginning of a migraine will *not* affect the pain.

Oh yes, please, tonight, dear! Forget that old excuse "Not tonight, dear, I've got a headache." When Southern Illinois University School of Medicine scientists studied women with migraine headaches, they learned that some got relief from pain by making love. Four of the 11 who said sex made a difference said that orgasm aborted the headache.

It wasn't simply a matter of a pleasant diversion to relieve the hurt, according to James Couch, M.D., professor of neurology at Southern Illinois. "We think the orgasm inhibits the progress of the migraine by stimulating the brain's limbic center," he explains. That means the orgasm short-circuits nervous system activity that's causing the pain.

Or it could have some effect on blood flow, says Patricia Solbach, Ph.D., codirector of the Menninger Foundation's Headache and Internal Medicine Research Center in Topeka, Kansas.

Warning: Intercourse is one of those "it works for some" remedies. For others, intercourse can trigger a headache— a dull pain that becomes more intense toward orgasm. Doctors at the San Francisco Headache Clinic say these headaches are related to having intercourse in a standing or sitting position.

See also:

- "Take the Pressure Off" on page 214.
- "Hot News about Heat and Cold" on page 219.
- "We're Not Just Blowing Smoke" on facing page.
- "Cut It On/Off with Caffeine" on page 226.
- "Poison Your Pain" on page 235.

▶ PREVENTION PAIN-RELIEF PROGRAM

Pain medication is not the only or even the best answer for treating the pain of chronic headaches, says Dr. Sheftell. First, see your doctor. Your doctor needs to rule out any serious underlying cause for your headache and may help you tailor a relief program specific to your needs, he says. "There is a whole slew of nonpharmacological ideas that can be used to treat and prevent chronic headache. That doesn't mean people with chronic headaches shouldn't take

Multipurpose Relief

For: Tension Headache, Migraine, Cluster Headache

WE'RE NOT JUST BLOWING SMOKE

You pour yourself a cup of coffee, light up a cigarette, and lean back in your chair to relax. But instead of relaxing, your head starts to feel as if someone just hit you with a bat.

That wasn't a bat. It was a butt.

Smoking may trigger a headache in some people and may even accentuate your pain after the headache has started.

Smoking pumps nicotine into your system and carbon monoxide into your lungs. When you stop smoking, you eliminate this headache-causing hazard, according to headache specialist Joel Saper, M.D., clinical associate professor of neurology at Michigan State University and director of the Michigan Headache and Neurological Institute in Ann Arbor.

medications from time to time. But people with headaches can do well for extended periods of time with no medication at all," he says.

Doctors search for those alternatives to medication. One recent study looked at triggers, or things that can set off a migraine. Researchers thought that if they could figure out what set off someone's migraines, then they could reduce or eliminate the attacks simply by advising people to avoid those triggers. They cited 127 different things that people with migraines said would provoke an attack. Included on the list were a lack of food, the wrong amount of sleep, head and neck pain, exercise, allergy, stress, and smoking.

Eliminating the triggers didn't stop the migraines, but it did cut their frequency in half for 19 of 23 people. (The number of attacks remained the same for the remaining 4.) If you can identify and eliminate your migraine triggers, you may experience substantial freedom from pain.

Doctors say that keeping a headache journal for a couple

of weeks can help you identify your personal triggers. In your journal, note the time of day your headache starts as well as what you were doing when the pain started. Also list what you ate that day. It may be your meals or snacks that bring on the pain.

Are You Feeding Your Headache?

Here's some food for thought: Pause a moment before you gulp down that hot dog, take a sip of red wine, or choose a chocolate bar for a midafternoon snack. Any one of these may cause a chemical reaction in your body that triggers a headache, says Dr. Diamond.

People can have heady reactions to certain foods. At least 25 percent of those people can eliminate their headaches simply by avoiding those problem foods, he says.

Specifically, Dr. Diamond says, headache-prone people should avoid foods that contain the amino acid tyramine. Tyramine is a chemical that causes the blood vessels to dilate or swell. Common foods such as aged cheese; smoked, pickled, or fermented foods; most alcoholic beverages (especially red wine); nuts; citrus fruit; and chocolate all contain tyramine. Additionally, chocolate carries another headache trigger, phenylethylamine, says Dr. Diamond, author of *Headache and Diet*, a cookbook for people on a tyramine-free diet.

Other foods, such as certain meats processed or cured with sodium nitrate—hot dogs, bacon, ham, and salami, for instance—may cause blood vessels to swell, setting off a headache. Some people have a low tolerance for monosodium glutamate (MSG), which is used as a meat tenderizer and as a flavor enhancer in Chinese restaurants. It, too, can trigger a migraine.

"Some people need the diet. Not everyone does," says Dr. Diamond. "I recommend most people try it for a year to see how it affects their headaches."

Nutrients That Make a Difference

The lack of certain nutrients in your diet also may trigger a headache. For instance, migraines may be triggered by a low level of magnesium in the brain, according to a study by neurologists at the Henry Ford Hospital in Detroit. Researchers found that magnesium levels were significantly different in the brain of those suffering migraines and in the brain of those not bothered by them. Magnesium levels seemed to be lower during headaches.

Although this is just a preliminary study, magnesium has been proven to influence some brain activities, including mood swings and brain-chemical release. Foods that contain magnesium include nuts, soybeans, whole grains, molasses, clams, and spinach. Just be sure to eat only those that fit into any other headache-free diet you may be following.

Women who experience migraines before their periods may benefit by taking certain vitamin supplements, according to Dr. Sheftell. "I recommend taking vitamin B_6 and vitamin E, especially around the time of the menses," when hormone levels fluctuate, he says. He recommends from 50 to 100 milligrams of B_6 and 400 international units of E daily. Check with your doctor before taking supplements.

On the other hand, too much vitamin A can *trigger* severe headaches, Dr. Sheftell warns. Women who use Retin-A, a vitamin A-based skin medication, for instance, may get more migraines than usual. Headaches may disappear when they stop taking the vitamin or using the face cream.

The sugar substitute aspartame may also trigger migraine headaches or make them worse. Researchers at the University of Florida compared the effect of aspartame with that of a look-alike compound in 11 people who had migraines. They found a significant increase in the frequency of migraines when aspartame was eaten. Also, migraines lasted longer when people were using aspartame.

Get Fewer with Feverfew

Feverfew is a daisylike herb that could be the solution to your painful migraines.

The herb was first used by the Romans, who believed it was a cure for fever. Ancient Greeks used the herb to treat

Multipurpose Relief

For: Tension Headache, Migraine

CUT IT ON/OFF WITH CAFFEINE

Caffeine is the Dr. Jekyll/Mr. Hyde of drugs, scientists say. On the good side, a couple of strong cups of coffee, or a glass or two of a caffeine-containing soft drink plus an over-the-counter medication, may halt a migraine or tension headache fast. The amount of caffeine you need depends on how much you ordinarily get. Some people will need the power of coffee, while some need just a small jolt from soda. Some over-the-counter painkillers even contain caffeine. Caffeine tends to help the body absorb pain medication.

But don't be too hasty, adds Fred Sheftell, M.D., a director of the New England Center for Headache in Stamford, Connecticut. Taking an analgesic with a caffeine chaser is an occasional option—to be used no more than twice a month. The treatment won't work for heavy, long-time caffeine users because they've built up a tolerance to this drug. Worse, drinking more than five cups of coffee a day can begin a painful cycle of on-again, off-again headache pain.

Researchers say there are two reasons for the up and down nature of caffeine-caused pain. Caffeine stimulates certain brain cells to secrete chemicals that relieve pain. If those brain cells are constantly stimulated, however, they get tired and become reluctant to release the chemicals. Without them, your head aches.

Also, caffeine causes your blood vessels to constrict, keeping pain at bay. But when the caffeine leaves the body, your blood vessels may dilate and trigger a migraine. This is one reason so many people with migraines may wake up with a headache in the morning.

To cope with the duplicity of caffeine, doctors advise that people who suffer from chronic headaches give up or reduce their intake of caffeine except for occasional use as a headache remedy. Specialists recommend no more than a cup of coffee per day. If you stop cold turkey, your headache cycle will probably be broken in two to four days.

headaches, stomachaches, and menstrual irregularities, and in childbirth. And while feverfew has only recently become available in the United States, the British have long used it as a medication.

In 1978 British scientists suggested that since feverfew was effective against migraines as well as arthritis, perhaps the herb contains some of the properties of aspirin. Two years later, a study confirmed this guess. Later studies showed that feverfew helps alleviate the frequency and pain of migraines, supposedly by making smooth muscle cells less responsive to body chemicals that trigger migraine spasms.

More recently, a group of British researchers at the University of Nottingham studied the effect of feverfew on 60 people with regular migraines. Every day for four months, half the headache sufferers took a feverfew capsule and half swallowed a look-alike capsule with inactive ingredients. Those who took the feverfew had 24 percent fewer headaches and reported fewer symptoms, such as vomiting, with the migraines they did get. Scientists think that feverfew may affect the production of serotonin, a brain chemical that specialists say is involved in migraines.

If you want to try feverfew, you can eat the leaves, according to herb expert Varro E. Tyler, Ph.D., of Purdue University. Try a small dose—three or four of the little feverfew leaves. That's 50 to 60 milligrams a day. Add the leaves to other foods to hide the bitter taste. If your mouth feels sore from chewing the leaves, you should discontinue use, cautions Dr. Tyler. Feverfew is easily grown, or you can buy feverfew capsules at almost any health food store, he says.

Get Up, Get Out of Bed

Like taking your daily capsule of feverfew, sticking to a routine can be more important than you suspect.

Monday morning: The alarm rings at 6:30 and you bounce out of bed and into the shower. You follow the same routine Tuesday, Wednesday, Thursday, and Friday.

Multipurpose Relief

For: Tension Headache, Migraine

GUIDING YOURSELF FREE

Your headache has been pounding and pounding, and now, in desperation, you call the doctor. She says, "Take two images and call me in the morning."

What? Not even an aspirin?

If you can use a little imagination, you may be able to stop a headache before it has a chance to get bad, says Seymour Diamond, M.D., director of the Diamond Headache Clinic in Chicago and executive director of the National Headache Foundation. He suggests using guided imagery to relieve the muscular tension that contributes to more severe headaches.

To do this type of imagery, you need a voice to take you through a sequence of calming images. You can have a friend read the script as you picture each scene, or you can write your own script and then record an oral description of the images that relax you. When the headache hits, you need only to find a quiet place to relax and a recorder to play back your tape.

Here's an example of one of the favorite guided trips among Dr. Diamond's patients that you can use as a basis for your script.

Lie down. Close your eyes. Focus your thoughts on your breath.

Begin to imagine being at the beach in minute detail: Hear the waves breaking and washing over the sand; see the white clouds against the blue sky as they float along; smell the salty air; hear the call of the seagulls as they dip and float on the wind; feel the warm breeze washing over your arms.

As you lie there, begin to be aware of the tension in your body. Picture a tiny, soothing wave—one about the size of your hand—rolling up on the sand toward your body. Feel the warmth of the water as it rolls over and into you, flowing directly to your tense spots. The wave laps at your tension, gathering it up as it slowly recedes, taking the tension out of your body. The wave flows down and back into the ocean, leaving you calm and relaxed.

Come Friday night, however, you don't pull the button to set the alarm, and Saturday morning you get the extra sleep you feel you deserve.

You also get that headache you don't deserve.

The wrong amount of sleep can trigger a vascular headache. Going to bed late, rising earlier than usual, or even an unaccustomed Sunday afternoon nap can trigger a headache, says Dr. Diamond.

Additionally, if you're used to grabbing a quick cup of wake-me-up java at 7:00 A.M., your body is going to protest when it doesn't get its customary dose of caffeine.

It's important to keep your body on a regular schedule, Dr. Diamond stresses. If you must get a little extra shut-eye on weekends, set your alarm clock for your workday rising hour and get up on time. Eat your usual breakfast. Then, if you still want to, you can climb back into bed for 40 more winks, says Dr. Diamond.

Imagine There's No Pain

Getting rid of a headache just as it gets started and before it gets a grip on your head can be as easy for some people as putting their imagination to work.

If you can conjure up a symbolic picture of your migraine pain—and imagine what might happen to that symbol when you feel the first symptoms of a migraine—you may be able to break the physical and emotional tensions that increase the pain. Experts say you may even be able to break the cycle that causes the pain.

Under the guidance of a trained professional, you can learn to use creative imaging exercises to discover where and how tension is being held in your body. You may get a better handle on reducing the pain when you have a better "feel" for it.

For instance, one woman who had migraines for more than 25 years imagined her headaches as a ball.

"I'd always had the sense that my pain was like a ball tilting in my head," she says. "I had no idea, however, that I could control the ball."

She became alert to the first few symptoms of her headache and pictured them as her ball beginning to tilt—to roll away from its pain-free spot. She learned to "see" that ball begin to move, getting ready to trigger a migraine.

As soon as she felt the ball tilting, she'd lie down, close her eyes, and through her imagination, pluck the ball from her head. Removing the ball released the tension in her head. Using visualization, she was able to reduce the number and severity of her headaches.

However, learning that kind of control is not an easy task. It's a process that takes practice. (See chapter 34.)

Music, Maestro

While visualization is a proven tool of migraine prevention, there is a relaxation technique that sometimes works even better: visualization combined with music therapy.

In a study at California State University in Fresno, 30 people who suffered regular migraines were divided into three groups: a biofeedback group, a music group, and a control group, which received no treatment at all. Both the biofeedback and the music groups learned a relaxation technique, gave themselves positive suggestions, and practiced a specific visualization. They practiced these techniques either along with biofeedback or while listening to music. They agreed to practice for two 40-minute sessions per week for a total of ten sessions.

A year later the group that listened to music had fewer migraines than the biofeedback group or the control group. And their migraines were shorter and less severe than those of people in the other two groups.

Why?

The music group spontaneously practiced more, researchers noted. When they listened to albums at home or songs on the car radio, the music was their cue to relax and practice visualization. All this practice helped improve their skills over the year.

You can try this yourself: When you hear music during the day, think peaceful thoughts and be conscious of having a pain-free head. Set aside 15 minutes each day as your time for relaxing. Turn on some soothing music and sit or lie down. Relax every part of your body, from your toes up. Let go of troubling thoughts. Rest and listen.

All Work and No Play Equals Pain

Speaking of relaxing, if you consciously add a little playtime to your full schedule, you may find that the frequency and severity of your migraines drop off.

A study reported to the American Association for the Study of Headache found that people with migraines who combine appropriate medication with a little time for fun can take the edge off their headache pain. It seems that those who get migraines, according to the scientists, tend to be hard-driving, responsible people.

Among a group of 40 people, those who spent time pursuing leisure activities and lightened up their perfectionist tendencies reduced the number of headaches from almost two to fewer than one per week. Pain intensity, they reported, was reduced by half.

Another study, done at the Northern California Headache Clinic in Mountain View, took a look at 40 people who had regular migraines. When they exercised 20 minutes, four times a week, and spent time pursuing art, music, or reading, they reported half the usual number of headaches.

PARTY PREP
It's the weekend. You're rewarding yourself with a fun night out. Good food. Good friends. A social drink or two to join in the party mood. However, you don't want to pay for that party with a hangover the next morning.

The Night Before
In addition to limiting alcohol consumption, there are plenty of things you can do to be sure it won't all go to your head.

Before you belt down that first brew, load up on vitamin C. It will counteract some of the effects of alcohol and will help speed it from your bloodstream. Other vitamins and minerals that help fortify your body against alcohol include B-complex vitamins, zinc, and magnesium.

Avoid the blue haze. Don't smoke—and avoid people who do. One hangover-causing substance called acetaldehyde is in both tobacco and alcohol. That means double trouble for the livers of those who smoke while drinking. But even standing in a smoky room can compound the misery.

Mix your liquor with citrus juice or water. Avoid the carbonated beverages because they increase the rate at which alcohol is absorbed.

Make it light. That is, the darker the color of the alcohol, the more likely it is to produce a hangover headache. Brandy, red wine, dark rum, sherry, and scotch will produce a headache more often than vodka, white wine, and beer.

Set a limit. Drink no more than one drink an hour, the rate at which most people metabolize alcohol.

Eat and be merry. Food, especially fat-rich party treats such as pâté and cheese, slow the absorption of alcohol.

The Morning After

As dawn breaks and you think about the day to come, here are some tips for avoiding aftereffects.

No hairy dogs, please. Don't fight your hangover with that traditional shot of more alcohol. It only dehydrates you more when your body is already bone dry.

Drink plenty of water and fruit juice. Water will rehydrate your body, but fruit juice, such as tomato, offers something more—fructose, a sugar that can lessen your hangover headache by speeding up the body's ability to burn alcohol. You might also spread honey, which is mostly fructose, on your morning toast.

Avoid aspirin. It irritates an already nasty stomach. Acetaminophen is a less irritating painkiller.

Medication Measures

For some people with severe migraines, doctors say the best preventive treatment starts with prescription drugs. Once the drugs begin to ease their pain, they can learn to control their headaches with alternative methods.

Prescription analgesics are usually reserved for people who have migraines more than twice a month or for those who shouldn't take drugs such as ergotamine, a powerful painkiller that's sometimes prescribed for migraines. They are also a logical choice for people whose headaches are predictable. (See chapter 26.)

CLUSTER HEADACHES

First it hurts. Then it doesn't.

It hurts.

It doesn't hurt.

It hurts.

It doesn't hurt.

It hurts.

It doesn't hurt.

Pity the person who has a headache that flashes on and off like a neon sign. This is the cluster headache—a migraine-like headache that explodes again and again only on one side of the head. You may get several of these vascular headaches in a single day and be done with it. More likely, your headaches may flash on and off for a week, three months, or even a year.

If you drew a picture of this headache, it would look like a mountain range. The pain builds gradually, relentlessly, to an agonizing peak and then sinks slowly toward the valley, only to build again. The valley between the mountains offers only a brief respite from pain.

This tends to be a man's headache—80 percent of people who have cluster headaches are men. They begin, usually, after age 20.

Each headache in the cluster lasts from a few minutes to 3 hours, although most average 90 minutes. The first in the series commonly begins between 6:00 and 8:00 P.M. A cluster headache may also awaken you from sleep early in the morning. In addition to the on-again, off-again pain, you may have tearing, nasal congestion, and flushing on the side of face where the headache occurs.

Doctors say the pain from these headaches is so intense that some people have been known to bang their head against the wall, trying to make the pain stop. This severe pain led ancient man to cut holes in the skull—surgery called trepanning—to let the "evil spirits" out.

Researchers aren't exactly sure what causes cluster headaches. It may be blood vessels dilating, inflammation, or

Multipurpose Relief

For: Migraine, Cluster Headache

POISON YOUR PAIN

You know that good things come in small packages. In the case of migraine and cluster headaches, good things come in strange packages.

One of the most effective drugs for migraine and cluster headaches comes from the black or purple fungus—ergot—that grows on damp rye grain. While the ergot is poisonous, the chemicals it produces have been refined into powerful painkilling drugs, including one called ergotamine (er-GOT-a-meen).

This chemical short-circuits the headache by narrowing the blood vessels.

A dose of ergotamine (Cafergot or Ergostat) will douse your headache quickly if it is taken at the onset, according to headache expert Joel Saper, M.D., clinical associate professor of neurology at Michigan State University and director of the Michigan Headache and Neurological Institute in Ann Arbor.

This drug, available by prescription only, can be taken by injection or as a suppository, an under-the-tongue tablet, a pill, or an inhalant spray. If it is taken at the onset of a vascular headache, it can diminish or stop the attack. Ergotamine should not be used on a daily basis, though, because it can cause rebound headaches. Doctors recommend taking ergotamine only every fourth or fifth day.

Side effects of ergotamine may include dizziness, drowsiness, nausea, and vomiting, as well as muscle aches and diarrhea.

pressure on the nerves behind the eye. Or the headaches could be triggered by a decrease in oxygen in the blood. Some experts say cluster headaches are caused by a sensitivity to the body's own naturally occurring histamine.

You may be able to forecast your tendency toward this kind of headache by looking in the mirror, researchers say.

People with cluster headaches tend to share certain facial characteristics, including deep furrows in the forehead, a square jaw, a cleft chin, coarse, wrinkled, ruddy skin, and a lionlike appearance. Men who experience cluster headaches tend to be Caucasian and have hazel eyes, and are taller than average.

Studies show that people with cluster headaches also tend to drink and smoke more than others, although stopping these activities doesn't seem to help.

▶ INSTANT RELIEF

If you are in a cluster headache cycle, your doctor can offer a few ways to help you get quick relief.

Get some oxy. A breath of pure oxygen is a potent pain stopper for many people with cluster headaches, says Dr. Diamond.

One doctor discovered that the oxygen levels in the blood dip just before the onset of this kind of headache. He began treating his patients with oxygen inhalers. He found that in up to 90 percent of the cases, breathing pure oxygen can stop a cluster headache within 15 minutes.

See also:

- "We're Not Just Blowing Smoke" on page 223.
- "Poison Your Pain" on page 235.

▶ PREVENTION PAIN-RELIEF PROGRAM

There are few things you can do to prevent a cluster headache, says Dr. Diamond. If you get cluster headaches, you should see your doctor so that help—oxygen and ergotamine—are never more than a phone call away. Long-range treatment is something that should be handled by a professional, he says.

There are no wonder drugs that can stop these headaches forever, says Marvin Hoffert, M.D., director of the Headache Research Foundation in Jamaica Plain, Massachusetts. Doctors may have you try several different medications

TWO HEADACHES IN ONE

What if your headache is a nonconformist? What if it sometimes pinches and squeezes like a tension headache—and yet sometimes pounds like a migraine?

Could be that you have what doctors call a mixed headache, says Fred Sheftell, M.D., a director of the New England Center for Headache in Stamford, Connecticut.

For years, doctors thought there were two distinct types of headaches: vascular and tension. Now many people are checking into headache clinics with symptoms that seem to fit both types.

"It's frequently dull to moderate pain daily or frequently, with several episodes per month of severe pain," Dr. Sheftell says. "And it can be compounded by rebound headache." Rebound headaches are *caused* by pain-relief medications.

Sometimes a person who has had one type of headache for many years begins to have a combination. Doctors think that this may be evidence that both muscle contraction headaches and migraines may have a common source in the nervous system.

Dr. Sheftell thinks a biochemical disorder may be behind mixed headaches. Something may go wrong with the chemicals in the brain that act as messengers—the neurotransmitters. Or it may be that the disorder allows an underproduction of the body's natural painkillers, the endorphins, compounded by taking too many pain relievers.

There are two types of mixed headaches. With one, a person who commonly has tension headaches starts having migraine symptoms, including nausea, vomiting, or sensitivity to light.

With the second type, a person who usually has migraines adds on a seemingly permanent tension headache. The migraines may continue once or twice a week, but the squeezing tension headache never seems to leave.

If you get mixed headaches, you should see your doctor for help. Many of the remedies that he or she may try will be pulled from standard remedies for both the tension and migraine categories. You may want to try some of the relief techniques that are common to both these headaches.

until they find one that works for you. Those medications may include lithium, verapamil, and other calcium blockers, which keep your blood vessels from changing in size. They also include the drug methysergide, which inhibits the effects of an important brain chemical, serotonin.

However, if you avoid some of the triggers that doctors say may touch off yet another headache during a cluster cycle, you also may avoid some of the pain.

Some of those triggers include strong sunlight, stress, naps, foods containing nitrites, and medications that cause your blood vessels to widen, such as histamine and nitroglycerin.

CHAPTER
9

JOINTS
AND BONES

Remember Darth Vader, the wondrous dark villain of the *Star Wars* films? The 6'6", 250-pound giant who played him, David Prowse, was stricken with arthritis following a weight-lifting accident. In a scant ten months, his mobility deteriorated to the point where he had to walk with a cane—proof positive that debilitating conditions of the bones and joints can strike even the mightiest of us.

Arthritis is a broad term that applies to some 250 separate maladies, and all but a few of them are painful, says Robert P. Sheon, M.D., coauthor of *Coping with Arthritis*. By age 70, fully 97 percent of the population has sustained sufficient joint deterioration from one or another form of arthritis for it to show up on x-rays, he says.

Osteoporosis, marked by progressive weakening of the bones, is more commonly found in women, says Roger P. Smith, M.D., associate professor and chief of obstetrics and gynecology at the Medical College of Georgia in Augusta.

Finally, overuse and repetitive movements lead to a number of painful disorders—including tendinitis and bursitis.

Fortunately, there is help available for all of these conditions—both tried-and-true treatments as well as some high-tech solutions recommended by the country's top physicians.

GET PROFESSIONAL HELP IF:

- You have any of the following with your joint pain:
    - warmth in a joint
    - limitation of joint movement
    - rash
    - abdominal pain
    - vomiting
    - fever not accompanied by cold or flu
- Your joint pain persists for more than a week
- Your pain is severe and limited to one joint
- Your pain results from an injury

ARTHRITIS

Every one of your joints is truly a wonderful and complex machine. It is made up not only of the ends of bones but also of ligaments, cartilage, lubricating fluid, and other bodily tissues.

Arthritis throws a monkey wrench into that exquisitely designed machine. Instead of moving freely, an arthritic joint will swell, stiffen, creak, groan, complain . . . and hurt.

Arthritis simply means "inflammation of the joint," and that's why the term can be applied to so many diverse conditions. The two most common forms of the disease are osteoarthritis and rheumatoid arthritis.

Osteoarthritis is so common, in fact, that most of us will develop it to some degree if we live long enough. It's a disease that results from wear and tear on the joints over the years. Specifically, what gets worn and torn is the cartilage that cushions the ends of the bones that meet inside a joint. Instead of slip-sliding past each other, those bones now may grind. Fortunately, that friction eventually polishes the bones smooth, and the pain eases.

What tips you off that you may have osteoarthritis? Age, for the most part. The condition is fairly common among older people. Signs of osteoarthritis include pain and stiffness. Usually the problem is localized in one joint—often the neck, back, knee, or hip. Sometimes (usually among women) the condition leaves its signature on your fingertips. Little hard bumps form at the outer edges of the end knuckle of your index or middle finger. They can cause some pain, but the biggest problem with them is that they're unsightly. And they signal to those in the know that you have this disease.

Rheumatoid arthritis is very different from osteoarthritis—and much more serious. Doctors cannot say for certain what causes the disease, but they believe the immune system somehow goes awry and attacks the body's connective tissue, internal organs such as the heart and lungs, and even

PAIN-FINDER CHART FOR THE JOINTS AND BONES

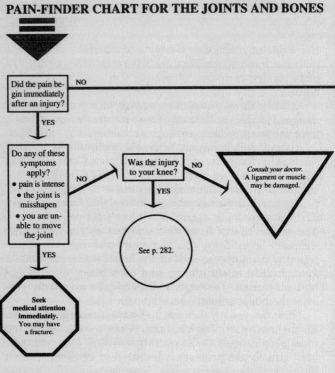

Did the pain begin immediately after an injury?

NO

YES

Do any of these symptoms apply?
• pain is intense
• the joint is misshapen
• you are unable to move the joint

NO

Was the injury to your knee?

NO

Consult your doctor. A ligament or muscle may be damaged.

YES

YES

See p. 282.

Seek medical attention immediately. You may have a fracture.

the eyes. No one knows precisely what signals this attack, but an unidentified virus is the primary suspect.

With rheumatoid arthritis, you'll experience some pain, along with a hot swelling, possible fever, sweating, insomnia, and weakness in the muscles connected to the arthritic joint. The disease can actually cause joint deformity, resulting in a loss of mobility. Fortunately, the joint doesn't hurt as much as you might imagine.

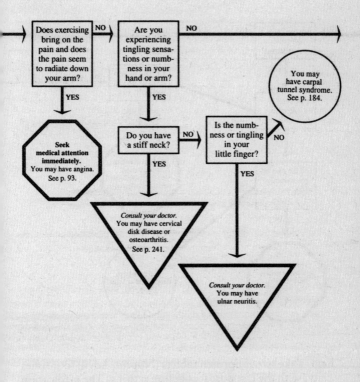

Does exercising bring on the pain and does the pain seem to radiate down your arm? — **NO**

Are you experiencing tingling sensations or numbness in your hand or arm? — **NO**

YES

YES

Seek medical attention immediately. You may have angina. See p. 93.

Do you have a stiff neck? — **NO**

Is the numbness or tingling in your little finger? — **NO**

You may have carpal tunnel syndrome. See p. 184.

YES

Consult your doctor. You may have cervical disk disease or osteoarthritis. See p. 241.

YES

Consult your doctor. You may have ulnar neuritis.

➡ INSTANT RELIEF

While arthritis comes in many forms, so does relief.

Banish the stiffness. If arthritis makes you wake up every morning feeling like your bones have been set in concrete, here's a tip from Lawrence Pottenger, M.D., Ph.D., associate professor of orthopedic surgery and rehabilitation medicine at the University of Chicago Medical Center, that may

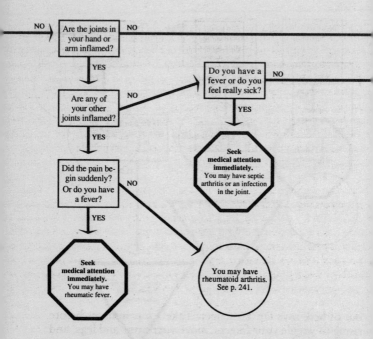

NO → Are the joints in your hand or arm inflamed?   NO →

YES ↓

Are any of your other joints inflamed?   NO →

YES ↓

Did the pain begin suddenly? Or do you have a fever?   NO

YES ↓

Seek medical attention immediately. You may have rheumatic fever.

Do you have a fever or do you feel really sick?   NO →

YES ↓

Seek medical attention immediately. You may have septic arthritis or an infection in the joint.

You may have rheumatoid arthritis. See p. 241.

help. Take two ibuprofen tablets (Nuprin, Advil) four times daily, with the last dose just before retiring. The medication will work while you're sleeping, helping to keep inflammation and swelling at bay. When you awake, your joints should feel a little more flexible and pain-free. As with any other over-the-counter pain reliever, ask your doctor about possible adverse reactions associated with long-term use of ibuprofen. (See chapter 26.)

Jump-start your bod. Another way to ease morning stiffness is to move and stretch those joints before you climb

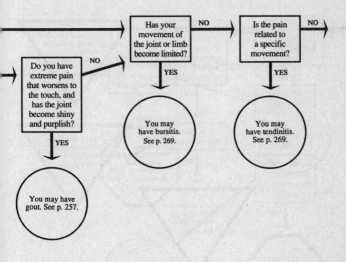

Do you have extreme pain that worsens to the touch, and has the joint become shiny and purplish?

NO →

YES ↓

You may have gout. See p. 257.

Has your movement of the joint or limb become limited?

NO →

YES ↓

You may have bursitis. See p. 269.

Is the pain related to a specific movement?

NO →

YES ↓

You may have tendinitis. See p. 269.

out of bed, says Dr. Pottenger. Take a few minutes before rising to wiggle your fingers, move your arms and legs, and stretch any achy areas.

Inject some relief. In some instances, doctors can give an injection of a corticosteroid to ease the agony of an arthritic joint. Ask your doctor if an injection might help your condition.

Extend yourself. When pain strikes the joints of your hand, try stretching them—gingerly. Not only will you relieve pain, but you'll also help keep the joints flexible.

See also:

- Chapter 21, on hot and cold therapy.
- Chapter 34, on visualization and guided imagery.

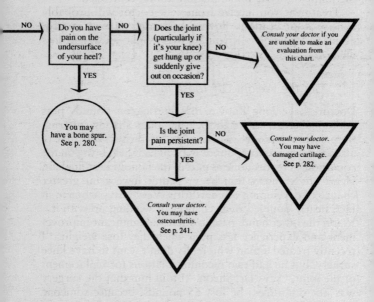

NO →

Do you have pain on the undersurface of your heel?

NO →

YES ↓

You may have a bone spur. See p. 280.

Does the joint (particularly if it's your knee) get hung up or suddenly give out on occasion?

NO →

Consult your doctor if you are unable to make an evaluation from this chart.

YES ↓

Is the joint pain persistent?

NO →

Consult your doctor. You may have damaged cartilage. See p. 282.

YES ↓

Consult your doctor. You may have osteoarthritis. See p. 241.

➤ PREVENTION PAIN-RELIEF PROGRAM

If you have arthritis, the most important thing you can do is to find a competent physician to supervise your treatment, says Daniel J. McCarty, M.D., professor of medicine at the Medical College of Wisconsin in Milwaukee.

"It is very important that the diagnosis be accurate and that measurements be taken at each visit to ascertain whether patients are getting better, worse, or staying the same," he says. "People should not be treating themselves, nor should they be going to physicians who are unskilled in the management of arthritis." Most people with arthritic symptoms can get relief by regularly consulting a family physician or a rheumatologist.

"If the inflammation in the joints can be brought under control, the pain will automatically be resolved," says Dr. McCarty. "Therefore, the fundamental treatment is resting the joints until the inflammation can be controlled."

Treatment you receive from your doctor will probably consist of medications, advice on starting an exercise program, and possibly—if you are overweight—a weight-loss diet.

Get the Weight Off Those Joints

Doctors have long known that putting on pounds puts additional stress on weight-bearing joints already suffering the painful symptoms associated with arthritis. Now they're also saying that extra pounds may, in fact, help bring on the condition. A report done as part of the famous Framingham Heart Study shows that heavy people have a far greater chance of developing osteoarthritis. Very heavy women, in fact, nearly doubled their chances of winding up with it.

On the other hand, people often see significant improvement and experience less pain when they lose weight. "I recently treated a man who really didn't want to have knee surgery, but he had two recommendations for replacement of the joint," says Dr. Sheon. "I told him that the surgery was not safe unless he lost 65 pounds, because someone who weighs over 180 pounds has a high risk of failure of the artificial joint."

The patient lost the 65 pounds. As a result, he felt such relief from his knee symptoms that he decided that he didn't need surgery, says Dr. Sheon.

Those people with arthritis who benefit most from weight loss are those who have arthritis in their weight-bearing joints, "particularly the knees, ankles, and feet," says Barry E. Koehler, M.D., former medical director of the Arthritis Society for British Columbia and the Yukon. Losing weight is less urgent for those with hip and upper-body arthritis, he says.

If you need to lose weight, ask your doctor to advise you.

Put Your Trust in Cod

A sensible diet can help you reduce pounds and thereby lighten the load your sensitive joints must carry. But unfortunately, medical science has not discovered any nutrients that will help you deal with arthritis pain directly—with a few possible exceptions.

In one early study, researchers found that taking supplements of fish oil reduced joint tenderness in people with rheumatoid arthritis by 33 percent. As an added benefit, people taking the fish-oil capsules also reported feeling less fatigued.

A second study done in the Netherlands found that fish oil helps reduce levels of leukotriene B4, a substance produced by the immune system that inflames joint tissues.

You don't have to take capsules to benefit from fish oil. Try tasty tuna steak instead. Other oil-rich catches of the day you'll want to reel in include salmon, mackerel, and halibut.

If you want to take supplements as well, talk to your doctor before doing so. (If you take cod-liver oil, you should be aware that amounts exceeding a teaspoon a day can build up toxic levels of vitamins A and D in your body.)

Another fatty acid—evening primrose oil—is on the horizon as a promising treatment for rheumatoid arthritis. In a study conducted at the Centre for Rheumatic Diseases at the Royal Infirmary in Glasgow, Scotland, evening primrose oil quieted symptoms in 90 percent of the people taking the supplement. More research needs to be done before the oil can be recommended as a treatment, researchers say.

Notable Nutrients

There may be reason to suspect that a diet rich in vitamins A and E may help ease the suffering of people with rheumatoid arthritis. In a Finnish study, blood tests done on people with the condition found reduced levels of both vitamins as well as reduced levels of zinc. Researchers believe these low readings are an effect of the disease rather than a cause but that low levels of these nutrients may add to the pain.

Vitamins A and E belong to a category of chemicals known as antioxidants. Antioxidants can neutralize free radicals—highly reactive molecules that can damage cartilage in the joints. The zinc link? This mineral helps form a "carrying protein" that brings vitamin A into the blood.

Some experts suggest that people who have rheumatoid arthritis may get some relief by eating foods rich in vitamin E, zinc, and beta-carotene (a plant substance that is converted into vitamin A in the body). Vitamin E is plentiful in almonds, margarine, and wheat germ; zinc, in low-fat meat and whole grains; and beta-carotene, in yellow-orange vegetables, such as carrots and winter squash, as well as in dark leafy greens.

Doubts about Dairy

If you want to start an argument among a group of medical specialists, ask them whether eliminating certain foods from the diet will curb the inflammation and pain of arthritis. Hoping against hope for a cure, people who have arthritis have tried every conceivable diet and have given up every conceivable food in an effort to coax the disease into remission.

Unfortunately, no evidence exists that *any* specific diet can cure the malady. However, a small study at the University of Florida found that a few people may develop arthritic symptoms because they are allergic to certain foods, particularly milk. This study, say researchers, is preliminary. But work in India seems to be leading in the same direction. Another small study done in New Delhi indicates that eliminating cereals, milk, and meat products from the diet may improve the symptoms of arthritis.

If you want to try eliminating these food products from your diet for a short time to see if you experience any improvement in arthritis symptoms, consult with your doctor first.

Medications Help You Manage

Dietary considerations aside, every arthritis program is likely to include medications.

There are two ways to look at the question of medications and pain control, says Arthur I. Grayzel, M.D., senior vice president for medical affairs and medical director of the Arthritis Foundation. With some forms of arthritis such as rheumatoid arthritis, the object is to control inflammation. "If you control the inflammation, you relieve the pain," he says.

For people with this type of arthritis, the current best treatment for pain and morning stiffness is probably aspirin, says Dr. Sheon. Aspirin gets at the pain by reducing inflammation and swelling, he says.

However, people who experience stomach irritation or internal bleeding should take over-the-counter or prescription alternatives to aspirin, such as ibuprofen (Motrin) or Arthropan, says Dr. Sheon.

There is yet another medication option for people with rheumatoid arthritis, at least. When milder prescription and over-the-counter medications don't relieve pain, doctors may prescribe any of a group of drugs that work by suppressing the immune system, says Dr. McCarty. These powerful drugs must be closely monitored because of their potential for toxic side effects, he says. Discovered during cancer research, these drugs include such tongue-twisters as hydroxychloroquine, methotrexate, sulfasalazine azathioprine, and 6-mercaptopurine.

"They are used either singly or in combination to achieve a true remission," says Dr. McCarty. People who achieve such remission have "no swollen joints, no tender joints, and no progressive loss of function," he says.

Whereas many patients decades ago resigned themselves to lost lives spent in wheelchairs, the goal of remission "can be achieved in the vast majority" of people today, says Dr. McCarty, "particularly if the drugs are administered relatively early in the course of the disease, before irreversible changes have taken place."

Where such a remission is not possible, these medications may at least alleviate symptoms and pain, he says.

These powerful medications should be used only by people who "don't respond to standard forms of therapy like aspirin, Motrin, and other agents like those," says Robert W. Bennett, Ph.D., associate professor of clinical pharmacy at Purdue University. However, these drugs need not be limited to people with the most severe symptoms, says Dr. McCarty. "The decision needs to be made by a rheumatologist, who then discusses the options and pros and cons with the patient," he says.

Osteoarthritis doesn't involve inflammation. "There the problem is basically relieving the pain," says Dr. Grayzel. Your doctor will steer you to the pain reliever appropriate for your condition.

Pain is not necessarily all bad, notes Dr. Sheon. People with arthritis could severely damage their sore joints if pain did not make them aware that they have a problem.

Get Moving

No matter what kind of pain-relief medications your doctor recommends, he or she is likely to add an entirely different prescription—exercise.

For many years, doctors advised people with arthritis to pack it in, rest up, reduce or eliminate physical activity. But new research demonstrates that such advice was probably counterproductive, depriving those with arthritis from enjoying active, vital lives and turning them into semi-invalids long before their time.

People with arthritis must exercise to keep their joints from freezing up. They need to work at keeping what range of motion they have—or even extending that range of motion, says Dr. Koehler. "From the point of view of function, it's highly desirable to keep your joints mobile," he says.

People who have arthritis, he says, should be doing two kinds of exercise: joint-specific exercises that involve muscle strengthening and improving range of motion, and aerobic exercise, such as walking or swimming.

Walk, Swim, Bike

Medical researchers now conclude that regular aerobic exercise not only boosts overall body health but also may directly benefit your joints.

Check with your physician about starting a low-intensity exercise program that can help you end fatigue, lessen pain, and feel more like your old self again.

Doctors often recommend walking, in particular, as a safe and effective aerobic exercise. Some doctors and researchers say that walking not only helps dump depression, it combats pain and helps your bones maintain essential supplies of calcium.

"Jogging tends to injure joints in older people," says Dr. Sheon. "Riding an exercycle is good if you don't have a lot of knee disease. Treadmill walking is excellent, and gentle aerobics are good."

Many elderly patients can benefit from swimming or bicycling as a form of exercise, says Dr. Sheon. If they've been inactive, he advises taking a regular walk in their local shopping mall to get back muscle tone.

"The level that people can undertake with aerobic exercise is quite variable," says Dr. Koehler. "I had a person who took up running marathons after he developed rheumatoid arthritis—he's an exception, obviously."

You may want to enroll at a health club to take advantage of such amenities as the swimming pool and stationary bicycles. Just make sure you steer clear of the StairMaster machines. These machines may be fine for people with healthy joints, but they are not recommended for people with joint disease, says Dr. Sheon.

"I don't like people who have lost cartilage from osteoarthritis using stairs of any sort," he says. "I expect those machines to keep me in business for ten years. Anyone with bad cartilage problems is going to feel pain right away on them and should be restricted from using them."

What about Weights?

However, if you have your doctor's permission, do take advantage of the free weights and Nautilus equipment that are de rigueur at most health clubs. Studies have shown that people with arthritis who participate in weight-bearing exercises can measurably increase their muscle mass as well as improve their mobility, says Dr. Sheon.

He once treated a woman in her sixties who had rheumatoid arthritis that had affected her knees for 20 years. The disease went into remission, but it left her with badly damaged knees. Bone rubbed against bone, and she constantly had fluid forming on the knee from friction.

"But after several months of treatment in which she lifted 20 pounds of weights gradually and progressively, she improved. For two years she has been walking 2 miles a day for exercise and taking no medicine," says Dr. Sheon. "I have many, many examples like that."

About a quarter-century ago, Dr. Sheon treated a remarkable patient who taught him a great deal about the value of strength training for people with arthritis. This woman had not been able to walk on her own for 35 years, he says, but she forced herself to get involved in a back program that required her to get down on the floor. In just six weeks, she walked without aid, and she kept getting better. Five years after beginning the program, she went on a walking tour of London.

"One of the things I realized from her outcome was that older people are just as capable as younger people in the development of strength," says Dr. Sheon. "I know from my experience that if you treated people in their seventies, eighties, or nineties exactly as you would a younger person, it would take longer but they could achieve the same end results."

Stretch That Joint

Along with a general exercise program, your doctor will probably give you some range-of-motion exercises to help keep your joints flexible and functional. Your doctor may even send you to a physical therapist or other health-care professional to tailor an exercise program to your specific needs. You can also consult your local chapter of the Arthritis Foundation for information about its self-help program.

Ask your doctor about range-of-motion exercises if these are not already a part of your program to banish arthritis pain. (See the illustrations beginning on p. 274 for some typical range-of-motion exercises.)

No matter what kind of exercise you choose, it's a good idea to make a habit of listening to what your body tells you. Stop if strong pain flares up or swelling increases, and don't overdo it the first couple of times out. For example, if you walk, increase the distance you cover by only 10 percent every two weeks.

Use common sense when it comes to deciding how much discomfort is appropriate, advises Dr. Koehler. Mild discomfort that settles down within an hour after exercising is likely to be worth experiencing, he says, but if you're still sore three days after exercising, that's obviously wrong.

Some people with arthritis may need to exchange their favorite sport or form of exercise for a less painful substitute if pain fails to subside, says Dr. Sheon. Joggers, for example, may need to find an alternate way to stay fit that isn't so hard on the knees—such as swimming. "I think water exercises are excellent," says Roland Moskowitz, M.D., chief of Division of Rheumatic Diseases at University Hospital in Cleveland. "They give you a nice, resistive exercise and good aerobic conditioning."

Make Lifestyle Changes

Your program to banish arthritis pain has a few more components. You need to become a sleuth to find them, however.

Look around you and see if there are any things you do on a daily or regular basis that contribute to your pain, says Dr. Sheon. If sweeping the dust bunnies out from under the bed leaves you with hours-long knee pain, maybe you don't *really* have to do it once a week, for example. Find some housecleaning shortcuts and make them part of your routine.

Another area to examine is your occupation, says Dr. Sheon. If you have chronic pain on the job that is making your life hell, don't quit, at least not until you analyze everything you do when *away* from the job, recommends Dr. Sheon. For example, a person who experiences pain from the repetitive motions involved in assembly line work may be doing some avoidable things outside work that are contributing to discomfort on the job, he says. Such motions as oversqueezing a steering wheel while driving, unconsciously clenching your fist, or participating in hobbies that require repetitive movements may also cause pain, and stopping these may permit you to continue working.

Straight Talk
In addition to being aware of your daily motions, you should also take inventory of your posture while sitting and standing, says Dr. Sheon. Emily Post was right: Good posture is important—particularly if you wish to rid yourself of excess pain. Even if your posture once was the envy of your charm school, pain probably has caused you to pick up some bad habits, Dr. Sheon says.

"Pain itself causes a guarding-type of posture, a fetal-type of posture," he says. "There is a slouching of shoulders, a leaning forward as if you're carrying the weight of the world on your back." As a result, you may have improper bone alignment and increased strain on your joints, he explains. "Therefore, posture correction is something that we find very helpful in virtually every patient with arthritis."

If you have back pain, for example, Dr. Sheon recommends that you practice sitting in a straight-backed chair, move your car seat closer to the steering wheel, and sleep on a firm mattress—further fortified with a bed board if necessary.

Sleep on the Problem
Medical experts say that one of the best ways you can reduce pain is to get sufficient sack time. Conversely, those who report being deprived of sleep have more pain distress. Early to bed and late to rise may wipe the pain lines from under your eyes.

Doctors also say that your birthday suit may not be the best outfit you can wear to bed if you have osteoarthritis. Some people who wear support garments such as stretch gloves, hose, and body stockings while they're sleeping find they have less pain and swelling.

Surgery: The Kindest Cuts of All

If arthritis pain and stiffness do not respond to other forms of treatment, your doctor may recommend surgery.

Treatments for arthritic joints, says Dr. Grayzel, range from using splints to help inflamed joints on up to actually replacing joints.

In cases where fingers, wrists, or other joints need stabilizing, splints often reduce pain, says Dr. Grayzel. They keep the joint rigid and absorb some of the stress by relaxing the muscles around them, he says.

One of the most exciting advances in this half-century is the development of artificial joints, which can replace those destroyed by arthritis, says Dr. Grayzel. Doctors "can operate on joints that are absolutely destroyed," allowing someone to walk again who years ago would have been confined to a wheelchair, says Dr. Moskowitz. He trained in rheumatology back in the late 1950s.

"It was not uncommon to have patients who lived wheelchair to bed," he says. "They were totally immobile. We rarely see that now. We now have better medical care, as well as the availability of surgical replacement."

If your doctor recommends surgery, it's always a good idea to get a second opinion.

GOUT

There's an eighteenth-century drawing that sums up the agony of gout. It depicts a man whose swollen foot is resting on a stool: "He's in obvious and severe pain, and there's a small horned devil driving his pitchfork into his great toe," says William Hunter, M.D., a Clemson, South Carolina, physician and former editorial adviser for *MD* magazine.

Both men and women are candidates for gout. Men typically develop the disease in their forties, while women typically develop it in their sixties or seventies. Gout doesn't happen overnight but sometimes takes a decade or two to develop.

Gout's reputation for striking the rich and . . . er, well-fed means that people who have it may take more than their share of ribbing. But feeding at the trough of human indulgence is not the only cause of this extremely painful disorder. A predisposition to it can also be inherited. Some people just can't process uric acid fast enough, says Dr. Hunter.

A gout attack is caused by uric acid crystallizing in the joints. People with excess uric acid in the blood—whether from dietary excess or from an inherited problem with processing this naturally occurring waste product—are at risk.

➤ INSTANT RELIEF

If gout has made one of your joints feel swollen enough to require a tow truck to haul it away, don't just sit there.

Use a footstool. If gout does, in fact, select your toe for its assault, elevating your foot ought to give it a bit of rest and relief, says Dr. Hunter.

If the shoe doesn't fit . . . pitch it! Minor insults to the foot can precede a major gout attack, says Dr. Hunter. Even shoes that pinch your big toe can cause a flareup, he says. A proper fit can prevent you from throwing an improper fit later.

➤ PREVENTION PAIN-RELIEF PROGRAM

Here's one piece of good news to motivate you if you have gout: You probably have the smarts to stick to your program. At least medical science suspects that you do. "In recent years some sharp doctor over in London measured the IQ's of gout patients against the IQ's of nongout patients and found that the gouty IQ's average 10 points higher," says Dr. Hunter.

While gout has plagued mankind for centuries, it is a disease that can be prevented. People often are unaware that they are potential candidates, says Dr. Hunter. But unless a suspicious doctor checks the uric acid level in a person's blood, there is no way of knowing that there is a gout attack waiting in the wings.

If an occasional bout of pain and swelling in a single joint leads you to suspect you have gout, discuss it with your doctor.

While classic gout strikes the area "where the big toe hooks into the foot," the problem can also strike your lower back, instep, hips, and assorted other joints, says Dr. Hunter. "Anyone who has chronic, recurrent bursitis ought to have their uric acid levels checked," he says.

Even a high uric acid reading is not a dead giveaway. Other conditions can cause elevated uric acid—including diabetes, advanced kidney disease, and taking diuretic medicines, says Dr. Hunter.

Where does all this uric acid come from in the first place? Uric acid is a waste product formed when the body breaks down chemicals known as purines that occur naturally in certain foods.

Pushing Out Purines

If your doctor determines that you have gout, he or she will probably recommend treatment for a few days with a nonsteroidal anti-inflammatory drug, such as Indocin, and with allopurinol to reduce purines to an acceptable level, says Dr. Hunter. Allopurinol is the drug most doctors prescribe, he says.

People who have gout or who are at risk need to be particularly careful with all their medications. Elderly women, for example, tend to develop gout if they have a history of taking diuretics, say experts. Diuretics taken for high blood pressure, for example, raise serum uric acid levels, says Dr. Moskowitz.

Make sure you mention to your doctor any medications that you may be taking.

Antigout Diet

Since gout attacks are caused by excess uric acid in the blood, and uric acid is produced by food chemicals known as purines, wouldn't it make sense to eliminate purines from the diet?

These days the first line of defense against gout is drug therapy, but many doctors still recommend a diet low in foods containing purines, says Dr. Hunter.

Since most foods that contain high levels of purines are also very high in fat, they should probably not be part of your diet anyway. Foods that are especially high in purines are anchovies, brains, gravy, kidney, liver, meat extracts, and sweetbreads. Other foods to avoid include raisins, rich desserts, canned and spiced meat, cocoa, peanuts, and chocolate, says Dr. Hunter.

Many high-purine foods taste good. But sticking your fork into them may lead to that naughty little devil sticking his pitchfork into you.

In addition to helping to control gout, avoiding these foods will help you keep your weight down. And people with gout do tend to be overweight. One Japanese study found that being overweight significantly raises serum uric acid levels.

So the bad news for people with gout is that they'll probably have to shelve their chocolate-covered raisins; the good news is that painful bouts of gout can be avoided or held to a minimum if they do so. Dr. Hunter says he had to give up cashew nuts himself—one of his favorite munchies—and switch to more acceptable snack foods.

One snack he does allow his patients is cherries. He is one of many physicians whose patients claim that cherries have helped their gout. At this writing no studies exist to prove or disprove the purported benefits of this delicious fruit, but if eating cherries seems to help you, there is no reason to stop enjoying them, says Dr. Hunter.

While we're on the subject of dietary restrictions, next time you visit a bar, tell the bartender to give you an olive, but to please hold the martini. If you persist in ordering drinks, you may get an unwanted twist with them. Too much alcohol also contributes to gout, warns Dr. Hunter. "Even small amounts of alcohol—beer, in particular—can shoot those purines up and lead to gout," he says.

Make Love, Not Uric Acid

Here's one final consolation. Even if banishing gout from your life means abstaining from a number of things you like, there is at least one worldly pleasure you can keep—sex. Frequent ejaculations may result in lower uric acid levels, according to one study that hit the medical journals several years ago. While an active sex life won't reduce uric acid levels in women, at least it won't hurt them.

OSTEOPOROSIS

Osteoporosis itself doesn't really hurt. In fact, many people don't even realize they have the condition until they fall and break a bone, says Georgia's Dr. Smith. Ask a frail, elderly woman who is convalescing from a hip fracture whether osteoporosis is painful . . . she'll tell you.

Women, in particular, tend to suffer osteoporosis—a condition that intensifies following menopause and causes their bones to thin out and turn brittle. As women reach their forties, their body increasingly begins to lose the calcium that normally is stored in the bones, explains Dr. Smith. Sometimes the bone is lost faster than their body can replace it. This loss can escalate to a dangerous peak when women reach their seventies, resulting in broken hips that often become life-threatening as well as wrist breaks that are debilitating, he notes.

"While women lose as much as 1 or 2 percent of their body calcium every year, their husbands who are the same age are losing only a tenth or two-tenths," says Dr. Smith. "Women between the ages of 35 and 65 have about a tenfold increased risk of forearm fractures, while men in the same age period have no increased risk."

This does not mean to say that men are not at risk for osteoporosis, however. Both men and women need to take steps to maintain their bones early in life to build a strong foundation for their elderly years.

➡ **INSTANT RELIEF**

There really isn't a quick fix for osteoporosis. The condition takes a long time to develop . . . and a long time to combat, notes Dr. Smith.

Bones are living tissue that is constantly building and rebuilding—not a substance that quits growing once you reach adulthood, says Dr. Smith. "Once that concept comes across, it's easier to understand why you have to keep bones fed and healthy," he says.

➡️ **PREVENTION PAIN-RELIEF PROGRAM**

Approximately 150,000 people suffer hip fractures each year, says Dr. Smith. From 12 to 33 percent of all people who suffer a hip fracture die within six months, often of such complications as pneumonia and pulmonary failure. Women who suffer their first fracture have already lost 30 to 40 percent of total body calcium, says Dr. Smith.

"It's very difficult, but not impossible," to rebuild total bone mass once a break has occurred, says Dr. Smith. "Some studies say that you may be able to bring back bone mass to some extent—but it's a slow process, just like it's a slow loss process," he says.

Fortunately, there are things you can do to stave off the onslaught of osteoporosis or to strengthen your bones if you already have the problem.

By eating and drinking right and exercising regularly, you may go into old age with your bones intact. If you've had an osteoporosis-related fracture already, you can reduce your chances of incurring another.

Bone Appétit

If you are in your teens or twenties, you are at the age when maximum bone mass is being established, says Dr. Smith. At this time of your life, "calcium in the diet is *very* important," he notes. And your need for calcium does not go away as you age.

"The American diet tends to be very low in calcium—about 500 milligrams—and you need between 1,000 and 1,500 milligrams a day," says Dr. Smith.

How do you go about getting that much calcium?

When it comes to building strong bones, a cow—not old Fido—is your best friend. One cup of protein-fortified skim milk provides 352 milligrams of calcium—an amount that goes a long way toward meeting your minimum daily requirement.

Fortunately for your arteries, you don't need to drink whole milk to take advantage of its bone-fortifying benefits.

Whole milk—high in fat and cholesterol—and skim milk "are essentially the same in calcium composition," says Connie Weaver, Ph.D., professor of foods and nutrition at Purdue University in West Lafayette, Indiana.

Other milk products—including yogurt, cheese, and whey—also are excellent sources of calcium, notes Dr. Smith. "If you order a hamburger, just have a cheeseburger instead," he advises.

The biggest problem many people have in getting enough calcium is that they can't handle milk, says Dr. Smith. If regular milk gives you stomach cramps and diarrhea, he recommends that you get your calcium from other sources. You might also try brands of milk that have a lactase enzyme added to make it easier to digest, says the doctor.

If dairy products are not exactly your favorite items on the menu, don't worry. There are plenty of other sources of calcium, says Dr. Smith. Calcium is in such foods as sardines, salmon, nuts, and tofu. "Every little bit helps," he says.

Based on that reasoning, he also recommends that people drink orange juice with calcium added and that if you feel you must use a stomach antacid, you should take a calcium-based antacid such as Tums.

Studies also indicate that a diet rich in leafy greens, legumes, vegetables, and certain fruits—apples, plums, pears, and grapes—may help you prevent up to a third of the calcium lost when you urinate. That's because these foods contain the mineral boron. While awaiting future studies on precisely why boron works so well, there's no reason why you can't eat the aforementioned healthy foods to do your bones a favor.

While eating properly is the smart thing to do, though, overdoing things can set you back. One leafy vegetable that you may wish to limit in your diet is spinach. Because spinach contains oxalic acid, it binds with calcium to form a very insoluble salt that cannot be absorbed, says Dr. Weaver. What's more, "if you eat spinach with milk, it will also decrease the calcium absorption of milk somewhat," she says. So although spinach itself contains calcium, don't count on it alone for your calcium intake.

Consuming a high-fiber diet is one of the best things you can do for your overall health. But fiber does have a downside—it can bind with calcium "to some extent," notes Dr. Smith. If you're at high risk for osteoporosis and are worried about binding, the solution is simple. "Just supplement your diet with a little extra calcium to make up for it," he advises.

If you are unable to get your minimum requirement of calcium from what you eat and drink, dietary calcium tablets can give you what you need, say experts. Calcium carbonate taken two or three times daily with meals is inexpensive and doesn't carry any risk of containing heavy metals—unlike calcium obtained from bone meal and dolomite, which can, say experts. (Talk to your physician before taking dietary supplements.)

One supplement you probably *don't* want to take is fluoride. For a brief time, the substance was touted as a possible miracle cure for osteoporosis, notes Dr. Smith. Unfortunately, while bone does absorb fluoride, "it isn't structurally as good as calcium," he says. "If you want to help your bones by using fluoride over and above your daily requirements of calcium, that's fine, but do not use it to replace true calcium."

Lighten Up

Also of value is vitamin D, which helps the body efficiently absorb calcium. Vitamin D is produced naturally in the body as a result of exposure to the sun. Doctors say that only 15 minutes of exposure to sunlight daily should give you the required amount of vitamin D, but you don't have to wait for summer to get enough of this important nutrient. Vitamin D is also found in dairy products and fish-liver oil.

Smoking, Drinking, and . . . Salting

It's also a good idea to stop smoking and drinking—or to at least limit yourself to an ounce of alcohol or less daily, advises Dr. Smith. (One ounce of alcohol translates into one mixed drink, 8 ounces of beer, or 4 ounces of wine.)

"Some of the biochemistry is unclear, but we know that both speed calcium loss from the bone or decrease the ability of calcium to go into the bone in the first place," says Dr. Smith. "Since men lose calcium, too, they are at risk to a certain extent as well as women—none of us is immune."

Finally, cutting back on salt may be a good idea. A Canadian study showed that women who increase their salt intake demonstrate a significant amount of calcium lost by being excreted in urine. Researchers fear that even "normal" salting of food could lead to a 10 percent decrease in calcium over a ten-year period.

Although confirmation in the form of additional studies has not yet come, you may wish to curb your use of salt.

Build Bones That Bear Up

Regular exercise that forces you to sustain your own weight—jogging, tennis, and aerobic exercises, for example—may keep fractures at bay for as long as 15 years, says Barbara L. Drinkwater, Ph.D., a Seattle-based research physiologist. "The operative word there is *may*," she says, noting that women on the low end of bone-density charts cannot get by with exercise alone.

But sedentary women with only average bone density certainly may give themselves "that winning edge" by exercising regularly, says Dr. Drinkwater.

The exercise "may increase bone density around 10 percent," she says. "And that 10 percent advantage may keep bones above the fracture threshold" for the rest of one's life.

How much exercise is enough? No study has been done to say with certainty how much exercise is sufficient to keep bones healthy. However, Dr. Drinkwater says, "one assumes if a sedentary woman exercises three times a week for at least 30 minutes, she's going to gain some benefit bonewise."

Anyone who decides to exercise must show some stick-to-itiveness. "We know that if you stop exercising, you're going to lose what you've gained," she says. "Women who intend to use exercise to protect their bones have to make a lifelong commitment to it."

Women should use their muscles every chance they get, and stronger bones will result, says Dr. Drinkwater. "The best advice I can give is to take the stairs instead of taking the elevator," she says. "Carry your own groceries out to the car, and carry your own suitcases."

But never overdo a good thing. "Make certain that your exercise is carefully constructed," says Dr. Smith. By "carefully constructed," he says he means it's important that the workout be supervised so that you don't fracture a bone in the process. He recommends that you consult a physician or sports therapist before you begin.

A Weighty Matter

Another way to build strong bones is to take up strength training, says Robert Marcus, M.D., professor of medicine at Stanford University and director of The Aging Study Unit at the VA Medical Center in Palo Alto, California. After nine months of strenuous weight lifting, undergraduate women showed an increase in spine mineral density—a sign that bones are building—of more than 1 percent. "This may not seem like a lot," says Dr. Marcus, "but virtually everyone in this study showed an increase in bone density."

Dr. Marcus is planning another study for women over 60. The younger women may not have increased their bone density to a greater extent because they already were in good condition, says Dr. Marcus. Older women who are less active may benefit more by beginning a strength-training program, he says.

You should attempt strength-training exercises only after getting the approval of your doctor to see if the benefits to your bones outweigh the risks, says Dr. Smith. Research indicates that a person with below-average muscle strength may be particularly at risk for developing osteoporosis.

Replace Lost Estrogen

One of the most effective long-term therapies to minimize bone loss is estrogen replacement, says Dr. Smith. Estrogen replacement halts the tenfold increase in the rate of calcium loss that occurs following menopause, he notes.

"What happens is that estrogen helps to hold calcium in the bones," says Dr. Smith. "It doesn't put calcium back in, but it does decrease the rate of loss, coming back out." This stops the rapid depletion of calcium reserves, he explains.

Hormone replacement, in fact, is likely the most effective way to combat low bone density following menopause, says Dr. Drinkwater. "A woman who has reached menopause should not count on exercise or calcium to protect her bones," she says. "That's a period in life where the loss of estrogen seems to be the most important factor."

Caution: Once you decide to go on the estrogen program, you should stay on it, say experts. "If you come off hormones ten years later, you'll suffer the same accelerated bone loss that you would have had ten years earlier," says Dr. Smith. "Somewhere down the road we may come up with a magic bullet that does a better job, but for now hormones must be taken indefinitely."

Using estrogen by itself apparently increases the risk of uterine cancer. To lessen that risk, physicians now prescribe estrogen in conjunction with progesterone, another female hormone, says Dr. Smith.

Monitor Your Medications

Some drugs can hasten bone loss from osteoporosis. These include steroids, thyroid hormone, and antiseizure drugs. If you're on these medications, talk to your doctor about whether you're at risk for bone loss and ask about the other preventive measures listed in this chapter.

Be aware that the Food and Drug Administration (FDA) no longer approves the use of anabolic steroids as a treatment for osteoporosis. Likewise, the use of massive vitamin D supplements has been discouraged because of possible toxicity and acute withdrawal symptoms when doses are halted.

Bone Futures

Certain medications may someday become even more valuable than hormone replacement in protecting people against fractures.

A Danish study has demonstrated that nasal-spray calcitonin is effective in delaying the disintegration of spinal bone in postmenopausal women. A second study indicates that the spray may also work in younger woman who have not reached menopause. The drug is now available as a prescription nasal spray in America.

New research also indicates that a medication for Paget's disease called etidronate (Didronel), when combined with calcium supplements, can reduce the number of fractures in high-risk women as well as result in denser bones. Once it becomes available, the cost may be as low as $15 per month, according to Charles H. Chestnut III, M.D., of the University of Washington in Seattle.

TENDINITIS/BURSITIS

Completing a double play in softball ... taking an extra five laps in the pool ... playing in a vigorous racquetball tournament ... even shoveling your driveway can lead to tendinitis, bursitis, or other forms of postactivity pain. Such pain is common in the joints of the shoulder, elbow, and knee.

Don't be too quick to assume that what's causing you pain is arthritis. Some stiff and sore joints actually may be caused by disorders of the body's soft tissue. People who overextend themselves in sporting events on weekends, as well as workers whose jobs require exertion, often experience pain in their ligaments, muscles, and tendons.

Tendinitis is one of the most common problems that you may encounter.

To understand the condition, remember that a tendon is a soft tissue structure connecting muscle to bone and that tendinitis is an inflammation of that tendon, says Donald J. Rose, M.D., an orthopedic surgeon at the Hospital for Joint Diseases in New York City who specializes in sports medicine and arthroscopy and is consultant to several professional ballet companies. "Tendinitis can result from a chronic irritating source such as a bone spur but usually results from chronic overuse—doing too much, too fast, too soon," he says.

One common form of tendinitis is tennis elbow. You don't have to be a court kamikaze to acquire this malady— only about 5 percent of those who have tennis elbow actually got it from playing tennis. Laborers who work on assembly lines or who use a wrench on the job are prone to it. It also plagues those who work with power tools.

Another cause of tennis elbow, fibromyalgia syndrome, occurs in 10 to 20 percent of adults, says William Chop, Jr., M.D., clinical assistant professor of family practice at the University of Oklahoma College of Medicine at Tulsa. The patient typically has tight, tense, tender muscles in the neck, shoulders, jaw, and scalp, and often in the lower back. Sometimes this tension is felt in the arms, especially affecting the elbow. "There seems to be a disturbance in the way the patient sleeps that perpetuates the problem," says Dr. Chop.

Another problem, although it's much less common, is bursitis. Simply stated, "it is an inflammation of a bursa," says John Baum, M.D., director of the Arthritis and Clinical Immunology Unit of Monroe Community Hospital in Rochester, New York. The knee, shoulder, and hip are frequent problem sites, he says.

A bursa is a sac, usually empty, that is found between the tendon and the bone or between the tendon or bone and the skin, says Dr. Rose. "If part of the bone—such as a bone spur—irritates the tendon, the bursa fills with fluid to protect the tendon" from the source of irritation, he says.

Bursitis is not the same problem as osteoarthritis, but the two sometimes mimic each other, says Dr. Baum. For example, "there is a particular bursa called the *pes anserina* bursa that is in a spot about an inch and a half below the knee on the inside," he says. "People who have pain in this bursa or in the tendons quite near this bursa sometimes wrongly think the pain is due to arthritis, but it has nothing to do with the joint itself."

People often discover that they have a damaged bursa when they get fluid in the area around the kneecap—a malady commonly called housemaid's knee, says Dr. Sheon. Now that scrubbing floors on one's knees has gone the way of the dodo bird, the malady usually strikes people who lay down carpet or tile for a living, he says.

Other forms of bursitis are two common types of shoulder problems that go by the colorful handles of Milwaukee shoulder and frozen shoulder.

Milwaukee shoulder—so named because Dr. McCarty, who discovered it, lives in that city—is caused by a crystal formation in the bursa of the shoulder, says Dr. Baum.

Frozen shoulder is a form of bursitis that results when the shoulder bursae become inflamed, says Dr. Baum. What happens is that the inflammation becomes so pronounced that the arm becomes almost impossible to move—hence the term frozen, he says.

Other common sites of bursitis are the hip and pelvic bones of the buttocks, notes Dr. Baum.

► **INSTANT RELIEF**

Since many soft-tissue injuries can cause a chronic problem if untreated, they should be evaluated by your doctor. But in the meantime, here are some things you can do to make those boo-boos temporarily all better.

Ice will suffice. For acute tendinitis, bursitis, and tennis elbow, experts recommend ice to stop your problem cold by decreasing inflammation. (See chapter 21.) Dr. Sheon recommends gently stretching the area while rubbing it with an ice cube. This technique will help stop adhesions from forming, he says.

Brace yourself. What if you have a minor-league variety of tendinitis and wish to engage in a strenuous activity today? Think twice, but if you have your doctor's approval, the appropriate brace may see you through. Special braces such as neoprene sleeves for the knee often are helpful in decreasing the symptoms of tendinitis, says Dr. Rose.

"They tend to reduce stresses to the tendon and give external support to the affected region," he says. In addition, he notes, "alignment problems that may contribute to tendinitis can be helped with a brace."

Ace elastic wraps have some of the same benefits as the neoprene braces, whereas rigid braces "usually are not helpful," says Dr. Rose.

While bursitis is less common than tendinitis, some people "find comfort with wraps," says James M. Fox, M.D., director of the Southern California Orthopedic Institute in Van Nuys.

Make certain that the brace or wrap isn't too tight and reapply it periodically so that you don't interfere with your circulation, says Dr. Fox.

Raise more than your spirits. Elevation is not particularly helpful with cases of tennis elbow, says Dr. Chop. While elevating the limb is usually not a factor in some types of tendinitis, says Dr. Rose, there is a tip that works on occasion. "High heels or lifts are very helpful for the treatment of achilles tendinitis by decreasing the strain on the tendon," he says, cautioning that one also needs to be seeing a physical therapist, who will recommend individualized stretching and strengthening exercises.

Try a cushion. If you have a painful bursa on your buttocks, a soft cushion may allow you to rest your bottom, says Dr. Baum.

Steroids may help. For bursitis, your doctor may recommend an anesthetic along with a cortisone injection until the pain and inflammation subside. "I've injected people who then got up, started walking around, and said 'The pain's all gone,'" says Dr. Baum.

➡ **PREVENTION PAIN-RELIEF PROGRAM**

Tendinitis and its less common cousin, bursitis, are treated pretty much alike—except that cortisone shots customarily are limited to bursitis treatment, says Dr. Fox.

Neither can be passively fought. As the very first step in your pain-relief program, you'll need to see a physician, who may also have you consult a physical therapist.

"If tendinitis is not addressed early and appropriately, it can and often does become chronic," says Dr. Rose.

The same is true of bursitis. Not all health problems disappear in time, and bursitis is a case in point, says Dr. Rose. "The irritating cause of the bursitis should be removed," he says.

People with bursitis or tendinitis who wait two to three months before seeing a doctor, without relief from home treatment, often find their symptoms especially hard to shake, says Dr. Chop. The person who tries to endure the pain, hoping that it will go away of its own accord, can wind up with chronic tendinitis or bursitis—a problem that can get bad enough to require surgery.

Once you see a physician, however, there are a number of things that you can do to tend your tender tendon or beleaguered bursa. However, bear in mind that all treatment should be individualized, suggests Dr. Rose.

Exert Yourself

Rule number one when it comes to exercise: If you know what caused your bout of tendinitis, refrain from that particular activity for a period of time while you heal, says Dr. Rose.

"For tendinitis, wait until the symptoms have greatly improved and the tendon is strong enough to withstand the activity without failing again," he advises. But while you need to temporarily stop the activity, "rest alone is not the answer, because it allows the muscles and tendon to atrophy."

The same advice is true of bursitis, although you may be able to modify your activity instead of cutting it out, says Dr. Fox.

An individualized exercise program is likely to play a crucial role in treating both tendinitis and bursitis, but the two conditions require a different approach.

Exercises to treat tendinitis should be of the stretching and strengthening variety, says Dr. Rose. Ordinarily, tendons—like bones or muscles—respond to increased stress or use by increasing their strength, says Dr. Rose. "But if a tendon's strength is not up to the task, tendinitis occurs," he says. "Appropriate stretching and strengthening exercises are specific to the region affected and must be under the direction of a medical doctor and therapist. The muscles and tendon must gradually build back their strength to prevent the tendinitis from recurring."

Overall, stretching is the most important way to manage tendinitis, says Dr. Rose. However, the use of light weights for controlled strengthening can play an important role, he says, adding that "heavier weight should be avoided until the later stages of therapy."

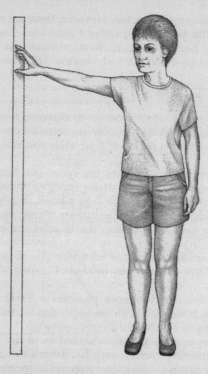

Stand with your side toward the wall, far enough from the wall so you can just reach it. Now walk your fingers up the wall, as high as you can go. Keep your arm straight and hold the position to a count of ten. Repeat ten more times, trying to go just a little higher each time.

Some Like It Hot

One advantage of visiting a physical therapist for an exercise program is that he or she can provide additional means of pain relief, including ultrasound, deep heat, and ice massage.

In some cases the physical therapist may relieve tendinitis by performing what is known as friction massage, says Dr. Sheon. "It involves rubbing across the grain of the tendon.

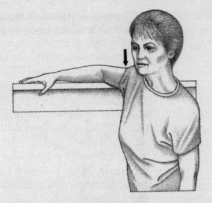

Here's a series of exercises to increase mobility in your shoulders. First, rest your forearm on a mantel or shelf above shoulder height. Now bend your knees or bend at the waist to give yourself a comfortable stretch in the shoulder. You can hold the position for up to a minute.

The individual fibers are massaged against each other to reduce scar tissue between the fibers."

Although ice is the preferred treatment for both tendinitis and bursitis, heat is useful in the later stages of tendinitis. Once you have your tendinitis on the ropes, your physician may allow you late in the healing process to use heat. It serves "to relax the tendon for easier stretching by increasing blood flow," says Dr. Rose.

Do not use heat for bursitis unless specifically advised by a doctor or physical therapist, he cautions. "Heat may actually exacerbate the problem by increasing the inflammation," says Dr. Rose.

Some therapists use alternating heat and cold treatments to achieve increased blood flow while decreasing the inflammation, he notes.

Putting Out the Inflammation

Healing from either bursitis or tendinitis is not going to happen overnight. In the meantime, your physician will

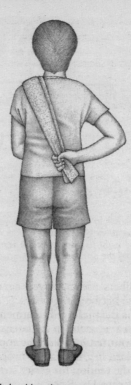

To stretch your painful shoulder, throw a towel over your good shoulder. Place the back of your hand on your back and grab one end of the towel. Pull down on the other end of the towel with your good hand. Keeping the hand on your back against your back the whole time, use the towel to lift it as high as you can without pain. Hold the position for 5 seconds. Repeat.

probably have you take nonsteroidal anti-inflammatory drugs, such as aspirin or ibuprofen (Nuprin, Motrin). They help in the treatment of tendinitis by decreasing the inflammation, pain, and swelling, says Dr. Rose.

Aspirin is preferable to acetaminophen (Tylenol). "Tylenol, while it decreases pain, has no anti-inflammatory effect," says Dr. Rose.

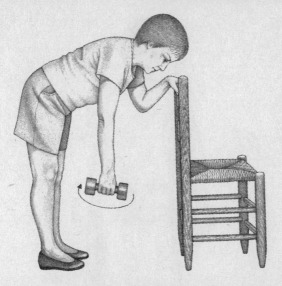

You'll need a weight for the next two exercises. Use a dumbbell that weighs 5 pounds or less or a plastic bottle filled with water. Bend over, keeping your back straight, and grab the back of a chair. Hold the weight in the affected arm and allow it to just dangle. Now rotate the arm slowly in one direction and then in the other direction. Rotate in each direction three to five times, making each circle slightly larger than the one before.

With tendinitis, the dosage for over-the-counter medications is often higher than that listed on the label, says Dr. Rose. "The level of medication needed to reduce inflammation should be prescribed by a physician," he notes.

For housemaid's knee, a common form of bursitis, ibuprofen may be taken for a week to combat pain, says Dr. Sheon.

Your physician may recommend other kinds of nonsteroidal anti-inflammatory drugs.

An antidepressant or a muscle relaxant may also provide relief from chronic tendinitis that's associated with fibromyalgia syndrome, says Dr. Chop. "They are not addictive and are fairly safe when used with care."

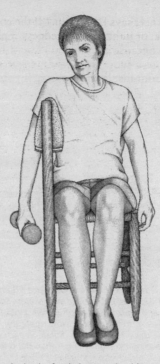

Drape a towel over the back of a chair. Now sit with your arm hanging over the edge of the chair and the weight in your hand. Relax and allow the weight to stretch your shoulder for up to a minute. Rest the arm on a table or your lap for 1 minute.

Doctors usually don't treat tendinitis with surgery "until several months of conservative management is undertaken," says Dr. Rose. In fact, he notes, "surgery is rarely necessary for tendinitis." With bursitis, your doctor may recommend surgery, says Dr. Rose, "to remove the inflamed bursa as well as—more important—the cause of the bursitis, such as a bone spur."

Surgery may also be required in some circumstances for

housemaid's knee, says Dr. Sheon. "If the condition persists beyond a week, or if there is any redness, a physician should be consulted, because an infection could have penetrated that bursa from a wood chip, splinter, or microscopic bit of fiberglass from insulation, causing an abscess," he says.

BONE SPURS

Time doesn't wound all heels—but some people's heels do suffer the agony of painful spurs. "A lot of athletes get them," says Dr. Baum, noting that former New York Yankee Joe DiMaggio is among them.

What is a bone spur? "Tendons attach to bone, and at the site of that attachment you can get inflammation," says Dr. Baum. When the body tries to repair itself, sometimes bone cells get into the act and start growing within the inflamed area. "On an x-ray you can see a little spur sticking out from the bone," he says.

While bone spurs can and do occasionally occur in other parts of the body, the heel is by far the most likely site.

Bone spurs can result from any number of causes, including several varieties of arthritis such as rheumatoid arthritis, says Dr. Baum.

▶ INSTANT RELIEF

Although a doctor's care is necessary to eliminate painful bone spurs, there is one thing you can do for immediate relief.

Cushion the blow. "Cut a hole out of a piece of padding and center the hole right over the spur," says Dr. Baum. "Sometimes the inflammation will go down. You still will have the spur but no more symptoms because you've protected it." The pad (such as Dr. Scholl's moleskin) keeps you from pressing down on the spur.

You also can buy doughnut-shaped commercial pads that go over the spur.

▶ PREVENTION PAIN-RELIEF PROGRAM

Taking nonsteroidal anti-inflammatory drugs such as aspirin may relieve pain because they reduce inflammation, says Dr. Baum. "Sometimes it may be all you need," he says.

Other times doctors get good results "with an injection

of cortisone into the area to reduce the inflammation," he says.

Bone spurs can irritate a tendon to the point that tendinitis results, says Dr. Baum. In that case, surgery may be required to remove the spurs.

KNEE INJURIES

The vast majority of all knee injuries can be classified as "overuse" injuries, says James G. Garrick, M.D., director of the Center for Sports Medicine at St. Francis Memorial Hospital in San Francisco. "Overuse injuries to the front of the knee are the single most common injury that we deal with," he says. "More often than not they are a result of knees not being strong enough for the level of activities people are pursuing."

Another common acute problem is torn cartilage in the knee, says Dr. Fox, noting that some people prefer to use the term cartilage instead of *meniscus*. In this acute condition the injury involves the "two small cushions between the bone's surfaces," he says.

Occasionally, people report that they have some actual tenderness and soreness on the bony surfaces of the knee—one of many conditions that are lumped together under the term "runner's knee," says Dr. Fox.

Although each of these conditions must be individually treated by your doctor, there are some short- and long-term solutions that these problems have in common.

▶ INSTANT RELIEF

When you've injured your knee, the smart thing to do is to stop the activity until you can seek medical help, says Dr. Fox.

Rely on RICE. Until medical help becomes available, remember the acronym RICE: rest, ice, compression, and elevation, says Dr. Fox. (See chapter 21.)

▶ PREVENTION PAIN-RELIEF PROGRAM

As more and more people took up exercise to lose weight in the eighties, knee injuries escalated. Then people started getting *smart*, as well as fit, says Dr. Fox.

"People today are more conscious of building their

strength and endurance slowly," says Dr. Fox. People are much more aware of the necessity of using quality footgear and of replacing that gear before it gets too worn and invites injuries.

Only your doctor can determine if you'll need to give up a particular activity for good after sustaining a knee injury, but don't despair—even if you do have to give up one activity, there are others that can take its place to keep your cardiovascular system fit, says Dr. Fox. "The idea is to use it, not abuse it," he says. "We're always looking for alternatives to running, for example. Running is beneficial for the most important muscle in the body—the heart muscle—but we get the same benefits from such wonderful alternatives as swimming and bicycle riding."

Building Strength

Often the best thing you can do for your injured knee is to do nothing, says Dr. Baum. "Sometimes rest is as valuable as anything else you can do," he says.

More often, however, your doctor—often in conjunction with a physical therapist—will try to help you build up your injured knee. Physical therapists may try to help people through such techniques as ultrasound, deep heat, and even massage, but most commonly they'll supply a commonsense exercise program that strengthens the injured knee.

Such programs can be quite lengthy and require a good deal of determination and stick-to-itiveness, says Dr. Fox. If you're not going to see it through, the therapy is doomed from the start.

"The therapist is like a phenomenally trained piano instructor," he says. "You can take piano lessons, but if you never practice, you're never going to get better."

One of the safest ways to get your knee back up to snuff is to swim and to perform knee exercises in the water, says Dr. Fox. He says that the water is ideal for people with overuse injuries because there is little impact that might reinjure the knee.

Whatever exercises you do, remember that strengthening is critical for the joint, because the muscles around the knee joint are like wires holding up a flagpole, says Dr. Fox. "If those wires don't have the appropriate tension, the flagpole will wobble and crack off at the base," he says. "But if the wires have appropriate tension, it stands up nice and straight and secure."

In other words, the thigh muscles really do take pressure off that joint surface, says Dr. Fox. "They really can alleviate some of the pressure within the joint and alleviate a lot of the discomfort and problems," he says.

When Surgery Is the Answer

A torn cartilage in the knee occasionally can heal back into place without surgery, says Dr. Fox. If the tears have a healthy blood supply, "there is a chance that the knee can go through its own healing process as long as it is protected," he says.

If rest followed by an appropriate exercise program does not do the trick, your doctor may recommend arthroscopic surgery, says Dr. Sheon.

Arthroscopic surgery involves looking into the joint, explains Dr. Fox. He tells his patients that the instrument used in the operation is very similar to the fish-eye lens they have on their front door. "If someone is ringing the bell in the dark, you put on the outside light and look through the lens to see who's there," he says. "The arthroscope has its own light source and its own lenses, so that we can magnify and look around corners." A television camera records what the doctor sees in the knee.

But seeing the problem is only part of the procedure.

"At the same time I can also make little puncture sites approximately 3 millimeters in length and insert small instruments to treat the problem," says Dr. Fox. He can remove portions of the torn cartilage or sew it back together, scrape bone surfaces, and take bone chips out.

Following surgery, you'll want to make doubly certain that you don't hurt your knee again. If the injury was sports-related, you may wish to have a pro check out your form to see if you've picked up potentially injurious bad habits, says Dr. Sheon.

In some cases, you may have to give up the sport that caused your injury and substitute a healthy but less demanding activity, says Dr. Fox.

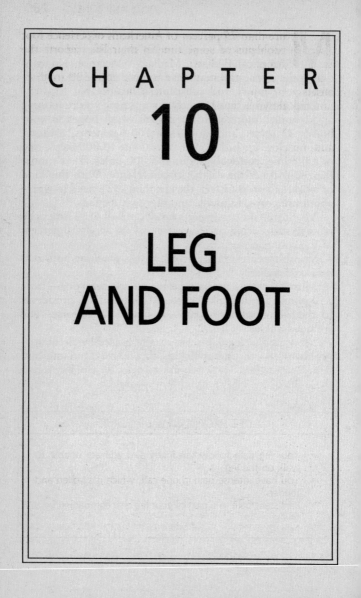

CHAPTER
10

LEG
AND FOOT

More than 75 percent of Americans experience foot problems at some time in their life, reports the American Podiatric Medical Association. No wonder. Podiatrists estimate there are more than 300 foot ailments.

Look down at your feet. Did you know you're looking at 52 bones (more than one-fourth of all bones in your body), 33 joints, and more than 100 ligaments, tendons, and muscles? Each day, you take about 10,000 steps, and in a lifetime, you walk about 115,000 miles. That's more than four times the earth's circumference. With this kind of workload on your feet, the last things you need to worry about are corns, bunions, and ingrown toenails.

Moving up the leg, experts say about half of all American women suffer from varicose veins, as do about 10 percent of the country's men.

Shinsplints are a pesky problem, too, plaguing both runners *and* walkers.

Muscle cramps probably have struck everyone—from 250-pound football players to 140-pound PTA presidents to their 65-pound students—as have charleyhorses and sprained ankles.

More serious leg pains are usually caused by circulatory problems, like thrombophlebitis, thrombosis, and intermittent claudication. These require a doctor's care. But for all these ills of leg and foot, relief is at hand.

GET PROFESSIONAL HELP IF:

- Your leg pain follows an injury and you are unable to walk on the leg
- You have intense pain in one calf, which is swollen and tender
- Persistent pain in a part of your leg is accompanied by a fever

PAIN-FINDER CHART FOR THE LEGS

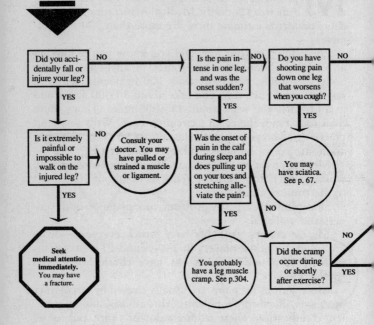

Did you accidentally fall or injure your leg?

NO →

Is the pain intense in one leg, and was the onset sudden?

NO →

Do you have shooting pain down one leg that worsens when you cough?

NO →

YES ↓

YES ↓

YES ↓

Is it extremely painful or impossible to walk on the injured leg?

NO →

Consult your doctor. You may have pulled or strained a muscle or ligament.

Was the onset of pain in the calf during sleep and does pulling up on your toes and stretching alleviate the pain?

You may have sciatica. See p. 67.

YES ↓

YES ↓

NO ↘

Seek medical attention immediately. You may have a fracture.

You probably have a leg muscle cramp. See p.304.

Did the cramp occur during or shortly after exercise?

NO →

YES ↘

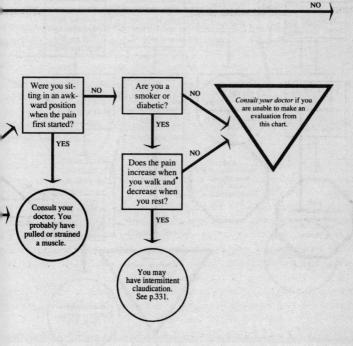

NO

Were you sitting in an awkward position when the pain first started?

NO

Are you a smoker or diabetic?

YES

Consult your doctor. You probably have pulled or strained a muscle.

YES

Does the pain increase when you walk and decrease when you rest?

NO

Consult your doctor if you are unable to make an evaluation from this chart.

YES

You may have intermittent claudication. See p.331.

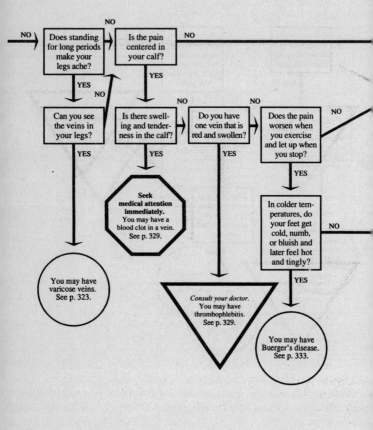

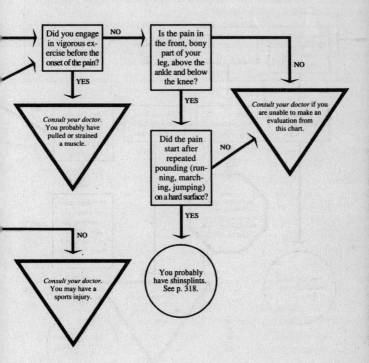

Did you engage in vigorous exercise before the onset of the pain?

NO

YES

Is the pain in the front, bony part of your leg, above the ankle and below the knee?

NO

YES

Consult your doctor. You probably have pulled or strained a muscle.

Did the pain start after repeated pounding (running, marching, jumping) on a hard surface?

NO

Consult your doctor if you are unable to make an evaluation from this chart.

YES

NO

Consult your doctor. You may have a sports injury.

You probably have shinsplints. See p. 318.

GET PROFESSIONAL HELP IF:

- Your ankle pain followed an injury and it is now impossible to move the joint
- You have a fever and both ankles or other joints are painful, red, and swollen
- You have injured your foot and the pain is worse when you walk or put your weight on it

PAIN-FINDER CHART FOR THE FEET

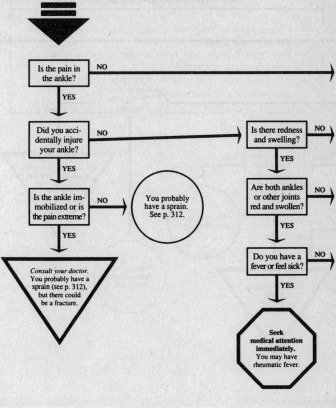

Is the pain in the ankle?

NO →

YES ↓

Did you accidentally injure your ankle?

NO →

Is there redness and swelling?

NO →

YES ↓

YES ↓

Is the ankle immobilized or is the pain extreme?

NO →

You probably have a sprain. See p. 312.

Are both ankles or other joints red and swollen?

NO →

YES ↓

YES ↓

Consult your doctor. You probably have a sprain (see p. 312), but there could be a fracture.

Do you have a fever or feel sick?

NO →

YES ↓

Seek medical attention immediately. You may have rheumatic fever.

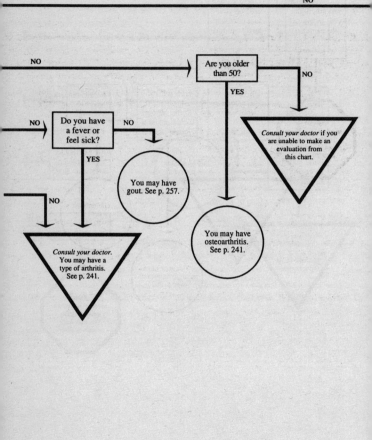

NO

NO

Are you older
than 50?

NO

NO

Do you have
a fever or
feel sick?

NO

YES

Consult your doctor if you
are unable to make an
evaluation from
this chart.

YES

You may have
gout. See p. 257.

NO

You may have
osteoarthritis.
See p. 241.

Consult your doctor.
You may have a
type of arthritis.
See p. 241.

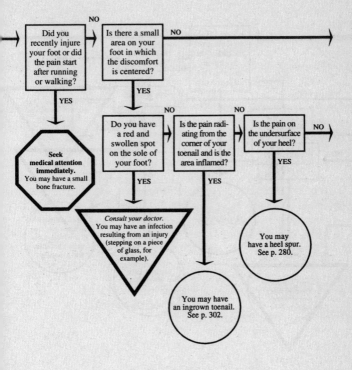

Did you recently injure your foot or did the pain start after running or walking?

NO →

Is there a small area on your foot in which the discomfort is centered?

NO →

YES ↓

Seek medical attention immediately. You may have a small bone fracture.

YES ↓

Do you have a red and swollen spot on the sole of your foot?

NO →

Is the pain radiating from the corner of your toenail and is the area inflamed?

NO →

Is the pain on the undersurface of your heel?

NO →

YES ↓

Consult your doctor. You may have an infection resulting from an injury (stepping on a piece of glass, for example).

YES ↓

You may have an ingrown toenail. See p. 302.

YES ↓

You may have a heel spur. See p. 280.

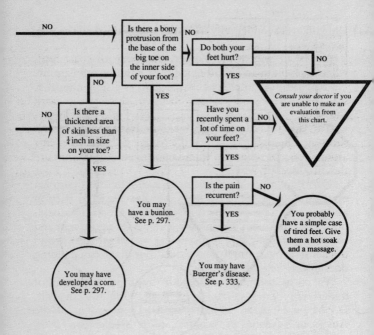

NO → Is there a bony protrusion from the base of the big toe on the inner side of your foot?

NO → Do both your feet hurt?

NO

YES

Consult your doctor if you are unable to make an evaluation from this chart.

NO

Is there a thickened area of skin less than ¼ inch in size on your toe?

NO

YES

Have you recently spent a lot of time on your feet?

NO

YES

YES

Is the pain recurrent?

NO

You may have a bunion. See p. 297.

YES

You probably have a simple case of tired feet. Give them a hot soak and a massage.

You may have developed a corn. See p. 297.

You may have Buerger's disease. See p. 333.

CORNS AND BUNIONS

Did you ever wonder why the littlest piggy cried all the way home?

Maybe he was at the market, shopping for roast beef, when his bunion and corns made even standing unbearable. His feet hurt too much to walk the grocery aisle for another selection. He winced and grabbed the closest bag: pork rinds.

You don't have to cringe, make undesirable choices on shortened shopping trips, or suffer such miserable moments afoot. You *can* relieve corn and bunion pain. But what are these things, anyway?

Corns are layers of compacted, dead skin cells that form on the toes or soles of your feet. They are caused by friction and pressure, says the American Podiatric Medical Association. The hard mass puts pressure on nerves in the skin and causes pain. Your skin is just doing its job when it grows thicker to protect you from pressure. But that extra padding doesn't feel very good.

Yet corns also may be caused by improper alignment of underlying bones in the toes, says William Van Pelt, D.P.M., a Houston podiatrist and past president of the American Academy of Podiatric Sports Medicine.

Bunions, which are a bigger problem, can also be painful. A bunion is a deformity or enlargement in the big toe joint caused by a bony protrusion that slants outward at the base of the big toe, driving it in toward the other toes, Dr. Van Pelt explains. Most people with bunions inherit the tendency, he explains. High heels, pointed-toed shoes, or just poorly fitting shoes do not cause bunions, but they can exacerbate the problem over the years, Dr. Van Pelt says.

"There's no doubt that the more pointed the toe, the higher the heel, the more force and pressure is placed on that part of the foot. The pressure is going to accelerate and intensify the pain," the doctor says. And while he sees more women for bunions, men also have the problem. "Women are more likely to seek treatment," he says. "Men are notoriously chicken."

▶ INSTANT RELIEF

You knew about the pain already. Let's look at some ways you can get relief.

Try a shot of hot, then cold. Use contrast baths to get circulation going again and to relieve bunion and corn pain, Dr. Van Pelt suggests. Sit on the edge of the bathtub with the affected foot under the faucet. Let hot water flow over it for 3 minutes, then cold water for 1 minute, then hot for 3 minutes, and cold for 1 minute. Then repeat one more time. Instead, you may begin with cold water for 3 minutes, followed by hot for 1 minute, repeating the procedure two more times. You may also soak the foot in alternate pans of hot and cold water. Contrast baths are an inexpensive, helpful remedy that "you can't OD on," Dr. Van Pelt says.

Slip yourself some skin. Moleskin, that is, and place it over the corn or bunion to protect the area. You'll find it at most pharmacies and grocery stores.

See also:

• Chapter 26, on medications.

▶ PREVENTION PAIN-RELIEF PROGRAM

If you don't want to suffer from corns and bunions, you'll need to pay careful attention to your shoes: Try the Goldilocks approach.

The fairy-tale girl picked her bed, bowl, and chair not by looks, color, or fashion: She always chose items that were a perfect fit. And when you slip on a pair of shoes, they shouldn't feel too big or too little, too soft in the sole, or too high. They should feel j-u-s-t r-i-g-h-t.

If you have corns, make sure your shoes are long enough and the toe area is roomy enough, Dr. Van Pelt advises. Buying roomier shoes may prevent new corns from forming.

For bunions, try to get a shoe that's shaped more like

the foot, Dr. Van Pelt recommends. Ask your podiatrist about orthopedic or molded shoes, a sometimes costly but helpful option. "Shoe manufacturers don't make shoes shaped for a foot with a bunion on it," he explains.

For bunion prevention, check an old pair of shoes before buying new ones. If you have a genetic predisposition to bunions, your ankles and feet tend to roll in, Dr. Van Pelt says. You can spot this rolling inward by looking at an old pair of shoes.

Shoes should wear evenly across the ball of the foot and on the outer back of the heel. If your foot is out of balance, a sign of rolling in of the ankles, you'll see an excessive, uneven wear pattern in both shoes, Dr. Van Pelt says.

"What you look for is a change in that wear pattern and also in a symmetry from one foot to the other," he says. "If your feet are in balance, your shoes are going to wear out the same. If they're different, you'll know it isn't right."

Or place a pair of your well-worn shoes on a counter and look at the heels. The seam running down the back of the shoe should be perpendicular to the ground. "If people pronate, or roll inward excessively, the seam or the imaginary line will lean toward the inside. The shoes will actually break to the inside," Dr. Van Pelt says. If you have these foot problems, be especially careful when selecting your shoes and consider seeing a podiatrist for advice. (To learn more about selecting well-made shoes, see "Be Sure You're Well Heeled" on page 316.)

Rock and Roll

Bunions and corns can prevent you from waltzing or jitter-bugging. But that doesn't let you off the hook when it comes to exercise. Exercise is fine, especially foot exercise, Dr. Van Pelt says.

If you've inherited a weak foot susceptible to bunions, the rolling in or collapsing of your foot overworks your foot muscles, Dr. Van Pelt explains.

"If you do a regular exercise program strengthening the muscles in your feet, then you will feel the fatigue less," he says. "You'll prepare your muscles to accept this extra work. That's how the exercises help. They won't stave off or prevent the deformity, but they will condition your muscles to do the extra work that's cut out for them."

Here is a particularly helpful exercise from Dr. Van Pelt. Standing barefoot, rise up on the toes of both feet, then roll to the outside borders of your feet, then simultaneously roll back on your heels. When you reach your heels, roll to the inside borders, then back up on your toes.

"You're doing a big circle," he explains. "This will efficiently and effectively exercise every muscle in your legs and feet."

Get Prescription-Perfect Support

You need to see a doctor to get the perfect foot supports (orthotics) for your feet. If you have a tendency for bunions and you notice a bump forming, orthotics may slow down the process, Dr. Van Pelt says. Even children are candidates for orthotics.

"I'm talking about toddlers just beginning to walk. If a child demonstrates a flexible flat foot, or if their ankles tend to roll inward, it's very important to wear good supportive shoes or orthotic devices to keep the foot from rolling inward," Dr. Van Pelt says.

You can purchase shoe inserts at drugstores or shoe stores. And while it's easier and cheaper to call on Dr. Scholl's over the counter than to make an appointment with a podiatrist, consider the chance you may be taking.

"You can buy a good pair of glasses down at the drugstore. And sometimes, if you're real lucky, you can hold them up to your eyes and find a pair that works," Dr. Van Pelt explains. "That's exactly the same with orthotics. Those that you buy off the shelf or at shoe stores are going to be a close fit, but they're not going to contain a prescription that carefully balances the foot. If a person has a family history of developing bunions or corns or tired feet, it's a good investment to get their feet examined and get a device that's made to their prescription, because this is a lifelong thing."

Once you pop those pads into your shoes, you'll feel the difference. You'll walk and stand with less fatigue, more like nature intended, Dr. Van Pelt explains.

Zapping Corns

You may be wondering about the effectiveness of over-the-counter corn removers. Dr. Van Pelt advises against these solutions, which are dabbed onto corns to dissolve them. The acid eats off the corn but can damage underlying tissues, he says. Plus, the corn will grow back if you rely only on the acid. Because your skin is doing its job by reacting to pressure placed upon it, the corn will reappear if the thing that caused it in the first place is still present. Scraping off a corn with a razor blade or pumice stone results in the same corn regrowth, Dr. Van Pelt notes.

If other methods have failed, corns and bunions may be surgically removed, Dr. Van Pelt says. If you have surgery for corns, ask your podiatrist to advise you about how to prevent their return, he advises.

INGROWN TOENAILS

You can paint them. Soak them. Pick at them. Curse them until the sun comes up and goes down again. But with ingrown toenails, you've got one thing to face. They hurt!

And guess what? They're inherited. Yes, you inherit the tendency for your nails to curl or become "dome shaped," Dr. Van Pelt says. This tendency causes the nail to curl down at the corners, then dig and grow into your skin. Other causes of ingrown toenails are poorly fitting shoes and improper nail trimming, he adds.

Ingrown toenail pain occurs when the toenail's sharp end grows into the flesh of the toe (usually the big toe). The condition is quite painful and there's a chance of infection, Dr. Van Pelt says.

➤ INSTANT RELIEF

You'll probably need to see a podiatrist if you have ingrown toenails, because they are almost impossible to get rid of on your own, says Dr. Van Pelt. Here are some ways to relieve their pressure and pain in the meantime.

Put your toe on the rocks. Application of an ice cube or ice bag to the toe can relieve pain, Dr. Van Pelt says.

Add a dash of salt. Dump Epsom salts into a pail of hot water and give your foot a long soak to ease swelling and relieve pain and pressure, Dr. Van Pelt advises.

Take the pressure off. Roll a piece of cotton to twice the thickness of a candlewick and place it between the skin and the ingrown nail tip. Place iodine on the cotton and wrap your toe with gauze and tape. Add a drop of iodine daily and change the cotton once a week. This technique stops the ingrown nail from piercing the flesh as it grows out from the surrounding skin, says California dermatologist Harold Fishman, M.D. He recommends that if the pain does not lessen after a few days, you see your doctor.

See also:

- Chapter 26, on medications.

➡️ PREVENTION PAIN-RELIEF PROGRAM

Toenail trimming—it's a delicate subject, usually not discussed in public. The only sounds associated with the act are the snip, snip, snip of a pair of toenail clippers. Although you probably don't realize it, you're making medically important moves with every squeeze on the clipper. Here's how to trim to prevent ingrown toenails.

Cut your nails straight across with clippers, Dr. Van Pelt advises. Do not round off corners. Your nail should project just past the end of your toe to protect it from irritation and pressure. Pressure may cause you to pick and risk irritation and infection.

"It's typical for teenagers to get ingrown toenails because they tend to tear and pick at their nails, and they'll leave a little hook. As the nail grows out, that hook presses into the skin and creates a puncture wound," Dr. Van Pelt says.

Older people may be prone to pick at toenails and risk developing ingrown nails because as they age, their toenails grow thicker, increasing pressure on the skin. But if you trim your nails properly and don't pick at them to relieve pressure, you should not have problems with ingrown nails as you age, the doctor explains.

Turn Your Toe Over to a Pro

The time may come when your ingrown toenails hurt too badly for you to manage on your own. "Once your nail grows in, it needs to be professionally managed," Dr. Van Pelt says. "That offending portion of the nail needs to be removed."

A simple in-the-office procedure may be performed, involving removing the side of the nail and the root, Dr. Van Pelt explains. The operation, which he describes as one of the best and most successful foot surgeries, is done in the office under local anesthesia.

MUSCLE CRAMPS

You're stretched out on the beach. All you feel is the sun's heat. All you hear is a nearby volleyball game and the ever-returning waves on the shore. Then it grabs you.

You bolt upright with a start and a throbbing lump in your calf.

You look all around. Where's the beach? And the waves, and the volleyball game, and . . .

The beach was a dream, but the leg cramp is a nightmare. As you lie in your bedroom, darkness all around you, reality is the knot of pain in your lower leg.

Doctors aren't exactly sure why people get leg cramps. They can arrive at night while you're sleeping. They can strike during exercise. They may even be a sign of intermittent claudication. (See page 331.)

If you are exercising on a hot day, you may get cramps for three reasons, says Randy Eichner, M.D., professor of medicine and chief of hematology at the University of Oklahoma in Oklahoma City. "Number one is dehydration. Number two is loss of sodium in the sweat. Possibly number three, though nobody really knows for sure, is low potassium," says Dr. Eichner. Fatigue and injury may play a role, he adds, giving the example of a football player leaving the field with cramps during the fourth quarter of a December game.

Night leg cramps most often are caused by stretching the muscle until it goes into a spasm and cramps, Dr. Eichner says.

▶ INSTANT RELIEF

No matter what the cause, one thing's for sure: You'll want relief *fast*.

Send the cramp the opposite way. You can relieve cramps by straightening your leg. Or try pulling your toes and the front of your foot toward your knee. Hold this position, which contracts the muscles opposite the cramped muscles. "You can stand up and hop around on it, too," Dr. Eichner says.

Knead that muscle. Massaging or rubbing the knotted muscle with one or both hands can relieve pain, says Steven Subotnick, D.P.M., a podiatrist and past clinical professor of biomechanics and surgery at the California College of Podiatric Medicine in San Francisco.

"Stop what you're doing and knead it like dough," Dr. Subotnick says. If you cramp while swimming, don't panic. "Just float and knead it," he says.

Try to knead up the calf muscle from the heel to the knee. In addition, try pressing your thumb or a loosely clenched fist on the particularly painful spot, says registered massage therapist Ralph Stephens of Iowa City, Iowa. If that doesn't work, release the pressure on the painful spot, then press again while moving your foot in circles, Stephens adds.

Pinch your upper lip. This technique involves placing the thumb and index finger of one hand just above the corners of your mouth. Squeeze the skin above the upper lip together tightly, using the sides of your thumb and finger, advises Chris McGrew, M.D., assistant professor in the Division of Sports Medicine at the University of New Mexico Medical School in Albuquerque. Dr. McGrew says the technique works for some people—he even used it himself when his legs cramped at night after running a marathon. Doctors aren't exactly sure why, but the technique is often successful. "It's worth a try," says Dr. McGrew. "It's certainly harmless."

See also:

- Chapter 21, on hot and cold therapy.

➡ **PREVENTION PAIN-RELIEF PROGRAM**

When you get a leg cramp during the night, you wake feeling panic and pain. It's a rotten feeling, and you never want to experience it again. Take heart. There are a few things you can do *in bed* to prevent cramping.

Try placing a firm pillow against the soles of your feet

before you go to sleep. The pillow can prevent your feet from extending into the pointed-toe position, which often brings on cramps.

If you like sleeping on your stomach, let your feet hang over the end of the bed, Dr. Eichner suggests. This prevents cramps because your foot won't be pressed against the mattress. If you like sleeping on your back, use lightweight blankets, he says, because the weight of heavy covers can pull your toes and foot down, bringing on cramps. Or sleep on your side, he suggests.

Before you hit the sack each night, make sure you've exercised *sensibly* during the day. Don't overdo and fatigue your muscles. Runners may want to add a longer training run once a week, without pushing too hard. This long run can teach nerves and muscles to tolerate fatigue better, reports exercise physiologist Marc Rogers, Ph.D., assistant professor at the University of Maryland. For walkers, an extralong walk is not necessary, Dr. Rogers says. "If you start walking gradually and don't increase too much, your muscles will adapt to new stress and lessen your chance of cramping," he says. Ask your doctor about sensible training levels for you.

Stretch Yourself

Regular stretching and massage may be one of your best allies in the fight against muscle cramps, most doctors and therapists agree. You may want to warm up muscles by walking or jogging easily before you stretch so you won't feel so stiff. One study involving 44 individuals showed that all were cured of night leg cramps after one week by performing brief calf stretches three times per day.

"If you can get people to stretch, it will keep their muscles looser," Dr. Eichner says.

What kind of exercises are best? Lunges and wall stretches can keep your calves from tightening and increase flexibility, according to Dennis Humphrey, Ed.D., professor in the Biomedical Sciences Department at Southwest Missouri State University in Springfield.

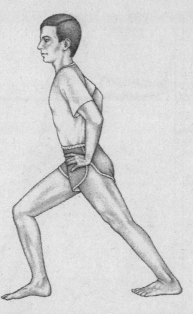

To stretch your calf muscle, step forward on one leg. Bend your knee, but don't bring your knee past your toes. Keep your rear leg straight. You should feel a comfortable stretch in that rear leg. Repeat on the other side.

Keep an Eye on What Goes Inside

Perhaps cramps are caused by something you did not do—like drink enough water or eat right—rather than by something you did—like play too much tennis. Doctors agree that the amount of water in your body during warm weather exercise is a factor. When you sweat you lose fluids and the minerals (electrolytes) they contain. These minerals are essential for proper muscle function.

"When there's less fluids in the muscle tissue and [the muscles] rub together [during exercise], they fire and it causes a spasm," explains Ken Murray, Texas Tech Univer-

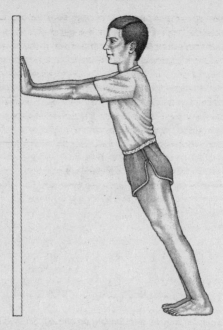

The second calf stretch involves standing a few feet from a wall. Place your hands flat against the wall and lean forward, keeping your heels on the ground and your legs straight. You should feel a lovely stretch through both calves. Hold the position for a few seconds.

sity assistant athletic director for sports health and a former Atlanta Falcons trainer.

So keeping fluid intake up is a must. Most experts recommend you drink water or a diluted sports drink. You need about 8 cups of water per day, says Evelyn Tribole, a California-based registered dietitian. Athletes should remember to drink an additional 2 cups of water to replace each pound of body weight lost through sweating, she adds. Drink small, frequent sips of water during competition (½ to 1 cup every 10 to 15 minutes), when you'd rather not have a gallon of water sloshing around in your gut.

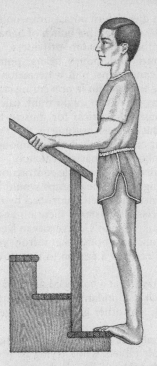

You can also use a stair to stretch your calf muscles. Stand with the balls of your feet on the edge of the stair. Lower your heels and hold. Now raise up on your toes and hold. For safety's sake, make sure you're holding onto the railing to keep your balance.

Minerals, Maybe

The role of potassium in the cramp equation is under debate, Dr. Eichner says. Potassium is very concentrated in muscles and serves a vital function. It zips across the membrane when muscles contract, the doctor explains. "The theory is if a person gets a little low on potassium, from taking water pills (diuretics) or because of poor diet, maybe somehow the muscle cramps because it's low on potassium. That's still pretty much a theory," says Dr. Eichner.

Still, eating a diet rich in potassium won't hurt. So next time you're at the store, grab a bunch of bananas, but don't miss nature's other potassium providers. These include dates; lima, pinto, and kidney beans; potatoes; prunes; winter squash; cantaloupe; and watermelon.

Is there a role for calcium in preventing cramping? Some say yes, some say no. "You might think calcium would be important because it's critical for muscle function," Dr. Eichner says. "But I've seen nothing on that in the literature, and when I hear cramps talked about among sports medicine doctors, nobody emphasizes calcium."

"Calcium is involved in muscle contraction. But calcium deficiency leading to muscle cramps would have to be severe, because calcium is well controlled by the body," explains Cindy Heiss, a registered dietitian and instructor in nutrition at Texas Woman's University in Denton. If you're lacking in calcium, your body takes it from your bones, she explains, so it's rare for a person to have low blood levels of calcium.

Once again, try to eat a balanced diet and include plenty of calcium, which is abundant in low- or nonfat dairy products, in broccoli and other green, leafy vegetables, and in sardines.

And finally, almost all doctors agree that you should steer clear of salt tablets while trying to prevent cramps. "Don't take salt tablets," Dr. Eichner says. "Most older people generally get more salt than they need in the standard American diet." However, young athletes may add a bit of salt to their food if they are bothered by cramps, especially during the summer, he says.

Rx from an M.D.

There's no sense fuming and kneading your way through nights and nights of leg cramps. See a doctor if you have recurring bouts with cramps.

"I find that an awful lot of people who have leg cramps have mineral deficiencies," says Stephens. "These people should see their doctor and be treated nutritionally."

Adds Murray, who's seen his share of leg cramps working with athletes during Texas summers, "If there's any question, especially with older people, they need to have a blood chemistry run to see what they are lacking."

Doctors may treat cramps with supplements, or they may prescribe quinine, which decreases the excitability of the nerves in the muscles. Quinine may relieve your cramps, but it has some undesirable side effects, including nausea, vomiting, and blurred vision, and it may be harmful for pregnant women.

"Quinine is widely given," Dr. Eichner states, "but I tend not to use it. I've found that the nonmedicinal sorts of therapy tend to work. Apparently it must be fairly innocuous for the large part, because it's so widely used. I'm just not big on it personally."

ANKLE SPRAINS

Ouch! Ouch! Ouch!

These were the first words out of your mouth that day last year when, while taking your regular afternoon walk, you put your foot down on pain.

Ouch! *%#&!@#$!!

Looking back on it, you couldn't figure out how it happened. Surely you didn't just trip over your own two feet, not with enough force to damage the ligaments in your ankle.

The sidewalk reached up and grabbed you.

That's the story you told yourself, but it wouldn't wash with your husband and kids. So you resigned yourself to the fact that you sprained your ankle while walking, performing the act we applaud when it's mastered by toddlers.

But what is a sprain anyway? Like remembering the difference between a stalactite and a stalagmite, between a thunderstorm watch and a warning, differentiating between sprains and strains can be confusing.

In reality, the difference is simple. A sprain involves damage to ligaments, while a strain indicates tendon injury, says Dr. Subotnick.

"A sprain usually happens because you twist your foot and it goes further than it was meant to go. The ligaments usually stop you from going too far. And if you go too far, you tear the ligaments," he explains. "It's usually painful immediately."

And how will you know you've actually injured the ligaments in your ankle?

"You know you've sprained it when you've hurt the joint and you have swelling immediately. You may get a big knot, and it will be very tender," says Murray, adding that ankle sprains are the most common sports injury he sees, far more prevalent than sensational knee injuries.

➤ INSTANT RELIEF

Here are a few things you can do for relief.

RICE to the occasion. That is, try rest, ice, compression, and elevation. *Rest* the injured area. *Ice* it for no longer than 30 minutes to control swelling. *Compress* the area by wrapping it with an elastic bandage, such as an Ace bandage, being careful not to wrap too tightly. *Elevate* the area, raising the injured ankle above the level of your heart to drain fluids with gravity's help.

Almost all doctors and health professionals agree that this procedure is important to follow as quickly as possible after the injury. Murray says that elevation is a very important part of the quartet because it decreases swelling, which hastens healing.

How long do you use RICE?

"The 'book' says about 48 hours," Murray explains, but adds that he's found an easier way to know than watching a clock. "If you put the back of your hand on one ankle, then the back of your hand on the injured ankle, if the injured ankle feels warmer, then you've still got bleeding and swelling." Thus, you should continue the routine until the ankle no longer is hot, he says. "It may be swollen, but when it's not warm, you can go ahead and start doing some other things." Be sure to resume your normal activities slowly, testing the injured ankle gradually after a day or more has passed.

Some tablets of relief. You can take aspirin, although Murray says acetaminophen (Tylenol) may be a better choice, since aspirin thins the blood and could increase bleeding. (See chapter 26.)

➤ PREVENTION PAIN-RELIEF PROGRAM

You've gotten over the initial shock of the ankle sprain and perhaps the embarrassment of how it happened. You've used RICE so long you've forgotten other purposes for frozen water and the sofa. Now it's time to move on to using heat. Actually, you're not off the ice block yet. But doctors advise that once swelling has subsided and your ankles are the same temperature, you may gradually mix heat and cold.

Here's how: Apply heat for 5 minutes, then switch to cold for 5 minutes, then go back to heat for 5, then go to cold for 5, and again, for a 30-minute total, Murray says. Try to do this at least two times a day.

"When you use hot and cold, you cause a pumping. You bring in fresh blood and with the ice, you cause vasoconstriction, causing you to push out blood," Murray explains. Epsom salt soaks are another warm option you may try once swelling has gone down, Murray says.

Hop to a Doc

In fact, if after 24 hours you still have to hop, you need to see your doctor. The joint should be able to take weight after about 24 hours of RICE.

"If you've sprained your ankle and it's not starting to heal up in a couple of days, you need to get an x-ray and get it checked out," Dr. Subotnick advises. Murray adds, "If you're having trouble bearing weight, you've got to be concerned about a fracture."

Your options for treatment at the doctor's office range from an Ace bandage to a splint or cast or surgery in some severe cases. Your doctor may refer you to a physical therapist for rehabilitation and follow-up care. Physical therapy treatments may include ultrasound, electrical stimulation, whirlpool baths, and application of moist heat packs or ice, says physical therapist Bill Grist of Lubbock, Texas.

"Once we've gotten the primary problems under control and the person can walk without assistance, we'll go on into dynamic exercise programs for improving the strength of the muscles surrounding the ankle," Grist explains. (See chapter 29 for more on physical therapy.)

You also may consult a massage therapist at your doctor's recommendation. This therapist will work on muscles of the calf and thigh to return circulation to the area and may work gently on the ankle after swelling has subsided, Stephens says. (See chapter 24.)

Build and Balance with Exercise

Think about putting on a swimsuit and taking a plunge to rehabilitate your ankle. That thought may sound as comforting as one more hour of ice bags, but consider the positive effects a pool may have on your rehab.

Specifically, Stephens says you should seek a flat-bottomed pool with cool water. Begin by walking on the bottom of the pool. Then bounce up and down lightly. Gradually work up to jogging in the pool, then see if you can build up to running in the water.

"The water makes you more buoyant, so there's less weight on the ankle. You have to go easy at first, but it's a real good way to build up a sprained ankle," Stephens says. Be sure to wait at least 72 hours after your initial injury to hit the pool, he adds.

"It's really important to the integrity of the joint to build those muscles back up again," Stephens says. "It's important for athletes to start training a little easier. Start at a reduced level of activity and gradually build up to where you were." If a person is not an athlete, it's important that they do a series of exercises to build that ankle up, he says.

One ankle-building exercise for dry land that Stephens recommends is walking on all four edges of the foot in different stages: Walk on your heels, then up on your toes, then on the outside of your feet, then on the inside, he explains. You also can walk with or lift marbles or golf balls under your toes for 20 minutes once or twice a day.

Perhaps the best way to prevent ankle sprains is to work on improving your balance. Then turning your ankle in the grocery store parking lot or in the aisle at church won't be as likely to happen. "If you are in a situation where you might sprain your ankle, you can correct that before you do it," Dr. Subotnick explains. But you need good reflexes.

Dr. Subotnick suggests the following exercises for bettering balance: Stand up and close your eyes. Now stand on one foot and practice balancing on it. Then try the other foot. This improves your sense of balance. You might also try jumping back and forth, side to side, and forward and backward, and running figure eights if you feel energetic, all to improve your agility and balance.

Stretching before exercise may also prevent ankle sprains, Murray says.

BE SURE YOU'RE WELL HEELED

You've been there before. You're standing in a shoe store trying to find a pair of heels to match your new dress. The party is tomorrow night, and you just can't wear those ugly old things you bought on sale years ago.

A pair in navy blue catches your eye. Their thin back strap looks luscious on the rack. You pick them up and they're nice and light. You find a chair and slip them on.

Then you stand. Then you step. Then you hurt.

Wearing shoes, a custom that's meant *civilization* for years in most of the United States, can be functional, pleasurable . . . or pure agony. Lace up a pair of tennis shoes with air or gel soles. You'll feel as if you're ready to run with angels. Then try on those high heels. You'll feel like you've been dancing in cement sneakers.

Many shoes look solid in the store. It's only after a month or so of wear that you find their looks were deceiving. While poorly fitting or shoddily constructed shoes usually won't give you foot problems, they can make underlying structural foot problems worse, says William Van Pelt, D.P.M., a Houston podiatrist.

Here are some guidelines offered by the American Podiatric Medical Association for choosing proper shoes.

- Take your time and try on several different styles and sizes. Sizes can vary with different manufacturers.
- Have your feet measured, while standing, each time you try on shoes.
- Shop for shoes in the afternoon. Your feet swell during the day.
- Try on both shoes. If one foot is larger, choose the shoes that fit the bigger foot.

- Allow a thumb's width between the end of your big toe and the tip of the shoe.
- Be sure that the ball of your foot fits well into the widest part of the shoe. The heel should fit snugly.
- Look for a shoe with a firm sole and a soft upper.
- Shoe soles should be flexible and move when your foot moves. Look for thicker soles to soften the pressure placed on your foot if you walk on hard surfaces.
- Avoid extreme, often uncomfortable styles.
- Choose shoes made of leather or any fabric that allows your feet to breathe and that lets the shoe conform to the shape of your foot.
- Select shoes that will match your activity, not your outfit. Try not to wear high-heeled shoes on a daily basis.
- When buying athletic shoes, be sure to wear appropriate socks to guarantee a good fit. And consider your sport and its unique foot requirements before making a selection.

Look for the seal of acceptance of the American Podiatric Medical Association on shoe boxes if you're prone to foot problems or if you want to make sure shoes are solidly and safely constructed, Dr. Van Pelt says.

Shoe Sense

Pick up your tennis shoes and look at the soles. Are your shoes as smooth as Don Rickles' dome? Now look inside. Is there any noticeable means of support? Are you walking or jogging on shoes that should be 6 feet under in the backyard?

"Footwear is very important," Murray says. "If you wear shoes that don't give you very much support, if they have a thin base and your foot can roll very easily, you may be in for ankle problems."

Look for comfortable, supportive sneakers with cushioning devices to ease the pressures that exercise places on your feet, the American Podiatric Medical Association advises. (See "Be Sure You're Well Heeled" on opposite page.)

SHINSPLINTS

Elizabeth was seven months pregnant when she left her home in Charlotte, North Carolina, and went on a week's trip to New York City to cover fashion shows for her hometown newspaper. She was braced for the Big Apple's crowded sidewalks, intersections of crisscrossing chaos, and, of course, Grand Central Station.

But she wasn't prepared for the pain.

One day after hitting the city, Elizabeth was engrossed not in fashion trends for the fall season but in the throbbing aches in her lower legs. When she walked, her shins hurt. When she sat at press tables, her shins hurt. When she collapsed in bed at night, her shins hurt. Even when she returned home, she hurt for weeks.

Shinsplints—what are these mysterious aches that can camp inside your calf and refuse to budge?

Shinsplints is not a specific condition. It is a general term encompassing several painful lower leg problems, according to William W. Briner, Jr., M.D., who has served on the sports medicine staffs at Ohio State University and UCLA.

While there's no clear answer to the question of what shinsplints is, we certainly know the answer to the question of how shinsplints feels. It hurts, usually on the front, lower portion of the tibia, the large bone of the lower leg. There may be swelling, as body fluids collect under the tears in the membrane and tendon tying the muscles to the front and side of the tibia.

While shinsplints usually announces itself with a dull, constant ache, it can sometimes cause sharp pains in the leg.

Shinsplints can be caused by repeated pounding on hard surfaces or by changing the surfaces on which you do your regular running or walking workout. It also may be caused by the foot turning in or out during exercise, Dr. Subotnick says. Overexertion without proper conditioning, running over uneven terrain, and exercising with inherent foot and arch problems may also cause shinsplints, according to Dr. Briner. It is common among runners, accounting for almost 20 percent of running injuries, according to several studies, and can also occur in walkers, Dr. Subotnick says. Women seem to be bothered with shinsplints more often than men, according to several studies, including one involving mid- shipmen at the U.S. Naval Academy. According to Dr. Briner, authors of the study believe that a woman's wider pelvis and greater joint laxity may be at the root of increased incidents of the lower leg pain.

▶ INSTANT RELIEF

What can women and men do for relief?

Stop! Call a halt to your walking or running and massage the sore area, Dr. Subotnick says.

Keep it short. Shortening your stride can help get rid of shinsplints, Dr. Subotnick adds. Try walking or running with a comfortable, shorter stride.

Try RICE. Give rest, ice, compression, and elevation a shot at relieving shinsplint pain, says Grist. Ice may be especially helpful, Dr. Subotnick says. (For more informa- tion on RICE, see the instant relief discussion in the section on ankle sprain on page 312.)

Give hot water a whirl. Take a warm bath and soak your sore legs, Dr. Subotnick says.

▶ PREVENTION PAIN-RELIEF PROGRAM

Few serious exercisers like this idea, but taking time off from your sport of choice may be the best option if shin- splint pain doesn't abate in a couple of days. "Very often the best treatment is avoidance of the traumatic activity," Grist says.

You may need two weeks to two months off, but don't panic. You'll still be able to fit into the running tights you got for Christmas, because you don't have to stop exercis- ing. Try biking or swimming, sports involving less pound- ing, while you're on the mend.

During this time-off or alternate-exercise period, try applying heat and cold to your legs, says Murray, who sees shinsplints often with Texas Tech's cross-country teams. Which should you use?

"Flip a coin. I've used both. It depends on what an individual feels is doing them good," Murray says. "An old rule of thumb is: Heat before you work out, ice when you finish a workout. Some people like ice the whole way. Some people like heat the whole way." (See chapter 21.)

Once you've rested and are pain-free, you may gradually begin running again. Just don't overdo it. "As a person begins recovering from shinsplints, often they can begin walking at a fairly moderate pace," says Grist. "Not too fast, just moderate, then gradually picking up."

Once you're back on the training road, make sure you work out sensibly, as training errors may cause shinsplints. Make certain you're walking or running with a comfortable stride, Dr. Subotnick says. Make sure your shoes offer support and cushioning. If your feet tend to flatten, says Dr. Subotnick, make sure you wear the right kind of shoes. Tennis shoes made with fairly rigid heel counters, arch supports, and firm midsoles are available to help this problem. You may want to try orthotics in your shoes to minimize pronation. Ask a podiatrist about this type of foot support, Dr. Subotnick recommends.

Surface Strategy

Walking or running on hard surfaces can also be a cause of shinsplints. "If you get off the hard surfaces and go to soft, that usually helps," Dr. Subotnick says. Switching surfaces can cause temporary pain, though, says Murray; so keep that in mind if you have lower leg pain and can't figure out why. Vary your exercise route, Grist advises, so that one leg is not always on the downside of the street. If you always walk the same route, for example, try taking it in reverse from time to time.

Make sure your muscles are warm and stretched before you work out. "We've found out with shinsplints, there

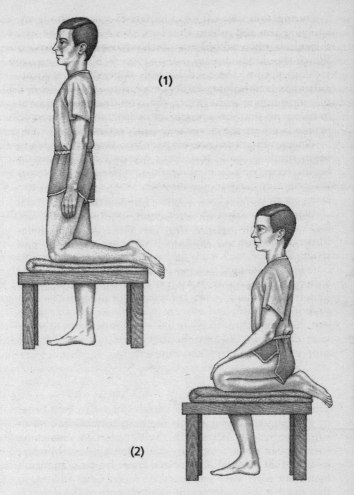

Here's a special stretch to help prevent shinsplints. (1) Stand next to a bench with one leg resting on the bench from knee to foot. You can let your toes dangle off the end of the bench if you like. (2) Now sit back on your foot and just relax. Hold for a count of ten, then repeat on the other side. You'll be more comfortable if you put a folded towel under your leg as padding.

are tightened heel cords. So you really need to work on stretching," Murray says.

If your shinsplints lingers like intestinal gas passed in a phone booth, see a doctor to rule out chances of a stress fracture. How long should you endure the pain? "It depends on how uncomfortable you are," Murray says. "I'd wait a few days, and if there still was pain, I'd see the doctor."

Your doctor will examine your legs and take x-rays, checking for a hairline crack or stress fracture of the tibia.

If shinsplints keeps recurring, you may want to see a podiatrist or sports medicine specialist, who can analyze your gait or running technique and spot any problem-causing flaws, Dr. Subotnick says.

Your doctor may refer you to a physical therapist, who'll probably treat you with ultrasound, whirlpool baths, ice, and massage on the sore area, says Grist. Massage therapists often work on shinsplints with great success, says Stephens.

"Massage is wonderful at getting the muscle reattached by working out the pooled fluids and getting the spasm out of it," Stephens says. "That's very good for it."

VARICOSE VEINS

Garbage pails and threats to national security. Burr haircuts given by real U.S. Marines and tattoos given by amateurs. A Christmas sugar loaf carried at the waistline. And varicose veins.

These are some of the things we love to cover up.

Varicose veins are twisted and enlarged veins close to the surface of the skin. They usually are in your legs, although any vein may become varicose (from the Latin *varus*, "twisted"). Far more women than men have them, and they can indeed be unsightly. Their telltale splashes of red, blue, and purple, or deep, lumpy little ropes stretched beneath the skin, can be awfully hard to hide. And they can hurt.

Varicose veins occur because of malfunctioning valves in the veins, says Robert Ginsburg, M.D., director of the Center for Advanced Cardiovascular Therapies in Palo Alto, California, and clinical assistant professor of medicine at the Stanford University Medical Center. Normally, the valves help push blood back up to the heart. When the valves malfunction and weaken, they are no longer able to close normally and blood pools in the veins. This pooling can happen along the length of the leg, trapping blood in the lower extremities. Then weakened areas of the vein bulge under the pressure of the excess blood and become twisted or varicose, Dr. Ginsburg explains.

"What happens chronically when the valves become incompetent is that you have a lot of swelling in the leg, so the leg feels very tight. It feels like it's dragging, like it can't walk, and it's extremely uncomfortable. You just can't do your normal activities," Dr. Ginsburg says.

Varicose veins usually are inherited, says John Bergan, M.D., a vascular surgeon and clinical professor of surgery at the University of California, San Diego. Some people may have a natural weakness in their vein walls. The normal cycling of estrogen and progesterone, the female hormones, may also be a contributing factor, Dr. Bergan adds. Pregnant women may develop varicose veins for several reasons, according to Luis Navarro, M.D., author of *No More Varicose Veins*. A pregnant woman has more blood in her circulatory system, forcing veins to expand to hold the extra blood.

"Veins are very thin vessels that are meant to withstand relatively low pressures. Anytime you put high pressure into the system, the veins are going to distend and the valves are going to become incompetent," Dr. Ginsburg explains.

Other causes of varicose veins linked to pregnancy include growth of the uterus, which increases pressure on the veins, increased body weight, and hormonal changes. Varicose veins can also result from being overweight or being physically inactive, with poor muscle tone.

▶ INSTANT RELIEF

Let's look at a few things you can do for relief.

Lift those legs. Raise your legs above hip level to ease discomfort. You may want to lie on the floor and prop your feet up on your bed or on your dresser for a little while, until your legs feel better. Raise your legs 12 inches while lying on your back.

Try doing periodic leg lifts if you stand for long periods at work, Dr. Ginsburg says. "Every hour or so, just lift your heels up and stimulate flow through your calf," he says. This will develop muscle tone and help reverse blood flow.

Take it off. Removing constricting clothing, such as a girdle, knee-high socks, or tight pants, can make you feel better, Dr. Ginsburg says.

Wrap on heat. Place a heating pad on sore varicose veins, the doctor adds. The warmth will make them feel better.

Take aspirin. If you can tolerate aspirin, take a few to relieve pain and help circulation, Dr. Ginsburg suggests.

▶ PREVENTION PAIN-RELIEF PROGRAM

Doctors disagree on whether you can do much to prevent varicose veins if they are part of your genetic makeup.

However, some doctors believe there are little things you can do—like not crossing your legs—that will help your circulation and make your legs feel better.

Keep It Free, Easy, and Supportive

When choosing clothing, try to avoid buying anything constricting like tight pants and undergarments, Dr. Ginsburg advises.

But do pick up a pair of support hose. (This advice applies to men as well as women.) While support hose will not prevent varicose veins, Dr. Bergan says, they can relieve pressure and pain. These hose range from support stockings and panty hose through heavy, surgical-weight elastic stockings to prescription stockings, Dr. Bergan explains. Begin with support stockings if you have pain, swelling, and achiness, he advises.

Along with wearing support hose, get into a routine of doing leg lifts every day. Try combining the power of gravity and support hose in this exercise: Pull on your support hose, then lie on your back. Now raise your legs straight up in the air, resting them against a wall. Hold this position for 2 minutes. Repeat this as often as possible throughout the day. The exercise allows blood to flow out of the leg veins back toward the heart.

Along the same line, avoid sitting in the same position for long periods. If you're traveling by car all day, stop frequently and walk around, Dr. Ginsburg says. Stretch your legs while filling up your gas tank.

"You should avoid anything that compresses blood flow. It's kind of intuitively obvious. It's sort of like a hose," Dr. Ginsburg explains. "You put any bend or kink in a hose, and nothing's going to come out. It's the same thing with a vein."

And while you're being careful not to sit too much, make sure you don't stand in one position all of the time, either. Why? You want to increase blood flow in the proper direction, Dr. Ginsburg says, which is toward the heart.

Keep Moving

Don't get the idea that the only way to treat varicose veins involves a lot of lying around with your feet in the air, however.

One of the most important things you can do to make your legs feel better and prevent your varicose veins from getting worse is exercise, says Dr. Ginsburg.

Put simply, walk. Walking improves circulation by helping the veins, and it prevents pooling of blood by strengthening the calf muscle that pumps blood up the leg toward the heart, according to Dr. Navarro.

Besides helping the veins pump blood back up where you want it, walking and other forms of exercise that use the legs improve muscle tone, Dr. Ginsburg says. Good tone is important because strong muscles do a better job of pumping blood from the legs to the heart.

The toned muscles themselves will be stronger and better able to act as a pump, according to Dr. Navarro. He goes on to cite a study showing that 75 percent of people who carry on with life despite varicose veins benefited from exercise that ranged from walking to swimming, from biking to belly dancing.

Quit Smoking

In another vein, don't smoke. A report from the Framingham Heart Study noted a correlation between smoking and the incidence of varicose veins. Researchers concluded that smoking may be a risk factor for those with a genetic tendency toward varicose veins.

"If you took two individuals with the same kind of venous problems and one smoked and one didn't, one would probably have a greater propensity toward developing blood clots than the other because smoking does increase your likelihood of clotting," Dr. Ginsburg says.

There's No Gain in Extra Weight

If you can take off extra pounds, you'll relieve yourself of extra pressure on those varicose veins. If you are overweight, your veins have to work harder. And if you are out of shape and overweight, they have to work still harder, without the extra help that muscle tone provides.

You may benefit from adding fiber to your diet if you are predisposed to varicose veins, according to Dr. Navarro. The reason? Straining to move the bowels can increase pressure on the venous system, even affecting the lower circulatory system. If you eat a balanced diet that's high in fiber, you'll have less chance of being constipated.

What the Doctor Can Do

If you feel you're on your last legs with varicose vein pain, see your doctor. Actually, it wouldn't hurt to have your doctor look at your veins anytime they start bothering you.

If you've been putting off that visit, relax. There's no reason to expect the worst: an old-fashioned vein operation called "stripping" that your mother or grandmother may have gone through years ago. Times have changed.

The first thing your doctor is likely to recommend is compression therapy. All that means is that you may need heavier, prescription stockings made especially for you, Dr. Bergan says.

Next, you may hear about an interesting development called "sclerotherapy." This nonsurgical technique involves injecting a solution—usually saline or sodium tetradecyl sulfate—into the vein. "The injection obliterates the veins," Dr. Bergan explains. He adds that it most often is used for tiny veins, especially those below the knee.

Finally, varicose veins may be removed by surgery, Dr. Bergan says. But it's not wholesale vein stripping. Today, "only the bad veins have to be taken out," Dr. Bergan explains. "In the 1920s and 1930s, the operations known as stripping were not as precise or selective. They were the best available then, but as more knowledge accumulated, the standard operations were abandoned for more precise operations for the individual."

Ask your doctor or a vascular surgeon about these options.

THROMBOPHLEBITIS AND THROMBOSIS

Swelling, heat, heaviness, pain, streaks of redness, a tender lump . . . these words describe what you experienced in your left leg after preparing Thanksgiving dinner for the whole family.

The trouble could be thrombophlebitis (more commonly called phlebitis), or even thrombosis.

When a clot and inflammation occur in a vein, you may have phlebitis, Dr. Ginsburg says. If the clot is not accompanied by swelling, you may have thrombosis, Dr. Bergan says.

In about 5 percent of cases, phlebitis is caused by inflamed varicose veins, according to Dr. Navarro. However, that does not mean that everyone with varicose veins needs to worry about getting phlebitis. "Doctors see patients with varicose veins and thrombophlebitis, but many hundreds of thousands of people never get thrombophlebitis," says Dr. Bergan.

Other causes of phlebitis are not really known, although it often occurs in patients receiving intravenous fluids, Dr. Bergan says.

Thrombosis, on the other hand, is a serious condition involving clots that may move without giving any warning signs, Dr. Bergan says. A clot that decides to move to the lung, for example, may be fatal.

Thrombosis may be a complication of phlebitis or may be caused by injury to a vein or by staying in bed for long periods of time, such as after surgery or an illness.

You should be under a doctor's care for either phlebitis or thrombosis.

➡ INSTANT RELIEF

There are some steps you can take to relieve pain while you're waiting to see a doctor.

Prop up those legs. Elevating your legs may offer relief, Dr. Bergan says. Resting the legs also will make you feel better.

Release the heat. Your legs will feel better if, early on, you use a heating pad, Dr. Bergan explains. Ice bags also may relieve pain.

See also:

• Chapter 26, on medications.

➡ PREVENTION PAIN-RELIEF PROGRAM

For superficial phlebitis, your doctor likely will treat you with heat, rest, ice, and elevation, says Dr. Bergan. "The greater the symptoms, the greater the need for medical care," he adds. So if those veins are really hurting, get in to see a doctor soon. Besides using these four treatments, the doctor may give you anticoagulant drugs to prevent additional clot growth. Surgery, involving removing or tying off veins, may be necessary in some severe cases.

For thrombosis, your doctor may prescribe anticoagulant drugs, Dr. Bergan says. The affected area probably will be immobilized to keep the clot from spreading or moving. To prevent further problems, your doctor also may compress your calf periodically—a technique known as intermittent calf compression—to increase the velocity of blood flow in your lower leg, Dr. Bergan says. Don't try massaging the area yourself. You need a doctor's special care and training in this case.

One more thing: If you have either phlebitis or thrombosis, your doctor will tell you to stop smoking, says Dr. Bergan.

INTERMITTENT CLAUDICATION

It's a fine Monday noon and you're out for a walk. Yow! You get a cramp in your calf, and you've only walked two blocks.

It's a too-perfect Tuesday morning and you're out for a walk. Ouch! You get a cramp in your calf, and you've only walked two blocks.

It's a dandy Wednesday evening and you're out for a walk. Jeepers! You get a cramp in your calf, and you've only walked two blocks.

It's a never-ending Friday afternoon and you're at the doctor's office. When he hears you get cramps in your calf when you've only walked two blocks, he'll examine you, but even before he makes the first test, he can make a pretty good guess at the diagnosis—intermittent claudication.

"Intermittent claudication is calf tightness or pain that shows up at the same distance or walking speed. It feels like a muscle cramp," says Dr. Bergan. "The term *intermittent* comes in because a person can stroll slowly or walk in a house or building and not get the pain. It always comes on with straight-line walking. It won't come on by walking slowly or if the walking is interrupted by standing."

That's why a person who has it may never notice anything while running errands or working around the house. And while the pain usually shows up in the calf, it can also hit the foot, thigh, hip, or buttocks.

Intermittent claudication is a sign that your leg arteries are partially blocked, says Dr. Bergan. When you have this problem and go for a walk, your leg muscles don't get enough blood and become oxygen-deprived. As a result, you get a cramp.

Take note: "Intermittent claudication is a symptom of arterial disease," Dr. Ginsburg says.

"It's hardening of the arteries down in the thigh or leg, but it's often associated with hardening of other key arteries," says Dr. Eichner. Like those affecting your heart.

▶ Instant Relief

There's one measure that will help the discomfort immediately.

Stop and don't go on. Resting for a few moments will make the pain go away, says Dr. Ginsburg.

▶ Prevention Pain-Relief Program

If you experience the characteristic pain of intermittent claudication, you must see your doctor. The doctor will examine you, check for signs of arterial disease, run blood tests, and probably hand you a brief prescription: Stop smoking, start walking, and lose weight.

"Stop smoking and keep walking," Dr. Ginsburg says. "In five words, that's the best thing you can possibly do."

Smoking causes the arterial blockage, says Dr. Bergan. "It is intimately linked with the blockage," he says.

Dr. Ginsburg agrees, adding that 99 percent of the people he sees for intermittent claudication are smokers. When you smoke, you're worsening a blood supply already limited because of intermittent claudication, Dr. Ginsburg says.

Walk Anyway

And now to exercise, the second part of Dr. Ginsburg's prescription. Why walk when walking causes pain? Walking apparently helps open up small blood vessels in the leg muscles that have been dormant. Some doctors believe that these vessels can take over work from clogged ones.

"Walking also teaches the muscles to get along with less oxygen," says Dr. Bergan.

When walking, don't push yourself past pain, Dr. Bergan advises. Just keep at it steadily. "Say a person can walk a block. Well, they should deliberately, every day, walk around the block. They can stop whenever they have to and rest, and then go on," Dr. Bergan explains.

And if the person has pain before going one block?

BUERGER'S DISEASE: RARE BUT WORTH KNOWING ABOUT

Buerger's disease. It's not something caused by too many pit stops at the local fast-food drive-in. It's not a mouth-watering urge that keeps Wendy's dad in new ties.

It's a very painful circulatory disease.

Named after American physician Leo Buerger, who identified its symptoms in 1908, Buerger's disease is a rare disorder causing tenderness and pain in the hands and feet. It occurs because of blockages in the blood vessels that supply these extremities.

Buerger's disease is more common in men than in women and can be linked to years of smoking or chewing tobacco. Thus, avoiding these substances can cure the problem in early stages. Left unchecked, Buerger's disease can lead to amputation.

While all this sounds frightening considering how many people smoke or chew, it's not as scary as it sounds.

"It's rarely ever seen in the U.S. population," says Robert Ginsburg, M.D., director of the Center for Advanced Cardiovascular Therapies in Palo Alto, California. "It's mostly seen in Middle Eastern populations. There's a lot of question as to whether the disease even exists anymore."

"I could be on a very busy vascular service for a year without seeing one new case," says John Bergan, M.D., a vascular surgeon and clinical professor of surgery at the University of California, San Diego. "That would be, say, one in 500. The condition, which is like Buerger described, is fairly common in India, Korea, Japan, and perhaps in Israel. But it is not common in this country or in Western civilization."

Why?

"I think it's some genetic factors," Dr. Ginsburg says. "I'm not even sure, and I think most people aren't even sure the disease exists."

Yet perhaps knowing about this condition and the one or two cases that do exist is one more good reason to avoid cigarettes and chewing tobacco.

"There's no point in tolerating pain. It doesn't matter whether the person stops and waits for the pain to go away or continues. It's probably best to wait, and then go ahead," Dr. Bergan says.

Pain will lessen gradually, and walking distance will improve 90 percent in about six months, he continues. "If they could walk one block, they'll be able to walk nearly two blocks without pain," Dr. Bergan adds. And while that may not seem like much, at least you'll be on the road to recovery.

Improved circulation through walking also is important because it provides infection-fighting white blood cells. These infection fighters are important because claudication can lead to foot infections and other foot problems, especially for diabetics.

"The risk of infection is extraordinarily high because you have poor blood flow to the foot. If you have claudication, make sure that you get your toenails professionally trimmed by a podiatrist, that you avoid trauma to the foot, that you wear well-fitting shoes, that you don't go out in the cold without warm socks, and that you don't let your feet get wet," Dr. Ginsburg cautions.

Forget Fat

You also need to watch your diet. If you weigh less, your vascular system has less of a burden. Switching to a low-fat diet is a wise choice because it will help you lose those extra pounds while preventing further damage to your arteries.

A low-fat diet won't reverse intermittent claudication blockages, but it can lower your cholesterol and make you feel better, says Dr. Ginsburg.

Your doctor or a specialist may be able to remove blockages surgically, using either lasers or a technique known as balloon angioplasty, Dr. Ginsburg says. In this procedure, a catheter (tube) is inserted into the artery and a balloon is inflated at the point of the blockage to open it up. The balloon technique has proven more effective than lasers, Dr. Bergan says, and works in about 85 percent of cases. Unfortunately, the balloon treatment benefits last only about two years, at which point arteries tend to clog again, he adds.

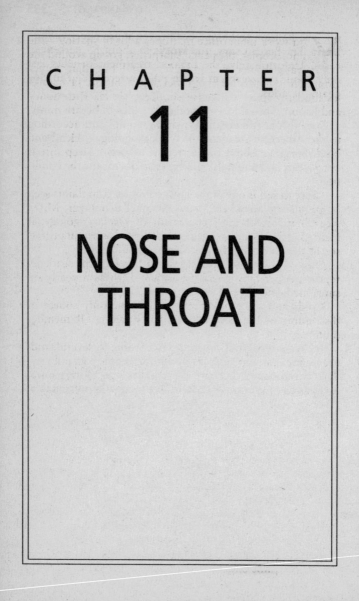

CHAPTER
11

NOSE AND
THROAT

You work in an office that does a lot of sharing—the photocopier, the pencil sharpener, gossip around the water cooler ... and every cold bug that comes along. The whole office starts sneezing in unison. Java junkies suddenly spurn coffee for soothing hot tea with honey and lemon. Throat lozenges take the place of breath mints.

Sore throat is a common medical complaint, according to the American Academy of Otolaryngology—Head and Neck Surgery. About one in ten of us gets a strep throat every year, and about 40 million see a doctor for the condition.

"Sore throat is one of the most common complaints seen by physicians anywhere," says Michael Benninger, M.D., vice chairman of the Department of Otolaryngology at Henry Ford Hospital in Detroit and clinical assistant professor at the University of Michigan in Ann Arbor.

Sinus problems are also widespread. In fact, the academy reports, Americans spend more than $1 billion yearly on sinus medicines.

Colds and sinus infections are not the only source of discomfort in the nose and throat, however. Remember mumps?

It isn't just for kids anymore. According to several studies, mumps cases are increasing among people past puberty. This is important, because the condition is more painful and has complications in adults. Yet mumps is preventable.

PAIN-FINDER CHART FOR THE NOSE AND THROAT

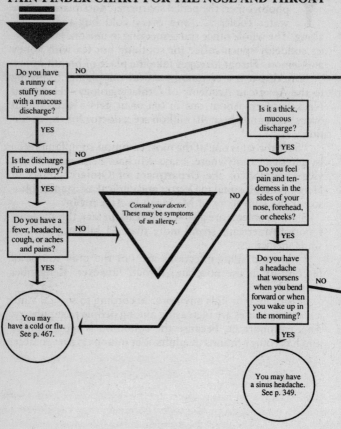

Do you have a runny or stuffy nose with a mucous discharge?

NO

YES

Is the discharge thin and watery?

NO

YES

Do you have a fever, headache, cough, or aches and pains?

NO

YES

Consult your doctor. These may be symptoms of an allergy.

Is it a thick, mucous discharge?

YES

Do you feel pain and tenderness in the sides of your nose, forehead, or cheeks?

NO

YES

Do you have a headache that worsens when you bend forward or when you wake up in the morning?

NO

YES

You may have a cold or flu. See p. 467.

You may have a sinus headache. See p. 349.

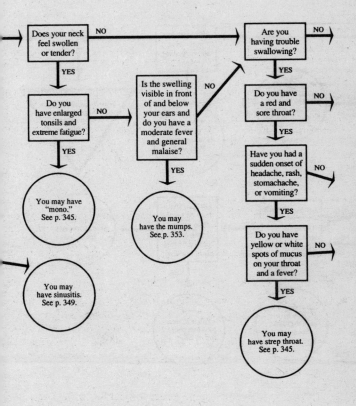

Does your neck feel swollen or tender?

NO → Are you having trouble swallowing? **NO** →

YES ↓

Do you have enlarged tonsils and extreme fatigue? **NO** → Is the swelling visible in front of and below your ears and do you have a moderate fever and general malaise? **NO** → Do you have a red and sore throat? **NO** →

YES ↓

You may have "mono." See p. 345.

YES ↓

You may have the mumps. See p. 353.

YES ↓

Have you had a sudden onset of headache, rash, stomachache, or vomiting? **NO** →

You may have sinusitis. See p. 349.

YES ↓

Do you have yellow or white spots of mucus on your throat and a fever? **NO** →

YES ↓

You may have strep throat. See p. 345.

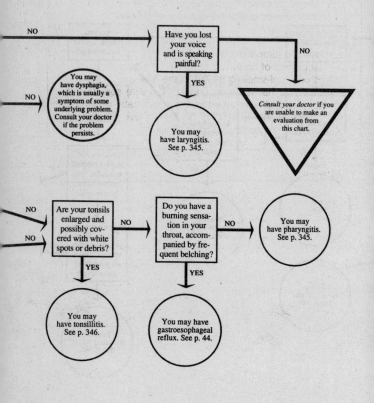

NO →

Have you lost
your voice and is
speaking painful?

NO →

You may
have dysphagia,
which is usually a
symptom of some
underlying problem.
Consult your doctor
if the problem
persists.

NO →

YES ↓

You may
have laryngitis.
See p. 345.

Consult your doctor if you
are unable to make an
evaluation from
this chart.

NO →

Are your tonsils
enlarged and
possibly cov-
ered with white
spots or debris?

NO →

Do you have a
burning sensa-
tion in your
throat, accom-
panied by fre-
quent belching?

NO →

You may
have pharyngitis.
See p. 345.

NO →

YES ↓

YES ↓

You may
have tonsillitis.
See p. 346.

You may have
gastroesophageal
reflux. See p. 44.

GET PROFESSIONAL HELP IF:

- Your sore throat is accompanied by any of the following:
  severe, constant headaches or earache
  stiff neck or persistent swelling in the neck
  fever
  rash
  chest and/or abdominal pain
  shortness of breath
  thick, foul-smelling mucus in the nose
- Your child has a sudden onset of severe sore throat, drooling, and fever and has difficulty breathing
- You are unable to swallow liquids or have a history of kidney infections or rheumatic fever

SORE THROAT

Finding the cause of a sore throat is as tricky as pointing a finger at the reason behind the national debt. There's no single culprit; rather, a whole group of offenders may have caused the pain.

Both bacteria and viruses can attack various parts of the throat. Their assorted nefarious efforts can produce a surprisingly wide variety of infections. You can treat some sore throats—the garden variety that accompanies the common cold—at home. Others are more serious and require a doctor's attention.

Here are just a few of the conditions that can produce anything from feather-light tickles to raspy rawness.

Pharyngitis—swelling of the pharynx—is particularly painful and can cause problems in swallowing. The pharynx is the whole back part of the throat, from the top of the nose back down to the level of the larynx, or voice box, explains Dr. Benninger.

Strep throat—caused by a strain of streptococcus bacteria—is more common in children than in adults. It is of particular concern because it can lead to rheumatic fever, which can in turn cause heart damage.

"The type of strep bacteria that results in strep throat normally does not colonize the back of the pharynx," Dr. Benninger says. "When the organism does colonize there, it results in infection and pain."

Although more common in children, tonsillitis—swelling of the tonsils—can occur in adults, says Charles P. Kimmelman, M.D., chairman of the Department of Otolaryngology, Head and Neck Surgery, at the New York Eye and Ear Infirmary at the New York Medical College in New York City. It normally feels just like a routine sore throat. In fact, you'll probably have the infection in the throat as well as in the tonsils, doctors say.

Laryngitis—inflammation of the vocal cords—causes scratchy throat, hoarseness, and sometimes pain.

Finally, sore throats may be caused by mononucleosis,

trauma (swallowing something that causes pain), or cancer in some cases, Dr. Kimmelman explains. Your environment may also play a role. Smoking, as well as breathing cigarette smoke or heated, dry air, can cause throat irritation, doctors say.

➡ INSTANT RELIEF

Here are a few things to try when you feel the first tickles of a sore throat.

Think liquid. Drink plenty of fluids. Warm tea with honey is comforting for many people.

Make a gurgling noise. Gargle several times a day with warm saltwater. Use ¼ teaspoon salt in ½ cup warm water. Doctors say this saline solution can help reduce tissue swelling.

Try a saltwater squirt. Here's a twist on salt gargles: Fill a rubber ear syringe (the kind you'd use to clean a baby's ears and nose) with a pint of warm saltwater. Lean over a sink and squirt the warm water against the back of your throat. This irrigates your throat and is better than gargles, says Charles Gross, M.D., professor of otolaryngology, head and neck surgery, at the University of Virginia.

"A lot of pain in the throat is due to muscle spasm," he explains. "So this relaxes the muscle spasm. It also dilates the blood vessels, which brings in additional body-protective mechanisms. Particularly if you're taking antibiotics, it'll increase the concentration of antibiotics in this area."

Get a little lozenge. Nonprescription throat lozenges can cool a sore throat. "These can numb the throat temporarily but don't change the course of the disorder much," says Dr. Kimmelman.

Spice it. Sucking on a whole clove (the kind you use for baked ham) can quiet throat tickles.

Close your mouth. Breathing through your nose sends a stream of warmed, humidified air past your throat. Cooler, drier air from mouth breathing can be irritating.

See also:

• Chapter 26, on medications.

► PREVENTION PAIN-RELIEF PROGRAM

A key part of your game plan against throat pain is similar to that of a student learning algebraic equations: You've got to know when to call for help.

If you have a sore throat with a runny nose, body aches, and mild fever, you probably have the kind of sore throat that routinely accompanies a cold. Keep yourself as comfortable as possible with plenty of fluids, gargles, lozenges, pain relievers, and rest. Your symptoms should resolve themselves in a week or so.

But if you have a sore throat for ten days to two weeks, or if you have a sore throat and no other cold symptoms, see your doctor, Dr. Kimmelman says. You should also see your doctor if your sore throat is accompanied by difficulty breathing, swallowing, or opening your mouth, or if you have joint pains, earache, rash, or a fever over 101°F.

"If you have a sore throat with redness and maybe tenderness along the lymph nodes in the neck, see a doctor," says Karen M. Kaplan, M.D., assistant professor of pediatrics at the Pennsylvania State University College of Medicine in Hershey.

Your doctor may take a throat culture—a procedure that involves wiping a sterile swab over the back of your throat. The resulting lab analysis of the culture reveals the cause of your sore throat. This test helps the doctor decide whether the infection is caused by a virus or bacteria.

Most sore throats are caused by viruses—the common cold variety, for example. Some are caused by bacteria, specifically streptococcus bacteria or "strep." The distinction is important, because bacterial infections get better when you take antibiotics, but viral infections do not.

The only course of treatment for a viral sore throat is "rest, fluids, and Tylenol," Dr. Benninger explains. Try to save your voice and your strength. In a week or so, your body will cure itself of the infection by building antibodies to destroy the virus.

But what about all those supersore throats, the ones with

the scary reputations and the special requirements in terms of treatment?

Oh, No . . . Mono

Infectious mononucleosis strikes fear in the hearts of boy-friends, girlfriends, and parents. Although "mono" is much more common in teenagers, it does strike others, Dr. Kim-melman says. The virus causes a severe sore throat; swollen glands in the neck, armpits, and groin; prolonged fatigue; and enlarged tonsils. It may also involve the liver. With mono, the pain lasts longer than other sore throats, says Dr. Kimmelman. And the older you are when you get mono, it seems, the worse it hurts.

The treatment for mono is the same as for viral pharyngi-tis, laryngitis, or tonsillitis. See your doctor, especially if you're having problems breathing or swallowing, and get plenty of rest. The doctor may give you antibiotics to fight secondary bacterial infections, Dr. Kimmelman says. Mostly, you'll have to ride it out as comfortably as possible. "Given time, it will resolve," he says.

Sore or Strep?

Strep throat is as often misunderstood as the directions for operating a VCR. Some people think that every time they have a sore throat, it's strep.

What's the difference between a sore throat and strep throat?

"That's a common dilemma we all face," says Gregory F. O'Brien, M.D., clinical associate professor of otolaryn-gology at Case Western Reserve University School of Medi-cine in Cleveland. "There really is not a firm clinical distinction between a sore throat and a strep throat. Our only reliable means of telling one from the other is with a throat culture."

However, he offers some general guidelines. A sore throat may be strep if

- Fever is greater than 102°F.
- Lymph nodes are swollen.
- White spots appear on the tonsils.
- These symptoms are not accompanied by cold symptoms.

These guidelines aren't perfect. Some early strep announces itself with only a mild sore throat, Dr. Benninger says. Because it can turn into rheumatic fever, it's important to see your doctor if you even suspect strep throat. Children are especially at risk.

"Penicillin is the treatment of choice for strep," Dr. Benninger says.

Tonsils: Not Man's Best Friend

Speaking of children, tonsillitis is a condition that is far more common among the school-age set. Tonsils are actually lymph nodes at the back of the mouth. When they get infected and swollen, they produce a sore throat that just won't quit.

"It is not very common to see adults with tonsillitis," explains Dr. O'Brien. "By late adolescence or early adulthood, the tonsils begin to shrink, so that by the time we have reached 17 to 21 years old, the vast majority of us have no significant tonsillar tissue." Adults who do get tonsillitis are likely to have severe cases, he adds.

To Yank or Not to Yank

Tonsillectomy (removing the tonsils) seemed a rite of passage 30 years ago, like getting braces on your teeth or wearing your boyfriend's letter sweater.

The thinking behind taking the tonsils out was fairly straightforward. Once children turn three years old, they probably don't need their tonsils anymore, according to the American Academy of Otolaryngology—Head and Neck Surgery. The tonsils' job of sampling bacteria and viruses to help build immunity is over by then.

These days, about 400,000 tonsillectomies and/or adenoidectomies are performed each year in the United States, the academy reports. And while this is still a significant figure—tonsillectomy is the second most common operation performed for children—surgery is no longer standard treatment. Times have changed.

"The latest figures indicate that in the decade of the 1980s, there was a 50 percent reduction in the incidence of tonsillectomies performed across the country," Dr. O'Brien says.

"Thirty years ago people felt that tonsillectomy was a risk-free operation. We know that's not the case," says Dr. Benninger. Bleeding and complications from anesthesia are risks inherent to the procedure. "If you don't have to do it," he says, "you don't risk those complications."

Earlier diagnosis and treatment with antibiotics have made for fewer tonsillectomies, says Dr. O'Brien.

When *is* tonsillectomy called for?

The operation may be called for, says Dr. Benninger, if

- Tonsillitis recurs four to five times in a single year or recurs several times over a number of years.
- The condition causes obstruction of breathing, including sleep apnea (disturbed breathing patterns during sleep).
- The condition hampers eating and drinking.

Tonsillectomies are performed about 90 percent of the time on children, and 10 percent on adults, Dr. Kimmelman says.

"It tends to be more painful for adults: They have a larger wound. And kids tend to heal faster," he says. "While kids are laid up for a day or two, adults usually are out of commission for about a week. They're very uncomfortable."

Pain and recuperation time may be lessened if antibiotics are given after surgery.

It's in the Air

What if bacteria and viruses are not to blame?

If you suffer from chronic sore throats, it's possible that

you are dealing with an environmental irritant. If that's the case, all the antibiotics and rest in the world won't make a bit of difference.

"There are a lot of people who have chronic sore throats that have to do with smoking, dryness of the air, and chronic mouth breathing," Dr. Benninger explains.

Doctors advise that you stop smoking and do your best to avoid others' cigarette smoke, that you use a humidifier to keep the air you breathe humid and moist, and that you breathe through your nose.

"Breathing through the mouth gives you a scratchy throat. At least part of the function of the nose is to humidify, warm, and clean the air we breathe," Dr. Benninger explains.

A humidifier, either a portable model you move from room to room or the type you attach to the furnace, adds moisture to the air at home, Dr. O'Brien says. He advises keeping the humidifier on all winter and setting the thermostat at 68°F or below during the day and at 60°F or lower at night.

"The hotter the air, the less humidity it can hold and therefore the more irritating it is. Conversely, cooler air is more humid and less irritating," Dr. O'Brien explains.

Other causes of chronic sore throat may be allergies, breathing industrial pollutants and chemicals, and overusing or straining the voice by yelling.

You should be under a doctor's care for allergies, but bring the sore throat to his or her attention. If you breathe pollutants or strong fumes at work, mention it to your doctor.

Try to avoid yelling or overusing the voice, Dr. Benninger advises. He often treats high school cheerleaders and ministers for chronic sore throats. See a voice coach, the doctor recommends, if you use your voice heavily. "Even Pavarotti has a voice coach," he jokes. Your doctor or a local university music department may help you find a suitable coach or voice teacher.

SINUSITIS

Unless you've got a doctor's skills and tools, you'll never see your sinuses, the tiny cavities inside your head that allow air to enter and secretions to exit.

"These openings into the sinuses are very small. A few millimeters for the bigger sinuses, and less than a millimeter for the smaller," says Dr. Kimmelman.

Sinuses can become inflamed when you have a cold, the flu, or allergies. They can also act up if you smoke, breathe others' cigarette smoke or other environmental irritants, or if you have a structural deformity of the nose that impairs proper breathing.

You may also notice sinus pain during airplane flights, especially if you already have nasal congestion, Dr. Gross says.

"It doesn't take much swelling to cause a blockage," Dr. Kimmelman explains. Once the openings are blocked, the air in the sinus is absorbed and fluid accumulates because it can't get out.

"The ostium [opening] is extremely sensitive to pain," Dr. Kimmelman says. Once you have inflammation, you'll have pain. You may feel it over the cheeks, eyes, or forehead or on top of the head, depending on which of your body's eight sinus cavities are involved, Dr. Kimmelman says.

"People think every headache is sinus in origin," Dr. Kimmelman says. "Only 10 percent or less are due to sinusitis."

Aside from the pain, you'll notice pressure, some green or yellow drainage from the nose, and perhaps a low-grade fever as other signs of sinusitis, Dr. Kimmelman says.

▶ INSTANT RELIEF

When sinus pain, pressure, and headache strike, here are a few things to keep in mind.

Steam it. "One of the old-fashioned remedies is to put some boiling water in a bowl, put a towel over your head, then breathe in the steam," Dr. Gross says. "This will help very frequently."

Try OTC decongestants. Getting your nose open is step one, Dr. Gross says. He recommends trying an over-the-counter (OTC) decongestant rather than an antihistamine.

"Antihistamines will make the secretions in the sinuses and nose dry up and become thicker. Most people think you want to dry them up, but you don't. You want to liquefy them and get them to flush on out," he says.

Get your nose open. You can also try a decongestant nasal spray, but only for a few days, doctors say. Prolonged use of nasal sprays irritates your nose and sometimes causes a mucous membrane to grow over the sinus openings, Dr. Gross says. "We've even had to operate occasionally to resect away the overgrown mucosa as a result of people misusing nasal sprays," he says.

Try a saline spray. A saline nasal spray is a good alternative to a decongestant spray, says Dr. Gross. You can make your own by mixing 1 tablespoon of salt in a pint of warm water. Commercial saline sprays are also available, he says.

Rub 'em open. Try massage to open blocked sinuses. With one hand over each eye, rub steadily on the bony ridge located right below and above your eyes. Then rub directly below your eyes and just above your teeth. This may chase pain away.

Soothe 'em with heat. Try warm compresses to relieve sinus pain. Although this treatment doesn't work for everyone, it won't hurt to try it, says Dr. Gross.

Water it. Drink plenty of fluids to help dilute secretions and keep mucus flowing.

▶ PREVENTION PAIN-RELIEF PROGRAM

If you've had no luck getting rid of sinus pain on your own, it's time to see a doctor. There are a few other symptoms that should also make you pick up the phone and make an appointment.

"If you've got fever or tenderness when you feel over the sinuses, or if you have any swelling, you should not bother with OTC medications and just see a physician," Dr. Gross advises. You'll probably be given a decongestant medication, he says. You'll probably also receive antibiotics to fight the infection, Dr. Kimmelman adds.

Your doctor may pack the nose with decongestants, a 10- to 20-minute procedure that sometimes breaks the congestion when nothing else will, Dr. Gross explains.

Surgery for Drainage

Your doctor may use an endoscope to diagnose and treat your sinus problem. The endoscope is a fiber-optic instrument that allows the doctor to see the sinus area.

Sinus surgery, usually indicated when a person has many bouts of sinusitis, may be performed with the endoscope, Dr. Kimmelman says. The idea behind the surgery is to make drainage and ventilation easier by making the opening larger.

One of the beauties of the procedure is that sinuses almost always return to normal after the surgery. "Even if it's in a fairly advanced disease state, sinuses can revert back to normal with proper care," says Dr. Gross. "Of the patients who have sinus headaches every now and then, probably one in a hundred will end up requiring sinus surgery."

Causes Surround You

There are ways you can avoid going under the endoscope's tiny spotlight. Start by looking around you.

"Sinusitis is really becoming much more prevalent all of the time because of our environment," Dr. Gross says. "All of the pollutants in the atmosphere have an adverse effect on the sinuses."

Your work environment may expose you to fumes that are irritating to sinuses. "We try to see what a person can do to change their job, perhaps moving to another department if they work in an area where the air is of questionable quality," Dr. Gross says.

Cigarette smoking—yours and others'—can also create sinus pain, Dr. Gross says. People who have mild sinusitis and smoke "will progress, in spite of treatment, to a more severe condition," he maintains.

Some doctors say you should also avoid alcohol because drinking causes blood vessels to swell, resulting in less drainage, more pain, and greater risk of infection. (Other doctors say alcohol doesn't have much effect.)

Wetter is Better

At home, try to keep the atmosphere humidified in a comfortable range. Use a humidifier all the time during winter months, when you breathe drier, heated air. If you don't have a humidifier, you can increase your home's humidity by keeping bathroom doors open during baths and showers, by keeping pots of water on a wood stove or radiator or near a fireplace, and by increasing the number of plants in your home. Keeping home air humid is important because a dry nose may be more vulnerable to infection, reports Lee E. Smith, M.D., assistant clinical professor of otolaryngology—head and neck surgery at West Virginia University.

MUMPS

Frankie has a problem, a problem that looms larger in his six-year-old world than the skateboard left in the driveway or the homework assignment he "forgot" about.

Frankie has mumps. That means Frankie's mom and dad may have a problem, too. They are trying really hard to get Frankie well without catching the disease themselves. If Frankie's parents had the mumps when they were children, or if they were vaccinated, they are immune to the disease. But if they are not immune, they risk catching a highly contagious disease that can have serious consequences in adults.

Frankie's mumps—a viral infection—have given him fever, a headache, and swollen, chipmunklike cheeks. Puffy cheeks, for which mumps are so famous, are caused by swelling in the parotid glands, located just below and in front of the ears, near the angle of the jaw, says Penn State's Dr. Kaplan.

Mumps usually occurs in children between the ages of 5 and 15 and is spread through direct contact with respiratory secretions. Frankie probably picked up the infection at school, when some other kid with the bug sneezed or coughed near him.

➤ INSTANT RELIEF

"Unfortunately, we have no specific medications to speed the recovery from mumps," says Dr. Kaplan.

So doctors and parents treat the symptoms (swelling, pain, and fever) instead.

Give it a rest. Summon all your available strength to fight the bug by taking it easy. You'll feel like resting, too, "because most people who have mumps feel sick," Dr. Kaplan says.

See also:

- Chapter 26, on medications.

➡️ **PREVENTION PAIN-RELIEF PROGRAM**

Frankie's parents have good reason to worry about catching their child's illness.

"As you get older, mumps can be quite significant," says Dr. Kaplan, who coauthored a study of a 1987 mumps outbreak among adults in Chicago. According to the study, out of 119 cases, 21 patients developed 23 complications and 9 were hospitalized. Only 3 persons had documentation of mumps vaccination. Costs associated with the outbreak were more than $120,000.

"The complications, both medical and social or economic, can be quite considerable," she adds.

Here's why Frankie's folks are worried.

If Frankie's dad gets mumps, he risks orchitis—swelling of the testes. The swelling may be very painful but only rarely leads to sterility, says Dr. Kaplan.

Frankie's mom, if she gets mumps, could develop oophoritis—swelling of the ovaries. And if she's pregnant, her pregnancy could have complications.

Both of them would be susceptible to problems like pancreatitis—inflammation of the pancreas—and meningoencephalitis—an infection of the central nervous system.

If adults catch the mumps, they clearly have more to worry about than fever and bulging cheeks.

"Adults can have such significant pain that it's not uncommon for them to require more significant painkillers. Sometimes they get admitted to the hospital for pain medication," says Dr. Kaplan.

A Shot at Prevention

Mumps should subside in a week to ten days, Dr. Kaplan says. But to her, that's too long.

"This is an eminently preventable disease," the doctor says. Mumps vaccine is thought to protect 90 percent of those who receive it, she says.

Anyone born in the prevaccine era is immune if they had mumps or were exposed to it when they were kids.

EPIGLOTTITIS: A CHILD'S EMERGENCY

Your grandson's face is flushed and shockingly warm to the touch. He tells you his throat hurts, and indeed, his voice does sound a little funny. So far, it sounds like a fairly common childhood illness. If there are a few other symptoms, however, you could have a full-blown medical emergency on your hands. A child having any of the following symptoms may have epiglottitis.

- A fever of 102° to 104°F
- Drooling
- Inability to swallow
- A muffled quality to the voice, but not hoarseness

Epiglottitis is inflammation of the cartilage covering the windpipe. Some adults may be predisposed to the condition, also called supraglottitis, if they have Hodgkin's disease, leukemia, or any disease that suppresses the immune system.

Caused by bacterial infection, epiglottitis is much more common in kids between two and five years of age. In children it constitutes an emergency because the throat area is so small that any swelling can make breathing very difficult.

"In hours, they can go from being normal to being on the verge of death. While parents are making arrangements to see the doctor, kids have died," says Charles P. Kimmelman, M.D., a professor and chairman of the Department of Otolaryngology, Head and Neck Surgery, at the New York Medical College in New York City.

If you suspect epiglottitis, seek emergency help immediately.

"Most adults born before 1957 are protected," Dr. Kaplan explains. "Having mumps infection or having the immunization gives you lifelong immunity."

Check your records to see if you were immunized, usually in the form of a combined mumps, measles, rubella (MMR) vaccine. If you weren't immunized or did not have mumps as a child, you may be susceptible. Doctors currently advise a second immunization for children born after 1957. And some colleges and universities are recommending second MMR vaccinations because of measles outbreaks on campus, Dr. Kaplan says.

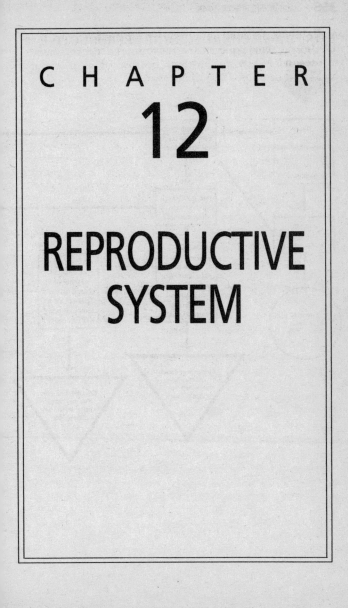

CHAPTER

12

REPRODUCTIVE SYSTEM

PAIN-FINDER CHART FOR THE REPRODUCTIVE SYSTEM—WOMEN

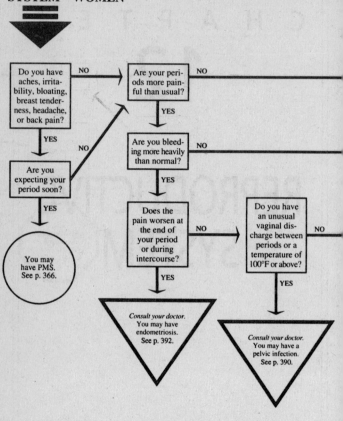

Do you have aches, irritability, bloating, breast tenderness, headache, or back pain?

— NO → Are your periods more painful than usual?

— YES

Are you expecting your period soon?

— NO →

— YES

You may have PMS. See p. 366.

Are your periods more painful than usual? — NO →

— YES

Are you bleeding more heavily than normal? — NO →

— YES

Does the pain worsen at the end of your period or during intercourse? — NO →

— YES

Do you have an unusual vaginal discharge between periods or a temperature of 100°F or above? — NO →

— YES

Consult your doctor. You may have endometriosis. See p. 392.

Consult your doctor. You may have a pelvic infection. See p. 390.

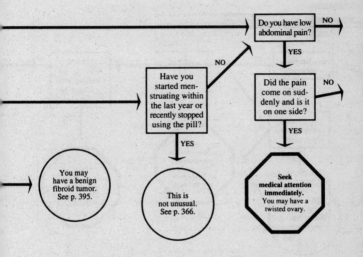

Do you have low abdominal pain? NO →

YES ↓

Have you started menstruating within the last year or recently stopped using the pill? — NO →

YES ↓

Did the pain come on suddenly and is it on one side? NO →

YES ↓

You may have a benign fibroid tumor. See p. 395.

This is not unusual. See p. 366.

Seek medical attention immediately. You may have a twisted ovary.

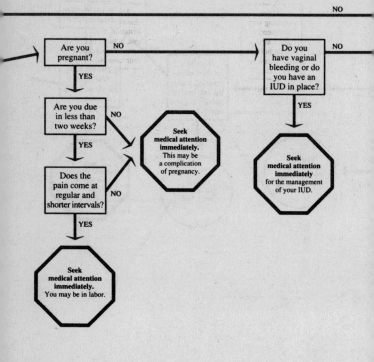

NO

→ Are you
pregnant?

NO → Do you
have vaginal
bleeding or do
you have an
IUD in place?

NO

YES

Are you due
in less than
two weeks?

NO

YES

Does the
pain come at
regular and
shorter intervals?

NO

YES

**Seek
medical attention
immediately.**
This may be
a complication
of pregnancy.

YES

**Seek
medical attention
immediately**
for the management
of your IUD.

**Seek
medical attention
immediately.**
You may be in labor.

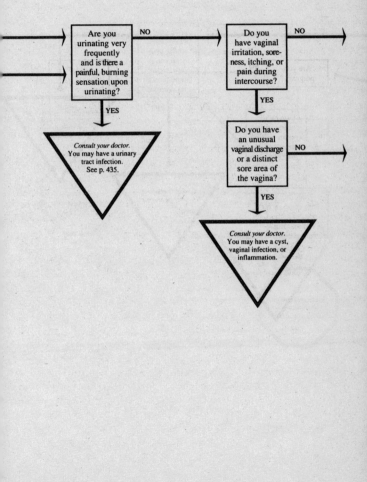

Are you urinating very frequently and is there a painful, burning sensation upon urinating?

NO →

YES ↓

Consult your doctor. You may have a urinary tract infection. See p. 435.

Do you have vaginal irritation, soreness, itching, or pain during intercourse?

NO →

YES ↓

Do you have an unusual vaginal discharge or a distinct sore area of the vagina?

NO →

YES ↓

Consult your doctor. You may have a cyst, vaginal infection, or inflammation.

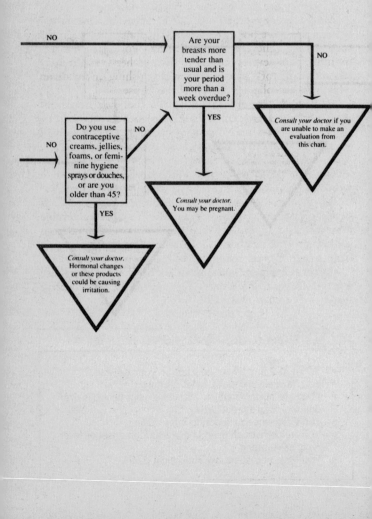

NO ──────────────────────────→ Are your breasts more tender than usual and is your period more than a week overdue?

NO →

Do you use contraceptive creams, jellies, foams, or feminine hygiene sprays or douches, or are you older than 45?

NO ↗

YES ↓

YES ↓

Consult your doctor if you are unable to make an evaluation from this chart.

Consult your doctor. You may be pregnant.

Consult your doctor. Hormonal changes or these products could be causing irritation.

Ask just about any woman of childbearing age and you'll find that below-the-belt tweaks and twinges are as common as rattles in an old car. And while disorders of the reproductive organs may be less common in men, they are certainly no less painful in men.

Almost every woman has had at least mild menstrual cramps. Half are bothered enough by cramps to use some sort of pain reliever. And about one woman in ten has monthly pain severe enough to disrupt her life. She may lose a day of work, say, or end up languishing on the divan when she had planned to reroof the house.

Women also seem be to more prone than men to painful disorders of the reproductive organs—such as endometriosis, fibroid tumors, and ovarian cysts. Both men and women are equally likely to pick up sexually transmitted diseases—such as genital herpes or gonorrhea—but women are more likely than men to go undiagnosed. That's because a woman's symptoms are often less obvious than a man's.

But men don't have *all* the advantages: Because their sexual organs are mostly external, they're more vulnerable than women to injury and trauma. Injury could come from sliding into the catcher's foot rather than home plate, or from a high-impact encounter with a bicycle crossbar.

Fortunately, there's one thing that men and women share when it comes to pain that's centered in the reproductive system—both can find relief.

WOMEN, GET PROFESSIONAL HELP IF:

- You notice any blisterlike sores on your genitals
- You have an unusual vaginal discharge
- You have abdominal pain and either your period is over-due or you are pregnant
- You experience pain during intercourse
- You are menstruating and have a sudden onset of fever, rash, or vomiting
- You have persistent low abdominal pain

PAIN-FINDER CHART FOR THE REPRODUCTIVE SYSTEM—MEN

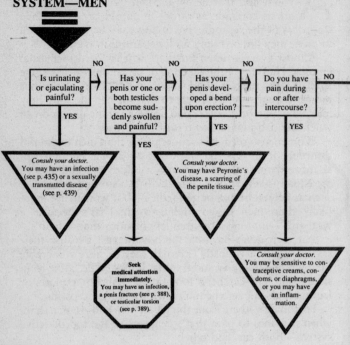

Is urinating or ejaculating painful?

NO →

Has your penis or one or both testicles become suddenly swollen and painful?

NO →

Has your penis developed a bend upon erection?

NO →

Do you have pain during or after intercourse?

NO →

YES ↓

Consult your doctor.
You may have an infection (see p. 435) or a sexually transmitted disease (see p. 439)

YES ↓

Seek medical attention immediately.
You may have an infection, a penis fracture (see p. 388), or testicular torsion (see p. 389).

YES ↓

Consult your doctor.
You may have Peyronie's disease, a scarring of the penile tissue.

YES ↓

Consult your doctor.
You may be sensitive to contraceptive creams, condoms, or diaphragms, or you may have an inflammation.

MEN, GET PROFESSIONAL HELP IF:

- You have sores on your genitals
- You have a discharge from your penis
- You have a swelling of the penis or testicles
- You have pain on ejaculation or urination
- You have low abdominal or penile pain with fever

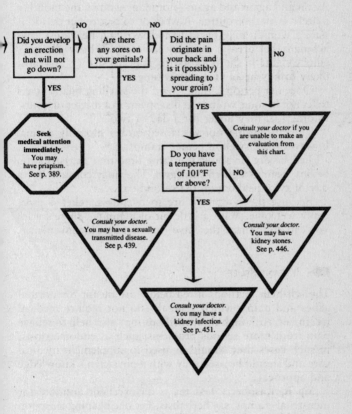

Did you develop an erection that will not go down?

NO

Are there any sores on your genitals?

NO

Did the pain originate in your back and is it (possibly) spreading to your groin?

NO

YES

Seek medical attention immediately. You may have priapism. See p. 389.

YES

YES

Consult your doctor if you are unable to make an evaluation from this chart.

Do you have a temperature of 101°F or above?

NO

YES

Consult your doctor. You may have a sexually transmitted disease. See p. 439.

Consult your doctor. You may have kidney stones. See p. 446.

Consult your doctor. You may have a kidney infection. See p. 451.

PREMENSTRUAL SYMPTOMS AND MENSTRUAL PAIN

Again and again and again—for many women the monthly pattern is all too routine. A week or so before her period is due, a woman may begin to feel swelling, heaviness, and aching in her breasts, legs, lower back, and belly. She may gain weight. If she is prone to migraines, they are most likely to pay her a visit at this time.

Once her period is under way, the swelling finally starts to let up. In some women, it disappears in a matter of hours. In others, it may linger for a day or two.

The curtain has not yet closed on her monthly drama, however. Exit swelling; enter cramps.

Just before or about the same time that menstruation begins, cramps tighten their grip. They may continue for a day or two, peaking on the second day.

Because the symptoms are so relentless, relief is especially welcome. With a little bit of planning, there's a lot you can do to turn "the curse" into a minor inconvenience.

▶ INSTANT RELIEF

The self-help methods listed below are meant for normal aches and pains, which generally do not require medical treatment. Although these methods may also help to relieve pain from more serious problems, such as endometriosis, in such cases they should be used to supplement medical care and should be used only with a physician's knowledge and approval.

Sip it. Raspberry leaf tea is an excellent antidote for menstrual cramps, say herbalists. Try one heaping teaspoon of dried leaves to a cup of boiling water. Steep for 3 to 5 minutes and enjoy.

Head for the door. Take a brisk 10-minute walk, letting your arms and hips swing freely and your breathing naturally ease into a rhythmic pattern.

How can something as simple as going for a walk help relieve something like menstrual cramps or premenstrual symptoms? Several studies show that one immediate effect of a quick stroll is an improvement in mood. Less anxiety and more energy may mean your pain bothers you less, explains Robert Thayer, Ph.D., professor of psychology at California State University, Long Beach, and author of *The Biopsychology of Mood and Arousal*. He suggests you schedule a walk just before or during those times of day you find most stressful. That way, you may derail your pain. Walking can also help reduce swelling by improving circulation in the pelvic organs and tissues, experts say.

Walk as though you're late for an appointment but not at a pace that leaves you dragging, Dr. Thayer suggests. If a fast clip wears you out or increases your pain, slow down to a comfortable speed. And walk for only as long as you can do so without increasing pain, recommends Linda Kames, Psy.D., a Massachusetts psychologist who specializes in the treatment of women with pelvic pain.

Pretend you're a belly dancer. Some people find that creating certain kinds of mental imagery eases pain and sometimes restores a body to normal. A few minutes of quiet time may allow you to come up with your own image, perhaps one of warmth, flowing, and calmness. If you draw a blank, you may want to try an image conjured up by a professional. (See chapter 34.)

For menstrual cramps, try this colorful scene offered by Gerald Epstein, M.D., assistant clinical professor of psychiatry at Mount Sinai Medical Center in New York City and author of *Healing Visualization: Creating Health through Imagery*. "Close your eyes and slowly breathe out and in three times. See, sense, and feel yourself to be a belly dancer, undulating back and forth, moving your pelvis in a rhythmical way. As you do so, see the menstrual blood flowing smoothly from you, and feel the muscles of the abdomen gently massaging the uterus. See yourself with transparent fingers gently massaging your uterus, knowing as you do so that the pain is disappearing."

Replay this mental image for 2 or 3 minutes every half

hour until your cramps stop, Dr. Epstein recommends. The trick is to make the images so real you can smell the Oriental perfume, for example, and feel the silk veils caressing your skin.

Vacation in the Sahara. For premenstrual water retention, try a visualization exercise called "Desert Sand," created by Dr. Epstein. "Close your eyes and breathe out and in three times. See yourself in a desert. In your mind's eye, cover your body with sand and feel the sun bake down on you. Sense the sand soaking up your internal water and the sun drying out the sand. Then open your eyes, knowing that the water is removed from inside you."

Do the sacral rock. You don't have to be a human pretzel to take advantage of yoga's wonderfully relaxing and calming poses, says Mary Pullig Schatz, M.D., doctor, yoga instructor, and author of *Back to Health: A Doctor's Program for Back Care Using Yoga.* She suggests certain simple-to-perform yoga poses as particularly good for menstrual cramps and lower back pain.

The "sacral rock" uses the floor to massage the painful muscles that are cramping and to stimulate acupressure points around your sacrum, the triangular-shaped bone at the base of your spine.

To perform the sacral rock, lie on your back with your knees bent and your feet parallel to each other on the floor, a few inches away from your buttocks. Place a folded pad behind your head and neck. Move your knees slowly to the left and back, then to the right and back. Repeat this at least ten times.

Then lie on your back and draw your knees up toward your chest. Support your legs by holding them behind the knees. Move your knees back and forth and from side to side, massaging your back muscles against the floor. Continue this gentle rocking motion for several minutes. To get up, roll all the way onto your side and push yourself up to a sitting position with your arms and hands. Getting up properly is very important.

Get humble. Yet another helpful yoga position is known as the child's pose. To perform this pain soother, kneel and

Multipurpose Relief

For: Menstrual Pain, Labor Pain, Discomfort During Pregnancy

PRESS YOUR PAIN AWAY

Ever grab a sore hand or arm and just hold it . . . hard? Like massage, acupressure is based on our natural instinct to rub, press, or hold an injured or cramped muscle.

Acupressure involves applying fingertip pressure to certain points to stimulate and heal a painful or injured area.

Pressing the right spots may first cause tingling, heaviness, or a dull ache. (Interestingly enough, the "right spot" to press for an acupressure treatment may be far away from the painful area.) But if you're pressing with an amount of pressure that's stimulating but not bruising, your discomfort may soon fade into the kind of relaxed, slightly tired, good feeling your muscles have after a workout, explains David Nickel, doctor of Oriental medicine and author of *Acupressure for Athletes*. Never continue to do a procedure that causes persistent pain, he cautions.

Try the spots shown in the illustrations.

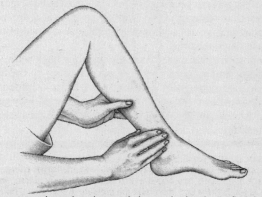

There are two leg points that can help ease back pain. To find the right point above your ankle, place your pinky on the center of the ankle bone's bump on the inside of your leg. If you hold your four fingers together against your leg, the sensitive point is right next to your index finger. There is also a sensitive point on the inside of your leg just below the bulge of the calf muscle. Press both for a full minute. Make sure you do both legs.

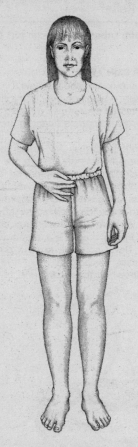

Acupressure can also help relieve PMS and menstrual cramping. Place two fingers two finger-widths below your belly button. Press in as you breathe out, then relax the pressure as you inhale. Do this for one minute or longer.

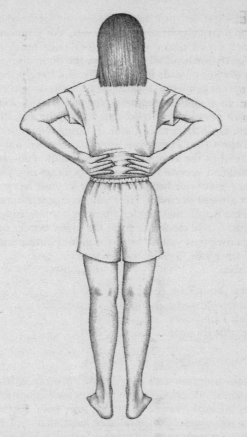

For back pain associated with menstruation, simultaneously press on both sides of your spine, just below the bottommost rib.

rest your chest on your thighs. Place your forehead on the floor, or turn your head to either side. For comfort, you can place a pad under your knees or your head. If you cannot get your head all the way to the floor, use pillows to support your head. Inhale slowly and deeply, holding your awareness in your abdomen and back. As you exhale, imagine your spine elongating. As you do this exercise, your back muscles will relax and your spine actually will lengthen, Dr. Schatz says. (*Note:* If doing this pose on the floor bothers your knees, you can place a folded washcloth in the bend of the knee to cushion the joint. You can also do a modified version from a sitting position in a chair. If necessary, rest your head on a pillow in your lap.)

Buzz around in circles. Here's a massage technique that may help. Apply this gentle, vibrating stroke using your fingertips. Circle clockwise from the lower border of your ribcage down past your navel to the pubic hairline and back up the other side, around and around.

See also:

- "Press Your Pain Away" on page 369.
- "Battery-Powered Analgesia" on page 393.
- "Melt Pain Away" on page 396.
- "Opt for Ibuprofen" on page 399.

➡ PREVENTION PAIN-RELIEF PROGRAM

Begin your program with your doctor's assurance that your pelvic pain is not caused by an undiagnosed condition that requires medical treatment. At that time your doctor may be able to suggest a medical treatment that will banish monthly pain from your life forever. Some women with premenstrual syndrome (PMS) respond to treatment with the hormone progesterone, for example. A woman with cramps may have a mild pelvic infection that should be treated with antibiotics.

A doctor can tell you what drugs, treatments, or surgery might help your condition. If you're also looking for a means of birth control, he or she may suggest oral contraceptives that reduce menstrual cramps.

Multipurpose Relief

For: Menstrual Pain, Labor Pain, Discomfort During Pregnancy

KNEAD IT

It's a natural tendency to want to rub sore, aching body parts. If you find yourself using your thumbs and fingers to dig into the muscles of your lower back, or pressing the palm of your hand on your lower belly, you've discovered one of the best hands-on ways to relieve menstrual cramps and pain during childbirth. For an even more relaxing experience, have your husband or a friend massage you. Or better yet, get a professional massage. (See chapter 24.)

"Women who are having problems with their pregnancy shouldn't get a massage without their doctor's okay," cautions Jocelyn Granger, a registered massage therapist and spokesperson for the American Massage Therapy Association (AMTA). The person doing the massage should use warm oil to reduce friction.

Here are some strokes that Granger recommends.

Stand or kneel at the head of the person receiving the massage. Use the palms of your hands and your thumbs to do long strokes along the back toward you from about the middle of the buttocks to just below the shoulder blades. Keep your thumbs on either side of the spine, about 3 inches apart, and the fingers pointing upward and out. Make big ovals, returning to the buttocks by moving the hands along the sides of the body back up to the buttocks. As you feel the muscles relax, slowly apply more pressure on the back.

Remain in the same position and use the thumbs and heels of your hands to do deep circular friction right in the area of the sacrum, the triangular bone at the bottom of the spine. Use plenty of oil. Slowly increase the pressure until you create warmth in the area.

If you want to get a massage while you're pregnant, you may be able to find a massage therapist with a special table that accommodates your shape. If not, you can straddle a chair backward, resting your arms on the top of the back of the chair, or lie on your side supported with pillows.

A pregnant woman may lightly rub the skin on her own ever-expanding belly with oil. But she should not have deep massage done on her belly or on her legs after her fourth month of pregnancy, Granger says. "That's because there's already a lot of pressure on the veins in the legs and belly, and you don't want to add additional pressure with your hands."

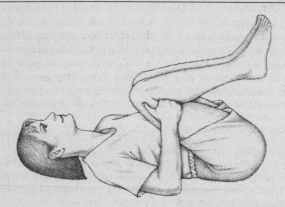

The discomfort of PMS and menstrual cramps often radiates pain into the lower back. For quick relief, try the yoga pose known as the sacral rock (left). Lie on your back. Draw your knees up to your chest and put your hands behind your knees. Then slowly and gently rock back and forth, in effect massaging your back muscles against the floor.

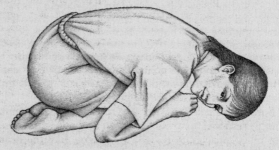

Another yoga pose to ease your lower back is known as the child's pose (right). Kneel and rest your chest on your thighs. Place your forehead to the floor or turn your head to either side. Inhale slowly, and as you exhale, imagine your spine elongating. If this pose bothers your knees, you can do a modified version in a chair. Place a pillow in your lap, bend forward, and relax.

A doctor can also make sure you are taking any over-the-counter (OTC) pain-killer properly. "I commonly find that a woman is not taking enough of an over-the-counter drug, or not taking it often enough to relieve her pain," says Andrea Rapkin, M.D., associate professor of obstetrics and gynecology at the UCLA School of Medicine. A doctor may supervise you while you take larger doses of ibuprofen, or switch you to a prescription medication. Anti-inflammatory OTCs should be taken at the very onset of pain or discomfort and repeated every 6 hours until the period of pain is finished, usually in a day or two, says Dr. Rapkin. Don't save the medication for times of peak pain, she advises.

Some doctors may prescribe mild diuretics to reduce bloating, especially if a woman gains more than 3 to 5 pounds of fluid each month. Diuretics increase urine output, which reduces the amount of fluid in your body. Once you've ruled out more serious medical problems, there are several things you can try to help you find relief.

Turn Down the Pressure

Stress reduction is a part of just about every chronic-pain management program, so it's no surprise to find that it's offered to women with chronic pelvic pain. "We suggest a full 20 minutes of relaxation twice a day, along with deep breathing four or five other times a day," says Dr. Kames.

Several different relaxation and stress-reduction techniques seem to help, including biofeedback (see chapter 17), progressive relaxation (see chapter 22), and guided imagery, or visualization (see chapter 34).

Both menstrual cramps and premenstrual symptoms seem to respond to stress reduction and to techniques that help relax muscles. After all, the uterus, like the heart, is mostly muscle.

Most relaxation techniques require a few sessions of training with a health-care professional, often a psychologist. But you can learn some of these techniques by practicing on your own.

Move Your Muscles

Relaxation by itself is not enough, however. You should probably *move* those muscles as well. Add exercise to your daily program to help banish PMS and menstrual pain and you'll find that you reap fitness and weight-loss benefits as well. Walking's a favorite exercise, along with swimming, biking, and yoga. Most experts say that regular exercise helps in several ways: relaxation, improved mental outlook, more stamina, and a body that is less likely to retain fluid.

Eat Well—It Matters

Be sure to consider diet in your program. Because there are only benefits and no risks in eating better, many doctors recommend that women with PMS symptoms improve their diet.

A typical PMS diet may attempt to eliminate caffeine and to reduce salt, sugar, and fat, especially saturated fat (fat that remains solid at room temperature). A PMS diet might also call for an increase in foods that are rich in magnesium, potassium, and fiber (such as dark leafy greens and whole grains). Some doctors recommend eating six small meals a day to counteract low blood sugar. Some diets emphasize the importance of eating complex carbohydrates the week before menstruation, in an attempt to improve mood. Complex carbohydrates include vegetables and starchy foods such as grains, potatoes, bread, and pasta.

Doctors who prescribe supplements are most likely to recommend B-complex vitamins, especially B_6, B_{12}, and pantothenic acid; vitamin E; magnesium; and calcium. They may also recommend evening primrose oil, which contains an essential fatty acid that some studies suggest may rein in raging hormones. Check with your doctor before taking any dietary supplements.

PREGNANCY

Even when it's a long-anticipated joyous event, being pregnant can be downright uncomfortable. After six or seven months the novelty starts to wear thin, and the aches and pains begin to set in. Those extra pounds you're packing can lead to backaches, swollen feet and hands, leg cramps, varicose veins, heartburn, constipation, and hemorrhoids, not to mention all those mysterious little twinges emanating from your ever-expanding belly as ligaments and muscles stretch and organs like your colon and bladder get the squeeze.

▶ INSTANT RELIEF

Lots of little things can make you more comfortable when you're expecting. Most fall under the heading of experience, the kinds of things that any woman who's had a couple of babies might recommend to her new-to-motherhood friends. Others are the result of scientific research.

Kick off your heels. High heels may exaggerate a swayback and concentrate pressure on the balls of your feet. While you're carrying your baby, you need what your grandmother called "sensible shoes"—those with low, firm, broad-based heels and lots of shock-absorbing sole. Walking or running shoes fit the bill. Shop for shoes late in the day, when your feet are their biggest, and always have your feet measured while you are standing up. And try on both shoes, suggests Glenn Gastwirth, D.P.M., director of scientific affairs for the American Podiatric Medical Association.

Head off potential foot problems at the pass. Pregnancy sets your feet up for trouble in two ways: You gain additional weight, and your body begins production of relaxin—the ligament-stretching hormone that prepares a woman's pelvis for delivery but also stretches the ligaments that support her feet. If your feet begin to hurt, not just feel tired, see a doctor, experts recommend.

Take a breather. Inhale normally. Then, at the end of your exhalation, pause for a second or two before inhaling again. You may notice a spontaneous, unforced continuation of the exhalation during this pause, which completes a true normal exhalation, explains Dr. Schatz, who is a student of yoga master B. K. S. Iyengar.

Deep breathing techniques are believed to help relieve stress and promote calmness. The same techniques you learn during your pregnancy to ease stress can be invaluable as pain relievers during childbirth, Dr. Schatz says.

Use a feather-touch. For swollen legs, it's best not to do heavy-duty massage. Instead, try a very light stroke, suggests Jocelyn Granger, a registered massage therapist from Michigan who is spokesperson for the American Massage Therapy Association.

Elevate one leg at a time. Starting at your toes (if you can still reach them), use 6-inch-long, smooth, feather-tip strokes to cover every square inch of your toes, feet, and ankles. Then do your leg to the knee and from the knee up to your groin, where the lymph glands for your legs are located. Spend 5 minutes on each leg, twice a day. "If you are faithful with it, you will see drastic improvement," Granger says.

When reaching the lower portion of your legs becomes too much of a stretch, recruit your partner—he's probably wishing there were a way he could help you feel better.

Find something to lean on. Sudden, excruciating calf cramps can strike at the worst moments when you're pregnant. And your awkward shape may make it hard for you to grab your toes to stretch the muscle out.

Try leaning into a wall. Step forward on the foot of the leg that's not cramped. Keep the foot of the cramped leg about 3 feet from the wall. Stretch your arms out in front, level with your shoulders. Touch the wall with your fingertips. If you can't keep the heel of your back leg on the floor, try to slowly lower it to the floor. Hold this pose until the cramp eases up. Doing this stretch regularly may also help prevent cramps, experts say. If pain continues in your calf for more than a few hours, contact your doctor: You may have developed a blood clot in your leg.

Sit in a sitz. Hemorrhoids, alas, often make their appearance at some point during pregnancy. To soothe pain and itching, ease yourself down into a shallow tub of warm water. Put some baby shampoo and water into a jar, along with ten drops each of cypress and chamomile—fragrant essential oils—shake it up, and pour the suds into the bath, suggests aromatherapist Judith Jackson, author of *Scentual Touch*. The sitz bath will soothe your hemorrhoids, while the fragrance soothes your soul.

Watch the sun rise. Being able to relax on cue could be a valuable skill to help you through any painful time, including childbirth. That's something Viviane Lind, M.D., a New York City psychiatrist and assistant professor at New York Medical College, found out when she was pregnant. She and several friends practiced a relaxation technique during their pregnancy that made their last few months more bearable if not actually blissful. Moreover, they were able to use the technique to rest between contractions while they were in labor.

"I teach women to relax, and during the course of the relaxation, we see if any image comes up," Dr. Lind explains. If the woman does come up with her own image, she uses that in the future as her cue to relax. If she doesn't, Dr. Lind suggests an eerily symbolic image that one of her patients conjured up: a sunrise.

"Imagine yourself sitting on the shore of a sandy beach on a clear day," Dr. Lind says. "See the sky lighten and become full of color. Watch as the sun first appears as a crimson sliver on the horizon, then slowly begins to fill the sky, filling your face and the world around you with its light."

Dr. Lind believes deep relaxation reduces stress on both mother and baby and helps maintain blood flow to the uterus during labor. Try the image several times and see how it feels. If it seems to help you relax, you can use it for quick relief, she says. You might also find someone who teaches biofeedback and relaxation who can work with you starting as early in your pregnancy as possible, she says.

See also:

- "Press Your Pain Away" on page 369.
- "The Ultimate Bath" on page 385.

➡ PREVENTION PAIN-RELIEF PROGRAM

Experts agree: One of the best ways to have a healthy, comfortable pregnancy is to clean up your act *before* you get pregnant and to work to stay in shape during your pregnancy.

If you need to lose weight, you should do so well before you become pregnant, so you have practice maintaining your new lower weight, says Valerie Hodenius, a certified nurse-midwife with Woman-Care of Cambridge, Massachusetts. Avoid crash diets that take off more than 2 pounds a week, she advises. They can lead to nutritional deficiencies that may worsen if the diet is immediately followed by pregnancy. Of course, all women should be eating nutritiously to ensure their own health as well as that of the baby. In terms of relieving the discomforts associated with pregnancy, diet is not likely to make a significant difference, with the exception of heartburn or constipation.

Putting Out the Flames

Heartburn is a common problem during pregnancy. Not only is your uterus crowding out your stomach, but hormones in your body are relaxing the circle-shaped sphincter muscle at the upper end of your stomach, allowing stomach acid to flow up into your lower esophagus. The escaped acid sears the esophagus and can make it go into spasms. The result: a cramping, burning sensation that feels like it's going to eat a hole through your chest.

Eating frequent, smaller meals and not eating for 2½ hours before bedtime can avert the worst of your heartburn, experts say.

"It's also very important to avoid certain foods," says Francis Kleckner, M.D., an Allentown, Pennsylvania, gastroenterologist. His no-no list includes coffee, tea, chocolate, mints, alcohol, and fatty foods. He also suggests you stop smoking (something every pregnant woman should do anyway!).

Avoid nighttime heartburn attacks by sleeping propped up on pillows or with the head of your bed raised 4 to 6 inches. You can put blocks under the legs of the bed or a wedge under the mattress.

Pregnant women can take moderate amounts of some antacids. Calcium carbonate types, such as Tums, or magnesium and aluminum hydroxide types (Mylanta or Riopan) are safe in small amounts, Dr. Kleckner says. You'll want to avoid bicarbonate of soda (baking soda), which contains too much sodium, and any antacid that also contains aspirin or large amounts of sodium.

Get the Right Moves

When you're pregnant, pain relief gets right down to the basics. Even the way you stand and how much exercise you get become important. And spending some time on these things is essential to your pain-relief program.

Heavy breasts and a protruding belly change your center of gravity. You'll tend to slouch, humping your shoulders forward, or to lean backward, exaggerating the curve in your lower back. Both positions can lead to back pain.

So, say the experts, stand up straight, with your weight evenly distributed on both feet, your buttocks tucked in, your stomach muscles slightly tensed, your head upright, and your shoulders in line with your hips. While maintaining this posture may seem tiring at first, it really does put the least amount of strain on your back muscles. You'll soon feel those muscles begin to unwind. This stance also allows you to breathe more deeply, a calming action that becomes harder to do as your pregnancy progresses.

Correct your posture, both standing and walking, while looking in a mirror. And do a frequent mental check of your posture as you walk or stand. When you sit, choose a firm, straight-backed chair. Overstuffed easy chairs and marshmallow sofas make it too easy to sink into a slouch (and impossible to get up without an extra hand).

CHILDBIRTH: YOUR PAIN-RELIEF OPTIONS

During the 1940s and 1950s, delivering a baby was more or less a "knock 'em out, drag 'em out" procedure. Women were given medications that made them oblivious to the painful process of childbirth. Unfortunately, these drugs also produced a doped-up baby and increased the likelihood of a forceps or cesarean delivery. The powerful drugs also meant Mom might be so blitzed that she would be unable to hold and nurse her newborn until hours later.

The "natural childbirth" movement developed in reaction to this overanesthetized experience. Women began staying home to have their babies, gritting their teeth against the pain and rejecting drugs of any kind. For many women, though, this experience was still far from perfect.

These days, a pregnant woman has more options: She can go to an obstetrician, a family practitioner, or a certified nurse-midwife and have her baby in a hospital, in a birthing center, or at home (this option is available only for low-risk pregnancies).

In terms of pain relief, there is a major difference between having a baby in the hospital and having one in a birthing center.

A certified nurse-midwife tends to take advantage of nondrug pain-relief techniques. A woman having her baby with a certified nurse-midwife will be encouraged to get up and walk around, change positions in bed (she may get on her hands and knees to relieve pressure on her lower back, for instance), take a warm shower or relax in a jacuzzi, moan, have a massage, or be distracted by music, television, or conversation. If she needs additional pain relief, she may get an injection of a fast-acting drug (Demerol or something similar) that will take the edge off her pain for 45 minutes to an hour.

A woman having her baby under the care of a certified nurse-midwife will (in the absence of complications) be able to assume any position she wants for the delivery, including a squat, rather than having to lie on her back. (Most certified nurse-midwives believe a flat-on-your-back position makes it harder for a mother to push the baby out, and studies show it presses on blood vessels and deprives the uterus and fetus of oxygen.)

In a hospital, things are different. At about midpoint in their labor many women receive an epidural block—an injection of a numbing drug near the spine. More of the drug can be injected at any time. An epidural does a great job of pain control, but sometimes at a price.

Depending on the strength of the epidural and the position of the needle, the woman's body can be numbed from her waist down to her feet. Her legs will be heavy and unable to support her weight. She will no longer feel pain, and sometimes she will no longer realize when she is having contractions. She may lose the urge to push. When she's required to push the baby out, she may find it hard to use the right muscles. This may necessitate a forceps delivery or vacuum extraction.

If the epidural is given too early in the labor, or too much of the drug is injected, labor may slow down or stop. The woman may have to wait until the anesthesia wears off or she may be given a drug to promote labor.

If she is in a hospital, a woman is also much more likely to have a fetal monitor strapped around her belly and to have an intravenous line inserted into her arm. That means she is tethered to the bed for the duration, allowed to get up and go to the bathroom only when someone unhooks her. It is hard for her to change position or to get up and walk to relieve pain during a contraction, even if she hasn't yet had an epidural.

"My experience has been that most women don't need a lot of heavy pain relief if they are out of bed and moving around, if they can change positions, be in and out of water," says Ruth Shiers, R.N., a certified nurse-midwife who is co-director of the Midwifery Center in Allentown, Pennsylvania, and a clinical instructor for the nurse-midwifery programs at the University of Pennsylvania, Case Western Reserve University, and Yale University. "These supportive measures make all the difference in the world. If you put that same woman in bed, strapped to a fetal monitor with an I.V. in her arm, she is probably going to need analgesics, if not anesthesia."

If a woman who is having her baby at a birthing center decides she wants an epidural, she can be transferred to a hospital. "But in nine years here, and almost 1,500 births, we've had to do that only three times," Shiers says.

Whether you opt for a hospital delivery or a birthing center, it's important to explore your options early, so you can find a healthcare provider you like and stick with him or her during your pregnancy, says Deborah Perlis, R.N., Ph.D., a certified nurse-midwife and acting director of the University of Colorado School of Nursing's Nurse-Midwifery program. Make sure you have a clear understanding of what kind of pain relief will be available and how any possible emergencies will be handled.

Hit the Pool

While regular exercise should be a part of any pain-relief program, there may be a special advantage to working out in a swimming pool while you're pregnant. Some fluid retention is normal during pregnancy, and it can become irritating and uncomfortable. Doctors usually suggest that a woman lie down with her legs elevated to help reduce swelling, and that soothing position does help.

But when researchers at the University of North Carolina compared the effects of 30 minutes of bed rest with the same amount of time in water, bed rest was all washed up.

"It's related to water *pressure*," explains Vern L. Katz, M.D., the study's main researcher. As any skin diver will tell you, being surrounded by water creates pressure on your body, forcing fluid out of tissues and ultimately into the bladder. The first thing many divers do when they emerge from the depths is hit the head.

According to Dr. Katz, you can use a swimming pool to add a little beneficial pressure to your life. The women he studied sat in an immersion tank with the water up to their shoulders. The water pressure removed more than twice the amount of fluid as did bed rest, and substantially more than sitting in a tub of waist-deep water.

"The equivalent would be exercising in a swimming pool," Dr. Katz says. He recommends half an hour at least three times a week of gentle water exercises in a pool that's between 80° and 90°F. That's about skin temperature. Avoid water above 100°, he says. It could overheat the baby. Water colder than 80° is okay, but most people have to be quite active to stay warm in water that cold, he says.

Different Strokes

What about other forms of exercise? "Our rule of thumb is that if you are in an exercise program, then carry on," Hodenius says. If you are starting an exercise program for the first time while you are pregnant, select one especially designed for pregnant women, she cautions. "It's physically and emotionally a wonderful thing, and it's safe." Of course, you should check with your doctor before beginning any exercise program during your pregnancy.

Will you be able to maintain your exercise program throughout your pregnancy? A woman who's been athletic before she became pregnant will understand when her body tells her to start slowing down, Hodenius says. "If a particular exercise starts to feel uncomfortable, that's your cue. Cut back or don't do it anymore."

Multipurpose Relief

For: Menstrual Pain, Endometriosis, Discomfort During Pregnancy

THE ULTIMATE BATH

A long, soothing soak feels like pure luxury, but you can tell everyone it's for . . . ahem, medicinal purposes only. Send your husband and the kids out for ice cream. Turn on the answering machine. Turn up the heat.

Draw the water comfortably warm, but not steaming hot. (Add more hot water as you need it.) If you're pregnant, you'll want to avoid water over 100°F. Try putting folded towels under your hips and head; better yet, get an inflatable pillow for your head.

Relax and breathe deeply in the water. When you get out of the tub, rub down with a fragrant moisturizer.

GENITAL HERPES

You have all the signs: a small group of tiny fluid-filled blisters or skin erosions on your genitals, fever, and aches that feel like the flu times ten. You know what it is—yet another bout of herpes—and you feel like you're stuck in an all-too-predictable rerun.

▶ INSTANT RELIEF

At our current level of medical treatment, genital herpes means forever. That knowledge may make the initial attack of this sexually transmitted disease *seem* like a lifelong contract with aggravation. But recurrences are usually mild, and there *are* ways to keep this nasty virus at bay.

Use warm water. Relieve pain during an initial herpes outbreak by running warm water from a shower over the affected area or by taking a warm bath, suggests Stephen Sacks, M.D., director of the University of British Columbia Herpes Clinic in Vancouver and author of *The Truth about Herpes.* Afterward, use a blow dryer set on low or cool, rather than a towel, to dry the area.

Divert the flow. Urine may make herpes blisters sting or burn. Redirect the flow away from blisters by using a bit of rolled toilet paper, Dr. Sacks suggests.

▶ PREVENTION PAIN-RELIEF PROGRAM

The very first step in your program to banish genital herpes is to see your doctor for a prescription.

Self-help treatments for herpes run the gamut from acidophilus to iodine, with none proven to work. Now, with acyclovir available, most of these home remedies have fallen out of favor, Dr. Sacks says.

Acyclovir (Zovirax) is a drug that stops the herpes virus from multiplying. Currently, it's the only drug on the market considered effective against genital herpes. (Other drugs are in development.)

Acyclovir is available by prescription as a pill or ointment and is sometimes even administered intravenously in hospitals for severe outbreaks. (Studies have shown oral and I.V. acyclovir to be much more effective than the ointment.)

"During your first episode, it's important to be treated with acyclovir, because it does substantially change the course of the disease," says Dr. Sacks. That initial outbreak, which normally lasts three weeks, hangs on for less than two weeks with oral or I.V. acyclovir, studies show. The drug also reduces unpleasant symptoms associated with herpes—urinary tract problems and swelling of lymph nodes in the groin.

Some people with herpes continue to take low doses of acyclovir to suppress frequent outbreaks. Studies show that acyclovir is helpful when used as a preventive. Other people keep acyclovir on hand to take when an outbreak occurs. It may reduce the length of a subsequent outbreak by about a day. Some people with herpes say acyclovir can completely avert a recurrence if the drug is started at the first inkling of symptoms.

Many people who have herpes say that stressful events in their life seem to provoke a recurrence. For that reason, stress reduction is sometimes suggested as a way to reduce outbreaks. "What I've found helps people most is to try to return to whatever they call normal," says Dr. Sacks. "Some people thrive on stress; others do better being laid back. People who continue to have problems after their initial episode may need help getting a perspective on things."

Rarely, a person may continue to experience pain in the genital area after a herpes attack has subsided. Similar to the burning, tingling pain that lingers after an attack of shingles, lingering genital herpes pain is treated the same way—with desensitizing creams or, sometimes, with antidepressants.

A MAN'S KIND OF PAIN

"It was the worst pain I ever had in my life." That seems to be the common denominator when it comes to injuries and disorders of the penis, testicles, or scrotum. No wonder men have contrived so many colorful phrases to describe the agony. Maybe laughter is the only thing that can take a guy's mind off his pain.

While women generally experience more diseases and disorders of the reproductive system, men's sexual organs are, for the most part, externally located in a highly vulnerable position. Besides accidental injuries—along the lines of being zonked by a baseball—there are a number of painful disorders that men may experience, according to Jack W. McAninch, M.D., professor of urology at the University of California, San Francisco, and chief urologist at San Francisco General Hospital.

Penis fracture. This is exactly what you think it is, a penis that has been fractured. Men often report hearing a crack or snap when it occurs. Afterward, their penis looks bent and hurts like the dickens.

Of course, penises don't contain bones. But they do have tough fibrous cylinders that fill up with blood to create an erection. Those cylinders can pop when an erect penis is suddenly bent or whacked. The result—and the cause of the pain—is torn tissue, plus swelling that in severe cases can be so extreme it's called "eggplant deformity."

Penis fracture occurs most often as a result of the penis missing its mark during sexual intercourse and striking the pubic bone, Dr. McAninch says. It's also been reported after rolling onto an erect penis, direct trauma from a second party (even from riding a frisky horse), bumping into a bedpost or nightstand, or forcing an erect penis into a pair of trousers.

"These guys go immediately to the emergency room," Dr. McAninch says. An ice pack and immobilization can relieve some pain, but quick help is needed. At the hospital a man may receive a shot of morphine to relieve pain. Then, within a few hours, he has surgery to repair the torn tissue and remove the pooled, clotted blood.

"Most guys are comfortable soon afterward and go home the following day," Dr. McAninch says. When they return two weeks later, most report no problems achieving erection and no abnormalities in the shape of their penis.

Men who do not have surgery are much more likely to have a permanently and painfully bent penis, Dr. McAninch says. "To be most successful, surgery should be performed no later than three or four days after the injury."

Testicular torsion. In this condition, a testicle rotates within the scrotum, cutting off its blood supply. The pain a man feels is his blood-deprived testicle screaming for oxygen, Dr. McAninch explains. Delaying treatment more than 6 hours could mean the testicle will die and have to be surgically removed.

It is possible to manually rotate the testicle without surgery. The problem, though, is that it's hard to tell which way to turn the testicle. "Obviously, turning it the wrong way makes the problem worse," Dr. McAninch explains. Surgery to correct the problem includes securing the wayward testicle to the scrotum with a few stitches. Since the other testicle is also likely to rotate, it too is stitched. Most men leave the hospital the next day.

Testicular torsion seems to strike athletic boys ages 10 to 16. But it can occur anytime, to any man. Wearing an athletic supporter or jockey shorts doesn't seem to help prevent it, Dr. McAninch says.

Priapism. You wished it would last forever. Now you wish it would go away.

Priapism is a persistent, abnormal erection, accompanied by pain and tenderness. It usually occurs initially with sexual excitement, but then it just won't let up. "Men keep thinking it will go away, so they may wait up to 12 hours before seeing a doctor," Dr. McAninch says. The condition is a result of blood that literally sludges up in the penis's erectile tissue, cutting off flow to or from the penis. It's most likely to occur in diseases that affect the red blood cells—sickle cell disease or leukemia. Street drugs like amyl nitrate or cocaine can also cause priapism.

The cure? An injection of epinephrine, a drug that relaxes blood vessels and makes normal blood circulation resume almost immediately, directly into the penis. If that fails, the treatment of choice is a "penis bypass" that shunts blood from erectile to nonerectile tissue.

PELVIC INFLAMMATORY DISEASE

Pelvic inflammatory disease (PID) is caused by a smorgasbord of microbes—gonorrhea, chlamydia, and what doctors call polymicrobia, a fancy term for "a bunch of different kinds of germs."

Like genital herpes, PID is frequently spread by sexual activity.

Symptoms cover a wide range. A person with a bad case of PID may have severe abdominal pain, fever, and other flulike symptoms, foul-smelling discharge from the vagina (or urethra in men), and pain and burning when urinating. Some women with PID never have such a gut-wrenching episode and so may not be diagnosed and treated properly. Instead, they have vague symptoms off and on for years—bad menstrual cramps, an occasional low fever, and what seems like a stomach virus or the flu.

Needless to say, someone with PID needs medical care, sometimes in a hurry. Medical care for this always includes antibiotics.

▶ INSTANT RELIEF

You've seen the doctor; you've gotten medication. While you're waiting the 24 to 48 hours for the drug to kick in, what can you do for relief?

Turn up the heat. Warmth is instantly soothing, and some experts maintain that heat applied to an infected area helps break up congestion and bring in medication-carrying blood. You could also enjoy sinking into a nice, hot tub. (See "Melt Pain Away" on page 396.)

Picture yourself healthy. In your mind's eye, see your uterus and fallopian tubes as pink and healthy again, and the nasty microbes retreating as the penicillin soldiers attack.

➤ PREVENTION PAIN-RELIEF PROGRAM

Drugs are the main defense against PID. Your doctor must do a culture of your vaginal discharge to see what organisms turn up, but if you're having bad pain she won't delay prescribing antibiotics. (She may switch or add antibiotics if necessary when the test results come back.) Antibiotics should have your fever and pain tamed in a day or two.

For the most up-to-date information and treatment, see a doctor specializing in sexually transmitted diseases (contact your local health bureau or Planned Parenthood) or a reproductive endocrinologist—a gynecologist with special training. PID can make a woman sterile if it's not treated promptly and correctly. In fact, it's one of the most common causes of female sterility.

Don't forget that you can be reinfected. Your sexual partner should be treated, too. Use condoms until your doctor gives you both a clean bill of health.

"We also advise women to take a 'pelvic rest,'" says George R. Huggins, M.D., chairman of Obstetrics and Gynecology at Francis Scott Key Medical Center in Baltimore. "That means no sex until their symptoms have cleared up." Sexual intercourse is often painful during this time, anyway, and can spread the infection throughout your pelvis and to your partner, he says.

Antibiotics often indirectly cause vaginal yeast infections, so ask your doctor for a prescription for a yeast-killing vaginal cream to use while you are taking the antibiotic, and perhaps for a time afterward. Antibiotics can cause diarrhea, too, because they wipe out helpful bacteria in your intestines.

ENDOMETRIOSIS

Not so long ago, a woman with endometriosis had a good chance of being told her pain was in her head, not her belly. Fortunately, these days there are good ways to diagnose and treat this very painful (and very physical) condition.

In endometriosis, the tissue lining the inside of the uterus somehow migrates and begins growing on other organs. It may find a foothold on the fallopian tubes and ovaries, even on the bladder and colon. Because it continues to respond to the hormonal changes of your monthly cycle, it acts just like endometrial tissue still in the uterus. That is, it builds up and bleeds each month, but blood inside the pelvic cavity has no place to drain. That buildup is what causes the pain.

Women with endometriosis sometimes have their worst pain toward the end of their menstrual period, not at the beginning. The pain can be bad enough that even fairly young women demand a hysterectomy. (Surgery does clear up their symptoms, but it's definitely *not* the treatment of choice for most.)

▶ INSTANT RELIEF

While you'll need to see your doctor for treatment of endometriosis, there are a few things you can do to make yourself more comfortable during the worst part of your cycle. See:

- "Battery-Powered Analgesia" on opposite page.
- "Melt Pain Away" on page 396.
- "Opt for Ibuprofen" on page 399.

▶ PREVENTION PAIN-RELIEF PROGRAM

The treatment program for endometriosis can be complex, with any number of options being tried at one time or another, depending on a woman's symptoms and age.

It *is* important to get a clear diagnosis. The Endometriosis Association suggests the best way for a doctor to diagnose this condition is with abdominal laparoscopy—a surgical procedure that peeks into your abdomen with an instrument that works somewhat like a miniature periscope.

"Doing laparoscopy is the only way you get an accurate assessment of how extensive the endometriosis is," says Dr. Huggins. And it's also the way to make sure you are not overlooking another condition that may be causing the same symptoms but which requires much different treatment, such as PID.

Antiprostaglandin drugs may help the pain, but they won't stop the growth of the runaway tissue. (Prostaglandins are hormones implicated in many pains that women experience as part of their monthly cycles.)

Multipurpose Relief

For: Menstrual Pain, Labor Pain, Endometriosis

BATTERY-POWERED ANALGESIA

Here's an electrifying treatment—better make that electric treatment—that can provide temporary relief from menstrual cramps, reduce the need for painkilling drugs during childbirth, and provide respite after abdominal surgery.

Transcutaneous electrical nerve stimulation, better known as TENS, makes use of a battery-operated device that blocks out pain messages with a gentle tingling sensation. Most types of TENS units will work as long as the unit is correctly placed on the lower abdomen, lower back, or both. (The transistor-sized battery pack can remain hidden under your clothes, clipped to a bra or belt.)

If your family doctor or gynecologist doesn't know much about TENS, he or she should be able to refer you to a physical therapist who can advise you. (See chapter 32.)

Although still uncommon, some obstetrics departments use TENS units during childbirth. If you're interested in trying this form of pain relief when you have your baby, you'll need to find a midwife or physical therapist who can instruct you.

Oral contraceptives help stop the pain and also inhibit the growth of endometrial tissue in some women, Dr. Huggins says. Oral contraceptives will not shrink the tissue that has already implanted itself, though. Drugs that do shrink implants are used in moderate to severe endometriosis. Because of side effects, most doctors limit their use to no more than nine months. Some doctors prefer to do surgery before prescribing these drugs, to remove as many of the tissue implants as they can. Laparoscopy—which uses miniature optics and tiny surgical instruments to remove implants through a tiny hole in the abdomen—is considered state-of-the-art surgery for endometriosis.

Both pregnancy and menopause halt the progress of endometriosis. Women who've had endometriosis when they were younger may develop symptoms anew if they take replacement hormones after menopause. If you're contemplating hormone therapy, make sure you mention any history of endometriosis to your doctor. Although medications and surgery are the most common treatments for endometriosis, there are other treatment options that may offer some relief.

Opting for Acupuncture

Acupuncture and electro-acupuncture may help ease the pain of endometriosis in minutes, and in some cases give permanent relief.

In one small study by researchers at UCLA, daily treatments with electro-acupuncture provided long-term pain relief to several women with endometriosis who had already received medical treatment for the problem. The women were treated 1 hour daily for six weeks. At the end of that time, all reported at least a 30 to 50 percent decrease in their pain. The women whom the study followed for three to five years reported themselves free of pain and without need of further medical treatment. (See chapter 16.)

Trigger-point therapy, sometimes called Western acupuncture, may also help. The technique involves injections of saline solutions into tender spots. (See chapter 33.)

FIBROID TUMORS

Just found out you have fibroid tumors? Well, join the crowd. About 20 percent of women develop these benign tumors of the uterus by the time they're 30, and most have few or no symptoms.

The tumors are usually discovered during a routine pelvic examination. Fibroids can range in size from as small as a grape to as large as a cantaloupe. Some women have whole clusters of fibroids; others have a single, albeit enormous, one.

When fibroids do cause pain, it's for one of two reasons: The tumor or tumors have grown so large they are pressing against other organs, or a tumor is growing so quickly it's outpacing its blood supply. A woman may have cramping, angina-like pain in her abdomen for months as a blood-starved fibroid tumor slowly degenerates and becomes scar tissue. Unless the tumor is very large, though, she'll likely have no other ill effects, Dr. Huggins says.

▶ INSTANT RELIEF

As with other kinds of pelvic pain, a few tried-and-true at-home tricks provide relief.

See:

- "The Ultimate Bath" on page 385.
- "Melt Pain Away" on page 396.
- "Opt for Ibuprofen" on page 399.

▶ PREVENTION PAIN-RELIEF PROGRAM

Long-term pain relief for fibroid tumors usually involves surgery and/or medication.

It is possible to have surgery just to remove the tumors, leaving the uterus intact. The operation, called a myomectomy, is a major procedure that requires a skilled surgeon. Some doctors suggest a hysterectomy when a fibroid has

Multipurpose Relief

For: Premenstrual Symptoms and Menstrual Pain, Pelvic Inflammatory Disease, Endometriosis, Fibroid Tumors, Ovarian Cysts

MELT PAIN AWAY

Ah, warmth. There's nothing like heat to soothe away menstrual cramps and other pains in the lower abdomen. Heat helps to relax muscles and increase blood flow to an area. Use a heating pad on your belly or lower back; make a heating pad sandwich, using one on your belly and one on your back; or use a wrap-around heating pad the same way. An advantage of the wrap-around pad is that you can use it while sitting in a chair.

Dressing properly also helps. During cold weather, wear a coat that comes down over your hips to keep your entire torso warm. Indoors, wear a long, thick sweater.

reached about the size of a grapefruit, especially when a woman is age 40 or older, but this surgery isn't always necessary and has its own risks, Dr. Huggins says. Explore your options carefully before you make a decision about any medical treatment. (You may want to read Lynn Payer's excellent book, *How to Avoid a Hysterectomy*.)

One drug that counteracts estrogen, nafarelin acetate (available as a nasal spray), can shrink fibroid tumors. "They come down very nicely, with often a 30 to 40 percent decrease in size," Dr. Huggins says. Unfortunately, once the drug is stopped (as it eventually must be, due to side effects), it takes only a few months for the tumors to grow back to their previous size. Usually this drug is used to shrink extra-big tumors prior to surgery.

Fibroids do tend to regrow, especially in women who have multiple tumors. A good way to minimize the risk of recurrence is to find a surgeon who agrees to carefully remove all the tumors he or she can find, even tiny ones. A reproductive endocrinologist may be your best bet.

Hormone replacement therapy can reactivate shrunken, dormant fibroids. You'll want to discuss this potential problem with your doctor before taking estrogen for menopause symptoms.

OVARIAN CYSTS

Each month, one of a woman's two ovaries naturally develops a fluid-filled cyst. Within a few days, the cyst bursts, releasing a tiny egg that is swept into the fallopian tubes toward the uterus. If it's lucky, somewhere along the way the egg hooks up with an eager, attractive young sperm with a fat bank account and a sports car.

Occasionally, though, a cyst does not burst. Instead, it grows larger and larger, creating pain that is sometimes mistaken for appendicitis or an ectopic (out-of-the-womb) pregnancy. It's this distinctive, fast-developing pain that sends a woman scurrying to the doctor or hospital emergency room, where she discovers she has a functional, or follicular, ovarian cyst.

▶ INSTANT RELIEF

Once your doctor is monitoring the cyst, there are a couple of things you can do to help you ride out the discomfort.

Chill out. You may want to try applying an ice pack directly to the painful spot. Some experts suggest putting crushed ice into a small plastic bag. Wrap the bag in a washcloth and apply, off and on, for a few minutes at a time.

See also:

- "Melt Pain Away" on page 396.
- "Opt for Ibuprofen" on the opposite page.

▶ PREVENTION PAIN-RELIEF PROGRAM

Most doctors agree that ovarian cysts bear watching. Treatment differs depending on your age. Doctors are less likely to take a wait-and-see attitude with older women, who are at higher risk for ovarian cancer.

Both younger and older women may be put on oral contraceptives for a few months to see if they help shrink

Multipurpose Relief

For: Premenstrual Symptoms and Menstrual Pain, Endometriosis, Fibroid Tumors, Ovarian Cysts

OPT FOR IBUPROFEN

Put the blame on prostaglandins.

The discomfort many women feel just before and during the first day or two of menstruation is due to a surge of these pain-provoking hormones. That's why pain relievers that block prostaglandins work so well to reduce these symptoms. Ibuprofen and—to a lesser extent—aspirin are the strongest nonprescription antiprostaglandin drugs available.

Begin taking the medication when your symptoms first kick in but before pain becomes intolerable, experts recommend. Take the drugs as long as you need them. Doctors warn, though, that for a normal menstrual cycle, you shouldn't need to take an over-the-counter pain reliever for more than three or four days. If you need more than this to relieve your pain, see your doctor.

Check with your doctor before using a pain reliever for endometriosis, fibroid tumors, or ovarian cysts. While these drugs may ease the aches that accompany such conditions, it's unwise to mask increasing pain that requires medical treatment. (See chapter 26.)

the cyst. In many cases, they do. In women ages 40 and older, if the cyst has not disappeared in two months, it may be removed surgically. (Make sure your doctor doesn't remove your entire ovary unless it's necessary—in the case of multiple cysts or cancer, for instance. Your ovary produces hormones that help protect you from heart disease and prevent loss of precious bone.) In younger women, some doctors wait months longer before considering surgery, to see if the cyst does eventually go away on its own.

Ovarian cysts can be monitored with ultrasound and pelvic examination. Continuing to take oral contraceptives will help prevent further cysts from developing, Dr. Huggins says.

Keep in mind: There are many kinds of ovarian cysts and tumors; the cancerous kind often aren't painful until they are quite large. Usually these tumors are first discovered during a pelvic exam that reveals an enlarged ovary. Women with a family history of ovarian cancer may want to have an ultrasound examination of the ovaries along with their yearly Pap smear.

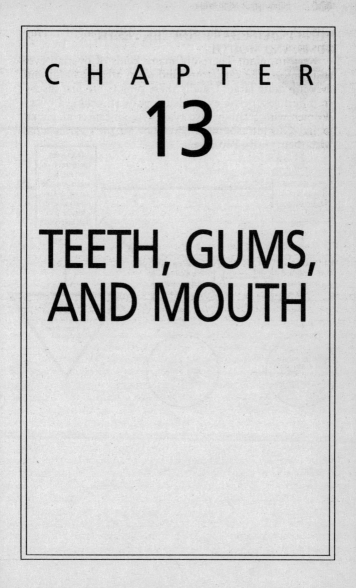

CHAPTER
13

TEETH, GUMS, AND MOUTH

PAIN-FINDER CHART FOR THE TEETH, GUMS, AND MOUTH

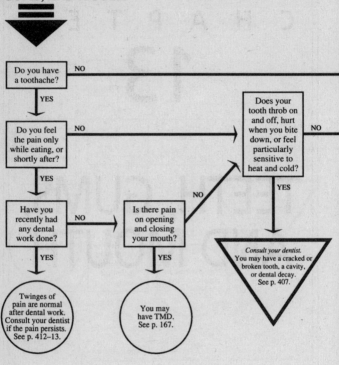

Do you have a toothache?

NO →

YES ↓

Do you feel the pain only while eating, or shortly after?

NO →

YES ↓

Have you recently had any dental work done?

NO →

YES ↓

Is there pain on opening and closing your mouth?

NO →

YES ↓

Does your tooth throb on and off, hurt when you bite down, or feel particularly sensitive to heat and cold?

NO →

YES ↓

Twinges of pain are normal after dental work. Consult your dentist if the pain persists. See p. 412–13.

You may have TMD. See p. 167.

Consult your dentist. You may have a cracked or broken tooth, a cavity, or dental decay. See p. 407.

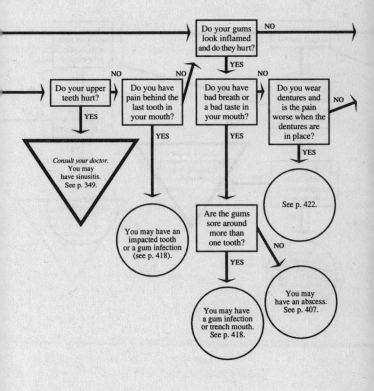

Do your gums look inflamed and do they hurt?   NO

YES

Do your upper teeth hurt?   NO

YES

Consult your doctor. You may have sinusitis. See p. 349.

Do you have pain behind the last tooth in your mouth?   NO

YES

You may have an impacted tooth or a gum infection (see p. 418).

Do you have bad breath or a bad taste in your mouth?   NO

YES

Do you wear dentures and is the pain worse when the dentures are in place?   NO

YES

See p. 422.

Are the gums sore around more than one tooth?

NO

YES

You may have a gum infection or trench mouth. See p. 418.

You may have an abscess. See p. 407.

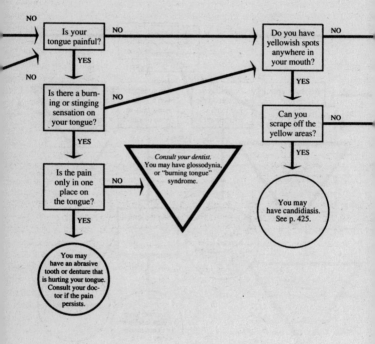

NO →

Is your tongue painful? — NO →

YES ↓

Do you have yellowish spots anywhere in your mouth? — NO →

YES ↓

Is there a burning or stinging sensation on your tongue? — NO →

YES ↓

Can you scrape off the yellow areas? — NO →

YES ↓

Is the pain only in one place on the tongue? — NO →

Consult your dentist. You may have glossodynia, or "burning tongue" syndrome.

YES ↓

You may have candidiasis. See p. 425.

You may have an abrasive tooth or denture that is hurting your tongue. Consult your doctor if the pain persists.

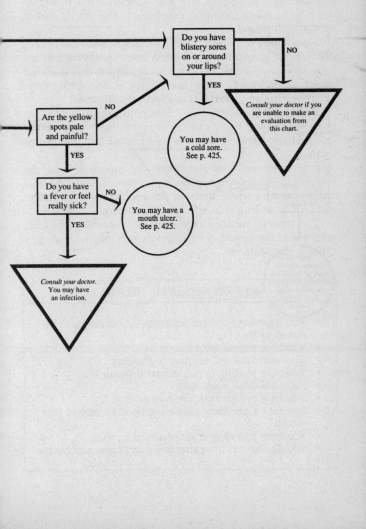

Do you have
blistery sores
on or around
your lips?

NO

YES

Consult your doctor if you
are unable to make an
evaluation from
this chart.

Are the yellow
spots pale
and painful?

NO

You may have
a cold sore.
See p. 425.

YES

Do you have
a fever or feel
really sick?

NO

You may have a
mouth ulcer.
See p. 425.

YES

Consult your doctor.
You may have
an infection.

L ife can be an oral obstacle course when it hurts to eat, talk, whistle Dixie, or plant a wet one on a pair of waiting lips.

Mouth pain is more than a nuisance—it can be life-threatening if it takes a bite out of your desire to eat. It needs to be taken seriously, especially in the elderly and in seriously ill people.

Mouth pain can occur when a tooth is sensitive, cracked, decayed, or impacted; when gums become inflamed or infected; when the delicate mucous membrane that lines the mouth is ulcerated; when the tongue is burned or raw; when lips become cracked, chapped, or blistered.

What causes mouth pain? Everything from neglect to viral infections, from cancer chemotherapy to sexually transmitted diseases, from drug-induced dry mouth to stress.

Like other parts of the body, the mouth reflects the body's general state of health. Sometimes, it's even the first visible site of a whole-body health problem such as leukemia, AIDS, a drug side effect, or a nutritional deficiency.

The type of medical treatment or at-home relief that works best for mouth pain depends very much on what's causing the problem.

GET PROFESSIONAL HELP IF:

- You experience loss of sensation or numbness in the mouth or lips
- You have pain when chewing
- Your gums are red, swollen, or bleeding
- You have swelling or pus around the gum line
- You have loose adult teeth
- You have persistent mouth pain or sores
- You find a persistent painless lump in or around your mouth
- You have a toothache accompanied by fever
- You develop any sores after beginning a new medication

TOOTHACHE

Let's face it. There *is* something worse than going to the dentist. The dull throb of a toothache, punctuated by sudden stabs of pain, is enough to drive even the most wide-eyed, sweaty-palmed phobic for help. And the sooner, the better. Wishful thinking aside, most toothaches don't go away by themselves, at least not for long. They're usually a sign that a tooth is in trouble.

A toothache usually means that acid-producing bacteria have etched away the tooth's surface enamel, exposing the underlying dentin—and eventually the nerve—to infection. The nerve can also be laid bare when a tooth cracks. Sometimes receding gums expose the softer root of a tooth, allowing fast decay. The pain can be worse when nerve infection develops into an abscess—a pocket of infection at the root tip.

An infected tooth may require root canal—major excavation that reams out the entire nerve of the tooth, replacing it with a rubber plug. Or the tooth may be so far gone it must be pulled and replaced with an artificial tooth.

Pain relief isn't the only good reason to see your dentist pronto. The sooner your aching tooth is treated, the more likely it can be saved, says Henry W. Finger, D.D.S., president of the Academy of General Dentistry. Teeth are like cancan dancers—when one topples, others are likely to follow, as teeth tip toward the space left by a missing neighbor.

➤ INSTANT RELIEF

These temporary measures can tame a torturous toothache.

Floss the spot. Flossing helps remove any particles of food that may be trapped in a cavity or between teeth and gums, says Dr. Finger. If floss doesn't do the trick, try your toothbrush or a water jet.

Anoint an ache. Over-the-counter toothache drops containing clove oil (eugenol) temporarily relieve most irritated

---

Multipurpose Relief

For: Toothache, Gum Disease, Dental Procedures

MODEST BUT MIGHTY

Don't underestimate the power of aspirin, acetaminophen, or ibuprofen to tame your pain until you can see a dentist. Any one of these over-the-counter analgesics can usually ease a toothache or inflamed gums well enough to allow you to go about your business until you are able to get help, says Henry W. Finger, D.D.S., president of the Academy of General Dentistry.

These drugs are also dentists' and oral surgeons' first choice when it comes to soothing pain after root canal or surgery to remove impacted wisdom teeth. Some dentists suggest their patients take two aspirin or ibuprofen (Advil or Nuprin) an hour *before* a dental procedure to reduce pain and swelling afterward.

Use the pain reliever according to package directions, Dr. Finger says.

Don't put a pill on your gum; even though doing so may seem to relieve tooth pain, aspirin and other pain-relieving tablets can cause a chemical burn that kills gum tissues.

---

teeth, says Dr. Finger. Clove oil is a nerve sedative that's been used since the days when a dentist was anyone handy with a pair of pliers. Put a drop on a bit of cotton packed next to the tooth, experts say. Then see your dentist as soon as possible.

Ice an acupressure point. Your hand may seem well removed from the pain in your mouth, but studies show that rubbing ice on a particular spot on your hand may help reduce the pain. You can find the spot, which is actually a traditional acupressure point, on the V-shaped area where the bones of the thumb and forefinger meet. Massage the point on either hand with an ice cube.

A study by one of the world's leading pain researchers, Ronald Melzack, Ph.D., of McGill University in Montreal, showed that ice massage at this point on the hand for 7 to 10 minutes eased dental pain in 60 to 90 percent of the people who tried it. "Surprisingly enough, it does work," says Dr. Finger.

See also:

- "Modest but Mighty" on opposite page.
- "Do the Saltwater Swish" on page 419.

➡ PREVENTION PAIN-RELIEF PROGRAM

If you have a toothache, make an appointment with your dentist without delay. Even though pain-relief techniques may chase the pain temporarily, you are guaranteed a return visit unless you have the cause of the pain removed. (See "Survival in the Dentist's Chair" on page 412.)

You are not helpless in the face of toothache, however. There's a lot you can do at home to prevent those infections that hurt so much. Proper brushing and flossing top the list.

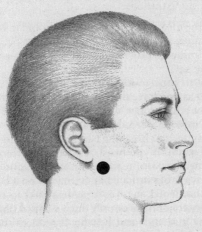

For temporary relief of toothache, you can massage the sensitive points just above the corner of the jaw on the affected side. Press the spots off and on, a few seconds at a time, to relieve pain.

Banish the Boredom of Brushing

Would you believe that even the supposed guardians of all that is sweet and clean and pure about our mouth might think toothbrushing is, well, boring?

"It's time-consuming, and most of us, dentists as well as patients, are not particularly excited about doing it," says no less an authority than Sigmund Stahl, D.D.S., an associate dean at the world's largest dental health facility, New York University's Kriser Orofacial Pain Center.

Dr. Stahl, by the way, admits he does little to try to spark it up. "I just put up with it," he says. On the other hand, with a little imagination, toothbrushing can be a great way to start and end your day. For instance, you could

- Post reading material on the bathroom mirror.
- Do ankle-strengthening exercises.
- Blast Bob Dylan on a boombox and pretend your toothbrush is a harmonica.
- Install a kitchen timer in the bathroom and time your mouthly ministrations.

You get the idea. The entire routine should take no more than 5 minutes, Dr. Stahl insists. "But most people spend only 2 to 3 minutes brushing, and even that seems like an eternity," he says.

It's okay if your toothbrushing is mindless, Dr. Stahl says, as long as you have the correct routine down pat. You should know the proper way to brush so well that you could do it in your sleep, he says.

Experts agree that brushing twice a day and flossing once a day is adequate. If you brush less often, bacteria start to "colonize" against your teeth. They form plaque that glues onto every available surface like barnacles on a boat. Once plaque has hardened, it takes a professional to remove it.

If you persist in brushing only once a day, doing it before bedtime may give the most benefit. It reduces the number of decay-producing bacteria at work in your mouth while you sleep. Since you swallow less frequently and produce less saliva while you're sleeping, plaque-producing bacteria usually have a field day.

Choosing the Right Tools

Use a soft-bristled toothbrush with rounded or polished bristles. It's much less likely to scratch or wear away gum tissue and tooth enamel, says Dr. Finger. Your dentist or dental hygienist can recommend the appropriate size for you. Some adults find a child-sized brush works best. Replace the toothbrush every three months, or whenever the bristles begin to splay out. Allowing the brush to dry out between uses discourages bacterial growth on the bristles.

Multipurpose Relief

**For: Toothache, Gum Disease, Mouth Sores,
   Denture Pain**

NUMB IT

Forget a swig of whiskey. There is a whole host of over-the-counter products that can temporarily ease oral pain without making you tipsy—pastes, drops, and mouthwashes, not to mention all the anesthetic sprays and lozenges used for sore throats. (They numb the mouth all the way down to the throat.)

These products may contain one of a number of active ingredients. Toothache drops may contain clove oil (eugenol) or benzocaine. Both can anesthetize a tooth nerve. Teething gels for babies usually contain benzocaine, but without alcohol. Some throat lozenges and sore throat sprays contain phenol or sodium phenolate, which are topical anesthetics. Anesthetic mouth gels or pastes may contain benzocaine or phenol. One—Zilactin—contains tannic acid, the same compound found in black tea.

Your dentist or doctor may be able to prescribe other pain-relieving mouth rinses or pastes for you if you need them.

SURVIVAL IN THE DENTIST'S CHAIR

No one enjoys going to the dentist. A minority find it terrifying and excruciating, but most people think they make out just fine at the dentist's office, surveys show. They may not view their visits as fun, but they don't experience unbearable pain.

About one in every seven dental patients has consistently bad experiences in the dentist's chair, however. For one reason or another, they don't get adequate pain relief for drilling or other dental work. Their tooth may not get numb when they are given local anesthesia. They may not respond to oral or intravenous antianxiety drugs, such as Valium, given prior to oral surgery. Nitrous oxide may leave them as anxious as ever. Anxiety, inflammation around a tooth, even a patient's own drug or alcohol use may contribute to problems of pain control.

Dentists May Belittle Pain

Most dentists are at loose ends when it comes to addressing these problems, says Peter Milgrom, D.D.S., director of the University of Washington's Dental Fears Research Clinic in Seattle.

"Dentists will say things like 'You shouldn't be able to feel that; I gave you a lot of anesthetic,' 'Hold on, this will just take a few minutes longer,' or 'Act like an adult,' " says Dr. Milgrom. The problem, he says, is that some dentists don't understand how unpleasant the painful experience is.

Dr. Milgrom works with both fearful patients and dentists who want to learn how to better treat such patients.

"The biggest thing a dentist has to learn is that when a patient says they have pain, they have pain," says Dr. Milgrom. "It's not useful for the dentist to second-guess a patient. It's the responsibility of the dentist to tell the patient he or she will do his or her best to stop the pain, and to do that, and then to question the patient about their comfort. The patient has to be assertive enough to insist the dentist stop if they're uncomfortable."

Insist on Slow Injections

Dentists also frequently need to learn how to give anesthetic injections properly, Dr. Milgrom says. Injections do hurt if the dentist injects the fluid too quickly. The stinging pain is the equivalent of a jet of water from the nozzle of a garden hose. An anesthetic injection should take about 30 seconds to do, Dr. Milgrom says. "But most dentists do them in 5 seconds or less."

Dentists, and doctors, frequently fail to prescribe adequate amounts of pain medications after surgery to keep their patients comfortable. "Part of this comes from their concern that patients will go to the dentist to try to get narcotics, but evidence is overwhelming that dentists and other health providers underestimate the pain," Dr. Milgrom says. He suggests you clearly state your preference as to what you want for pain control.

"Some people do fine with no drugs; others know they want drugs," he says. "Work to establish a relationship with the dentist so you are seen as part of his practice. Talk with him sincerely about your experience so he understands how you want to be treated."

After the Ordeal

Studies from the National Institutes of Dental Research show that a full therapeutic dose of a nonsteroidal anti-inflammatory drug, such as aspirin or ibuprofen, taken before the dental appointment provides the maximum amount of relief from dental pain after the procedure. Some dentists also use long-acting local anesthesia such as bupivaocaine or etidocaine, which can provide relief from surgical pain for up to 6 hours after a dental procedure—twice as long as lidocaine, the most commonly used anesthesia. Be aware, notes Dr. Milgrom, that the anesthetic effect varies a lot from one person to the next.

Besides picking a dentist they trust, what's the most helpful thing patients can do for themselves? Breathe, and breathe again, Dr. Milgrom says.

"Anxious, nervous people tend to hold their breath. They may not breathe at all during an injection, and breathe very shallowly during the procedure," he says. This just makes things worse because it creates more muscle tension and anxiety. Start doing deep, slow breathing on the way to the dentist's office and continue to concentrate on your breathing throughout the procedure, he suggests. Also, try to think of yourself as a rag doll, keeping your muscles as relaxed as possible.

If you find them helpful, use water-jet devices or mouth-washes in addition to brushing and flossing, but *not* as substitutes, Dr. Finger cautions. Plaque holds on for dear life; it needs to be scraped or brushed off.

And don't get the idea that fluoride toothpastes and rinses are just for kids. A study by researchers at the University of Iowa College of Dentistry found that people over age 54 who used a fluoridated toothpaste for a year had 41 percent less tooth decay and 67 percent less root decay than another group using a nonfluoridated toothpaste. Another study showed that 63 percent of people over age 65 have root decay, largely because gums tend to recede with age.

Don't Forget to Floss

Brushing should be followed by meticulous flossing. Un-waxed floss is preferred, but it doesn't make much difference what kind of floss you use as long as you floss, says Dr. Finger. Waxed floss may be a bit easier to use if your teeth are tightly spaced or if the floss shreds on fillings.

If you're not sure how to brush or floss correctly, ask your dentist or dental hygienist for a demonstration the next time you have your teeth cleaned. You might also ask for "disclosing" tablets, chewable pills containing a red dye that temporarily stains areas your toothbrush has missed. Some dentists also provide cheap plastic dental mirrors that let you easily see the backs of your front teeth and your rear molars, two stops the Toothbrush Express frequently leaves off its schedule.

"People frequently brush some parts of their mouth just fine but miss other areas," says JoAnn Gurenlain, president of the American Dental Hygienists' Association. "And some people only floss their front teeth, because their back teeth are too much trouble. Regardless of the difficulty involved, it is important to brush and floss between all your teeth."

When you're done with your teeth, turn your attention to your tongue, Dr. Finger suggests. This velvety appendage is home base for much of the bacteria in the mouth. Scrub with a toothbrush or ask your pharmacist for a tongue scraper. You'll be amazed at how much gook comes off and how clean your mouth feels when your tongue is scrubbed. (Who knows? You may even find a few of those missing socks you were blaming your clothes dryer for devouring.)

Using an over-the-counter mouthwash, such as Listerine, or a prescription one, such as Peridex, at bedtime may help reduce plaque buildup by killing acid-producing bacteria. (Mouthwashes that reduce plaque contain one of four essential oils, most commonly thymol. Look for a product that has the American Dental Association's seal of acceptance.)

And if you snack on sweets or starches during the day, follow the treats with a tooth-scrubbing, saliva-producing food such as carrots or sugarless gum.

Call on the Pros

See a dentist or a dental hygienist at least twice a year for a professional cleaning. Depending on how encrusted your mouth is, a good cleaning will take anywhere from 45 minutes to several hours, spread out over a few weeks. It will include scraping plaque above and below the gum line of each tooth and between teeth, polishing the flat surfaces of all teeth with an abrasive cleaner, or, in some cases, using tiny abrasive strips to remove stains from between teeth.

If you have arthritis, Parkinson's, or some other condition that makes it hard for you to brush well, consider more frequent professional cleanings. Your dental hygienist can also recommend brushes and floss holders that are easier to handle.

Finally, don't use chewing tobacco or snuff. Besides eroding your gums and cheeks, both of these products contain sugar. Frequent use is a sure way to develop gum-line cavities, not to mention bad breath and oral cancer. Chewing tobacco and snuff are just as addictive as cigarettes. If you can't stop on your own, ask your dentist or doctor where you can get help. Local cancer societies and other organizations sometimes sponsor low-cost programs to break the chaw habit.

ROOT CANAL: OHHH, NOOOOO

Some dentists would like to blame Johnny Carson. "Any time something hurts, his joke writers have to compare it with root canal," says one disgruntled endodontist. Insists another: "People are already in pain when they see us. We don't make them hurt any worse." Both point out that very few patients have a pressing need to have work done on a root canal that doesn't *already* hurt.

The fact is, root canal does have the reputation of causing more pain than most other dental procedures. And that's no joke.

A root canal involves removing the infection from a decay-damaged tooth, explains Peter Milgrom, D.D.S., director of the University of Washington's Dental Fears Research Clinic in Seattle. If the nerve is not completely dead—and often it isn't—it's exquisitely sensitive. That's why a numbing drug—anesthesia—is injected around the root of the tooth before work is started.

But if infection is bad, inadequate analgesia can be a problem, says Dr. Milgrom. "Even with potent new anesthetics, inflamed tissue around the root of the tooth can make it difficult to anesthetize fully," he says. The infection interferes with the action of the anesthesia. Using more anesthesia, adding nitrous oxide, or putting anesthetic drops directly on the tooth's nerve can all help to relieve pain.

After the procedure, when the anesthesia wears off, you'll be experiencing pain both from the dental work and from the remaining gum or bone infection, which may take a few days to calm down. If you're concerned about pain during this time and want pain-relieving medications, talk with your dentist, advises Dr. Milgrom. He or she may recommend over-the-counter nonsteroidal anti-inflammatory drugs. If you're still not getting adequate pain relief, call your dentist for a prescription pain reliever, says Dr. Milgrom.

Dr. Milgrom does something most endodontists don't do: He sometimes sends people home without working on them.

"Often a patient shows up looking like a wet dishrag. They are in pain, they didn't sleep the night before, they haven't eaten for a few days, and they don't have an appointment," he says. "The dentist tries to squeeze them into an already busy day, and the treatment ends up being uncomfortable."

Dr. Milgrom may give truly miserable patients antibiotics and sleep and pain medications, and send them home for some R&R. "Usually in a day or two the pain settles down, then we have them come back, teach them some simple breathing and relaxation exercises, and then do the root canal procedure in a calm way."

GUM DISEASE

Like a bad love affair, most forms of gum disease are deceptively painless in their early stages. Unless we recognize the symptoms—pink toothbrush bristles, puffy gums, breath that smells like a corroded car battery—we remain blissfully ignorant until the dentist gives us the bad news.

But there are cases in which early gum disease hurts enough to top the torture of any toothache. In a condition popularly known as trench mouth (named after the World War I soldiers who brought it home), the gums become ulcerated and begin to slough away.

Even normally painless periodontitis (inflamed gums) can flare into abscesses and pockets of infection, involving tooth roots and even the bone of the jaw if it's not treated promptly.

Gum disease that becomes bad enough—due to neglect and severe malnutrition—may lead to gangrene of the mouth, a condition once seen only in starving people in Third World countries but now occasionally noted at inner-city dental clinics treating the poor and homeless.

Gum disease is caused by hordes of invading bacteria and is usually the result of poor oral hygiene, general poor health, or a sugar-coated diet. Trench mouth (you don't have to be in a trench to get it) seems to crop up most often in young people burning the candle at both ends. Students cramming for final exams are typical victims.

Pregnant women sometimes get mild gum inflammation that disappears soon after they give birth, and people with AIDS, acute leukemia, or uncontrolled diabetes may be more likely than normal to develop gum disease. Usually they are treated by periodontists, dentists specializing in the treatment of gum disease.

▶ INSTANT RELIEF

Dentists often suggest these at-home helpers.

Brush with a feather-touch. A gentle brushing with a

soft-bristled toothbrush dislodges debris and bacteria around the gums. Try dipping your toothbrush in a plaque-reducing mouthwash occasionally while you brush.

See also:

- "Modest but Mighty" on page 408.
- "Numb It" on page 411.
- "Do the Saltwater Swish" below.

➤ PREVENTION PAIN-RELIEF PROGRAM

Seeing your dentist or dental hygienist on a regular basis should keep gum disease at bay; but if you should experience gum puffiness, bleeding, or pain, make an appointment immediately.

Multipurpose Relief

For: Toothache, Gum Disease, Mouth Sores, Denture Pain

DO THE SALTWATER SWISH

Dentists frequently recommend saltwater rinses as a primary line of defense for mouth pain. Why? For starters, everyone has salt and water at home. It's not something you have to go out and buy, says Henry W. Finger, D.D.S., president of the Academy of General Dentistry. For another thing, it works.

"It's soothing, it rinses away bacteria in the mouth, and it contains nothing that could irritate the mouth," he says. Many prepared mouthwashes contain alcohol, which can sting already irritated tissues and make a dry mouth even drier.

If you want to take advantage of this readily available, dentist-approved home remedy, rinse your mouth vigorously with a solution made from ½ teaspoon of salt dissolved in a cup of warm water. Spit it out; don't swallow it. Rinse as often as you want, but don't delay seeing a dentist, Dr. Finger says.

The best way to prevent gum disease is plaque removal, says Dr. Stahl. That means following the same brushing and flossing routine that keeps your teeth tiptop, and especially flossing every one of your teeth every day, no matter what!

If you already have gum disease, it probably will also mean you'll need to have plaque professionally removed from your teeth, including plaque that has worked its way *below* the gum line and lodged on sensitive tooth roots. This procedure, called scaling and tooth planing, involves scraping the tooth root with a tiny metal instrument (and sometimes a vibrating ultrasonic scaler). It can take a long time to do, and it can be uncomfortable, especially if you have sensitive tooth roots.

Whoever does the cleaning—usually a dental hygienist—should be prepared to see that you get pain relief in the form of topical or injected anesthesia or nitrous oxide as soon as it becomes necessary. Usually this means summoning the dentist to administer relief. Don't hesitate to insist upon it.

Some dentists do what's called intensive conservative treatment. They may clean your teeth every month for up to six months or more to give gums a chance to heal. This process cleans the areas you might not be able to reach yourself—the deep pockets around a tooth's root.

If gum disease persists after a round of cleanings, you may need to take oral antibiotics, usually tetracycline, to finish it off. Or your dentist may prescribe antibiotics from the start if your gum infection includes a fever, fatigue, and swollen lymph glands or if you have trench mouth or juvenile periodontitis, says Max Goodson, D.D.S., Ph.D., director of the Department of Pharmacology at the Forsyth Dental Center in Boston.

"Antibiotic therapy has been proven useful in the more advanced forms of adult gum disease," he says. "In milder forms of gum disease, however, results of studies are mixed. Some show a benefit; others do not."

Anti-Gum Disease Diet

Some dentists and periodontists take a strong interest in their patients' nutrition. Most, however, seem to think that unless someone is obviously malnourished, diet has little to do with preventing or treating gum disease.

Several intriguing studies, however, suggest that good nutrition can help gums withstand bacterial attack, resist bleeding, and recover more quickly from extractions or injuries, according to Rima Bachiman, D.D.S., a dentist specializing in older patients and a professor at New York University's College of Dentistry.

Vitamin C rates as the nutrient most often studied. It may boost immune function and help in the production of collagen, a connective tissue found in most parts of the body, including the gums, says Dr. Bachiman. Bioflavonoids, nutritional components usually found with citrus sources of vitamin C, may also play a part in maintaining healthy gums.

Because protein, B-complex vitamins, beta-carotene, zinc, and other nutrients are involved in good gum health, it's important to eat a healthy diet, not just take vitamins, says Dr. Bachiman. Even osteoporosis, a disease in which nutrition plays a significant role, can play a part in gum disease. The teeth can become loose when bone density decreases in your jaw and can contribute to fractures of the jawbone.

Is poor nutrition aggravating your gum problems? That might be the case if you eat fewer than three vegetables and two fruits a day, an amount recommended by the U.S. Department of Agriculture and the National Academy of Sciences to meet requirements for nutrients like vitamin C and beta-carotene.

Dr. Bachiman frequently calls in her patients' medical doctor and a nutritionist when she sees that they need a program to improve their oral health.

"We look at everything," she says. "And that includes their current health problems, the drugs they are taking, what they are eating, and what they can and should be eating."

DENTURE PAIN

Ain't nothing like the real thing, and that goes for teeth, too.

Dentures take some getting used to—or perseverance, as one denture manufacturer puts it. They need to be fitted properly and adjusted periodically to be comfortable. Mouth or tongue pain usually means a denture plate isn't fitting right anymore, for one reason or another. It needs to be adjusted. Or it may need to be relined, which means that the part of the denture that fits against your gums may need to be recast. If the fit is way off, the entire denture may have to be remade. How the teeth fit together—the bite—is also crucial. If it's off just a bit, it can cause denture pain, experts say.

Most people get used to dentures within a few weeks and no longer have sore spots. They frequently say their gums "harden up," but the gums don't actually develop calluses or hard spots, says Gerald O'Keefe, D.M.D., a maxillofacial prosthetics specialist at Prosthodontics Intermedica and associate professor at Hahnemann University in Philadelphia. "People simply learn how to use their dentures," he says.

▶ INSTANT RELIEF

If going toothless seems like a better deal than fiddling with a recalcitrant set of choppers, try these interim solutions. See:

- "Numb It" on page 411.
- "Do the Saltwater Swish" on page 419.

▶ PREVENTION PAIN-RELIEF PROGRAM

New dentures almost always need to be adjusted, sometimes several times, before they become comfortable. Material may need to be removed to relieve sore spots, or the teeth in a denture may need to be ground to adjust the bite.

"No matter how well a denture is made, it needs adjustments," Dr. O'Keefe says. "In the past 20 years, I've seen two sets of dentures that didn't need adjustments, and I've seen lots of dentures in that time."

A major problem with new denture wearers, he says, is that "the vast majority take the attitude, 'Here are my dentures, I never have to go back to the dentist again.' " The result: mouth sores and a set of dentures that, like good china, is used only when company's visiting.

See your dentist once or twice a year to have your mouth and dentures checked. The dentist will look for irritated spots on your gums, tongue, cheeks, and palate. He or she can also make adjustments in your dentures if necessary, says Dr. O'Keefe.

Beware the Bone Robbers

Don't rely on over-the-counter denture pads or liners to adjust your fit, warns Dr. O'Keefe. Although these products do put a soft cushion between your tender mouth and the denture, they also reduce the bite space—the distance between the upper and lower teeth—and thus put undue pressure on the jawbone. That pressure can lead to rapid bone reabsorption, a destructive process that destroys the jawbone.

"People who use over-the-counter denture liners are playing Russian roulette with their bones," Dr. O'Keefe says. "With time, they won't have any jawbone left."

Denture adhesives, on the other hand, can be appropriate. "Some people just don't have the anatomy to maintain a proper anchor for a denture, so they need to use an adhesive," Dr. O'Keefe says.

Soft acrylic dentures may be appropriate for some people—those who've had radiation treatment to their mouth, for instance, or who have an irregularly shaped jawbone. These dentures have more cushioning than the regular variety. Their disadvantages: They are harder to adjust and to keep clean. Also, soft liners wear out faster than hard denture materials.

Clean Dentures Carefully

Plaque, a sticky bacterial film that's constantly forming in your mouth, also forms on dentures. For this reason—and to prevent staining—dentures should be brushed thoroughly with a denture toothpaste. Follow your dentist's directions or the directions on the denture cleaner package.

When plaque accumulates, it hardens to form tartar on dentures and is difficult to remove without soaking first or scraping. Soak dentures in a solution of 1 tablespoon of white vinegar to 8 ounces of water. Or use a commercial denture cleanser. When they're not in your mouth, keep your dentures in water. If they dry out, they can warp, ruining their fit, says Dr. O'Keefe.

Dirty dentures may not cause mouth sores, but they can certainly contribute to the problem, says Dr. O'Keefe. Fungal infections are common; they appear as sore white patches on the gums and the roof of the mouth and are more likely to develop in people who wear their dentures to bed. Treat sores caused by fungal infection with antifungal creams applied to the affected areas. And use an antifungal solution to soak dentures at night, advises Dr. O'Keefe.

Once a day, brush your tongue, rinse with saltwater, then take a gauze pad dipped in salt water and wipe your gums, cheeks, and the roof of your mouth. Then rinse again, he advises.

When your dentures are causing discomfort, be particularly aware of the foods that seem to cause you trouble. Some people who wear dentures can eat anything they want. Others, though, find they need to fine-tune their foraging. They realize they can't bite down hard with their front teeth on something like a bagel or an apple. Leafy greens may pose a particular challenge, Dr. O'Keefe notes.

MOUTH SORES

Feel like your mouth is ground zero for a SCUD missile attack?

Many of us get an occasional raw spot in our mouth that simply comes and goes. We may get one to five small, pale ulcers, called canker sores, inside our cheeks or lips. Or we may get cold sores—virus-induced blisters that erupt to form painful ulcers if they're inside the mouth or ugly scabs if they're on the edge of the lip or somewhere else near the mouth. We may even get a collection of small white pimples that eventually join up to form a lacy patch on an inside cheek or the side of the tongue. This condition—lichen planus—causes pain only in its erosive form.

Some people develop fungal infections in their mouth. The most common infection—yeast, or candidiasis—causes creamy yellow, slightly raised patches that turn red and sore when they're rubbed. Denture wearers, those taking antibiotics, diabetics, and people who are immune-suppressed—AIDS patients, for instance—are most likely to develop yeast infections, says Barry Rifkin, D.D.S., Ph.D., chairman of the Department of Oral Medicine and Pathology at New York University's Dental School.

Sometimes cells inside the mouth react to protect the mouth from the constant irritation of chewing tobacco or a rubbing denture. They form a thick, rough, white or red surface, called leukoplakia or erythroplakia. Initially painless, these patches should still be seen by a doctor.

People can develop many other semi-mysterious problems with their mouth, tongue, and lips. Itching, burning mouth can be a sign of diabetes, nutritional deficiencies, or, in older women, low estrogen levels. Cracks around the corners of the mouth can mean a B-vitamin deficiency or a yeast infection. A raw, cracked, or "balding" tongue can point toward nutritional deficiencies, chronic dry mouth, infections, or reactions to drug use.

➡️ **I**NSTANT **R**ELIEF

Can't wait for the pain of a canker sore to wind down on its own? Waiting to see the doctor? Try these temporary tactics.

Take a tea break. Hold a wet tea bag to a canker sore, some doctors suggest. Black tea contains tannin, an astringent with pain-relieving power that's also found in some over-the-counter remedies.

Suck an antacid tablet. Antacids neutralize digestive juices and acids in the mouth that may aggravate sores or raw spots. Swishing a liquid antacid around your mouth will do the same.

TEETHING PAIN MAKES YOU CRY
Your baby is crying and fussing. He is drooling and gnawing on anything he can get his grubby little fists on. He must be cutting a tooth.

Actually, you can hardly miss with this diagnosis, says Stephen S. Moss, D.D.S., a New York University College of Dentistry professor of pediatric dentistry. Between the ages of six months and three years, your child "cuts" 20 teeth, so there's hardly a time when there's not a tooth coming into the mouth.

Teeth don't actually cut through the gums, Dr. Moss insists. Tooth eruption is a slow, gradual process many dentists believe is painless. The pain, if there is any, usually comes from inflamed gums around tiny new teeth, a result of the same bacteria that cause gum disease in adults, Dr. Moss says. "You can see the redness and puffiness in a baby's mouth, just like in an adult's."

He and other pediatric dentists teach parents to clean their kids' teeth twice a day. "Take a gauze square, and with about as much pressure as if you were removing nail polish, wipe the gums and wipe the erupting teeth," he recommends. "Parents clean one end of the baby with a great deal of glee and gusto. We dentists want equal time for the other end."

Dab it with a styptic pencil. Styptic pencils have a core of alum, a drying agent that helps stop bleeding from minor shaving cuts. Alum also helps to dry up blistery canker sores.

See also:

- "Numb It" on page 411.
- "The Chill Factor" below.

▶ PREVENTION PAIN-RELIEF PROGRAM

Most minor mouth sores simply fade away within two weeks or so. Those that persist deserve a doctor's attention, Dr. Rifkin says. You need to make sure you do not have

---

Multipurpose Relief

For: Toothache, Mouth Sores

THE CHILL FACTOR

Ah, ice. If nature hadn't invented it, some mad scientist would have, making a zillion bucks from its cooling properties.

There are a number of ways to use ice to lessen mouth pain, says Henry W. Finger, D.D.S., president of the Academy of General Dentistry. Press an ice chip onto tender canker sores or cold sores, or suck on ice to cool a burning tongue.

Some teeth recoil at the least hint of cold, but others calm down. Try ice massage on the *outside* of the jaw that contains the aching tooth.

Ice packs are invaluable for reducing swelling after root canal or dental surgery to remove impacted wisdom teeth, suggests Dr. Finger. Apply a bag of crushed ice or an ice pack to your cheek as soon after the surgery as possible, and use it off and on for 10 minutes at a time, he says. Be careful not to leave it on too long if your face is still numb from the anesthetic injection—you could get frostbite! Ice will also help to reduce pain once the anesthesia has worn off.

oral cancer, an infection, or a disease that is making itself known via your mouth.

See a dentist, Dr. Rifkin suggests. They are better trained to identify oral lesions. Some can do biopsies, but some may refer you to an oral surgeon for the biopsy. Antibiotics, topical steroid creams, or antiviral or antifungal drugs may be indicated, he says.

Blood tests may be warranted if a whole-body disease such as leukemia or diabetes is suspected. Blood tests may also reveal certain nutritional deficiencies, says Dr. Rifkin.

It can take some skill on a doctor's part to pinpoint the cause of your mouth problems. And sometimes the problem ends up being "managed" but not cured. Your symptoms are made tolerable, perhaps with something like a topical steroid cream, but they just seem to hang around. That kind of problem can be frustrating. If you're concerned about your treatment, says Dr. Rifkin, you may do well to make an appointment with an oral pathologist or faculty member in the department of oral medicine at a university-based dental school.

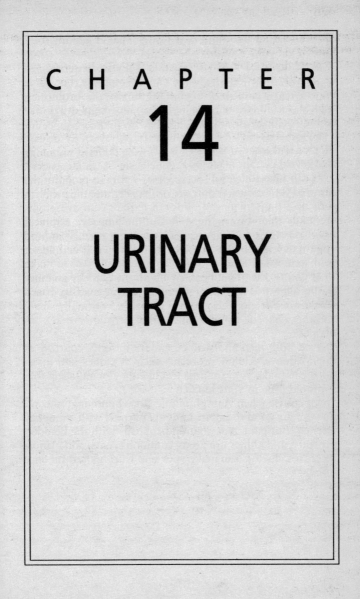

CHAPTER
14

URINARY
TRACT

Everyone knows how frustrating it is to have problems with your plumbing at home. Five minutes before Super Bowl kickoff you find out that a spectacular water show your spouse calls Old Faceful has erupted in your kitchen sink once again. Eventually the problem is solved, of course, but not before you've vented a lot of frustration and torn out enough hair to make a toupee for Telly Savalas.

That's how it is when things go wrong with the plumbing inside of you—your bladder, your kidneys, your prostate. All your life you've taken your internal faucets and pipes for granted, but when they act up, they're a pain in the . . . well, you know.

Other than squirming and shifting uncomfortably in your seat back in grade school until the teacher noticed your hand waving desperately in the air, you've had no problems. Until now.

If you're a woman, problems with the bladder and urethra are lumped together under the general heading of urinary tract infections. If you're a man, it's a normally small, chestnut-shaped gland—called the prostate—that's to blame.

And both men and women endure miseries courtesy of their kidneys. Kidney problems such as stones and infections can make your innards feel like they're imitating that ruptured pipe in your kitchen.

Of course when your plumbing stops humming, it won't do you any good to call in a plumber armed with a monkey wrench. But panic not. Painful problems with the bladder, prostate, and kidney are pretty common events, and in most instances, doctors can make your Old Faithful faithful once more.

GET PROFESSIONAL HELP IF:

- Your urinary symptoms are accompanied by:
    blood in your urine
    persistent fever
    chills or vomiting
    pain in the back, abdomen, or groin
- You have urinary problems or pain and you are pregnant

PAIN-FINDER CHART FOR THE URINARY TRACT

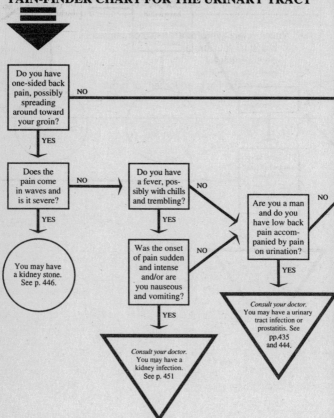

Do you have one-sided back pain, possibly spreading around toward your groin?

NO

YES

Does the pain come in waves and is it severe?

NO

YES

You may have a kidney stone. See p. 446.

Do you have a fever, possibly with chills and trembling?

NO

YES

Was the onset of pain sudden and intense and/or are you nauseous and vomiting?

NO

YES

Are you a man and do you have low back pain accompanied by pain on urination?

NO

YES

Consult your doctor. You may have a urinary tract infection or prostatitis. See pp.435 and 444.

Consult your doctor. You may have a kidney infection. See p. 451

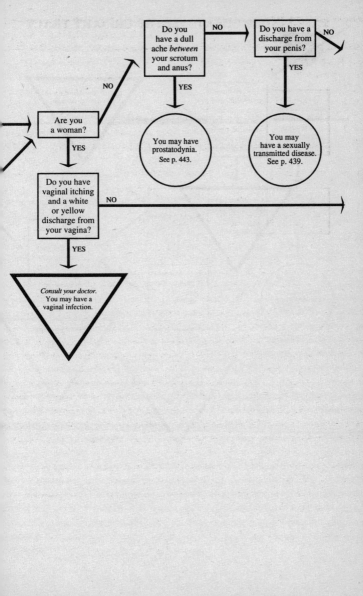

Do you
have a dull
ache *between*
your scrotum
and anus?

NO

Do you have a
discharge from
your penis?

NO

YES

NO

Are you
a woman?

YES

YES

You may have
prostatodynia.
See p. 443.

You may
have a sexually
transmitted disease.
See p. 439.

Do you have
vaginal itching
and a white
or yellow
discharge from
your vagina?

NO

YES

Consult your doctor.
You may have a
vaginal infection.

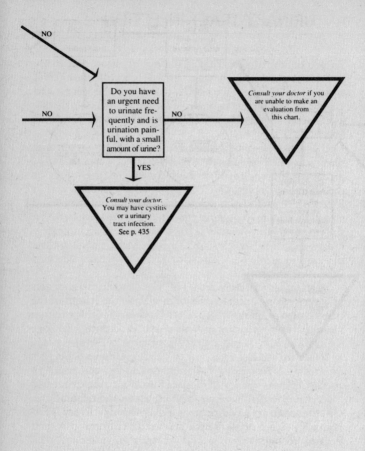

NO

NO

Do you have an urgent need to urinate frequently and is urination painful, with a small amount of urine?

NO

Consult your doctor if you are unable to make an evaluation from this chart.

YES

Consult your doctor. You may have cystitis or a urinary tract infection. See p. 435

URINARY TRACT INFECTION

To pee or not to pee. That is the big question that many people ask themselves when a urinary tract infection (UTI) strikes ... whether 'tis nobler to endure the slings and arrows of agonizing pain upon urination or to risk distending the bladder by holding the urine inside you till it hurts.

If you're a woman, the first tipoff of a UTI is that burning sensation when you urinate, says Richard J. Macchia, M.D., professor and chairman of the Department of Urology at the State University of New York Health Science Center at Brooklyn. Other symptoms may include incontinence and a need to urinate frequently. Pain in the waist area, between the ribs and hips, is not a UTI symptom; it may indicate a kidney infection, says Joseph Corriere, M.D., professor and director of urology at the University of Texas Medical School in Houston.

Men under 65 rarely get UTIs "because the prostate acts as a very strong antibacterial organ," and the length of the penis is also a deterrent, says Dr. Macchia. (For information about painful urination in males, see "Prostatitis" on page 441.) However, as men age, they also get these infections.

You'll never feel so alone as when you have a bladder infection—it isn't exactly something you like to confide to even your best friend or spouse. But don't think that Ma Nature has singled you out for these trials and tribulations. On the contrary, you're in good company. Every year, about 5 percent of all the women in this country visit their doctors to fight the pain and frustration caused by UTI, says Dr. Corriere.

Some women have a single infection and never have a recurrence, while others endure repeated episodes, he says.

Not even doctors know all the reasons that women get UTIs, says Bruce Block, M.D., medical director of the Shadyside Hospital Family Health Center in Pittsburgh. Sometimes UTIs are transmitted sexually, but something as common as wearing panty hose also can lead to infection, he says.

Plenty of other things also cause problems, says Dr. Corriere. People with diabetes seem to have an increased risk of UTI because diabetes leads to abnormal bladder functioning and urine retention, which in turn lead to bladder infections, he says.

As yet, medical science doesn't know why bacteria that occur naturally on a woman's vagina and anus wind up getting into the bladder and causing infection, says Dr. Corriere. Here's another unanswered question: Since studies show that some bacteria go up the urethra in most women, why do bacteria colonize and cause an infection in *some* women and not in others? When science finds an answer to those burning questions, perhaps UTIs will be gone PDQ.

➡ INSTANT RELIEF

Urinary tract infections are also a pain in the purse, says Dr. Corriere. UTIs are the second most common infectious disease after respiratory infections and are more expensive to treat, he says. The only redeeming thing about them is that they're fairly easy to treat with "an effective antibiotic," he adds. There are a few things you can do on your own, too.

Drink to your bladder's content. You can get some temporary pain relief by drinking plenty of fluids, thereby washing away some unwanted bacteria, says Dr. Block. Extra fluids "won't help if the infection is in the genital tract, but if it's in the urethra or bladder it will certainly help," he says. It may benefit some individuals to drink large quantities of juices rich in vitamin C (such as orange and cranberry juice) because they produce acidic urine, which can inhibit the growth of some organisms, says Dr. Macchia.

Stop Sudafed. In some cases, people who take decongestants like Sudafed for their sniffles can have a reaction resembling a UTI, says Dr. Block. "The medication can

MOCK UTIs

When is a urinary tract infection not a urinary tract infection?

This is not a funny riddle. The fact is that many women have an urgent need to urinate, a sense of incomplete voiding, allergies, and the pain and discomfort that traditionally come with a UTI—but they don't have one, says Richard J. Macchia, M.D., professor and chairman of the Department of Urology at the State University of New York Health Science Center at Brooklyn.

For lack of a precise term, Dr. Macchia calls this condition the lower tract irritability syndrome (LTI). He is trying to convince other physicians to adopt the term to spread awareness about this common ailment which he's identified in the United States, Africa, the Soviet Union, and "all over the world."

If a visit to the doctor rules out UTIs and "at least 30 other possible causes," a person may very well have LTI, says Dr. Macchia.

If a person has LTI and there is no identifiable cause, all the physician can do is try to help relieve the symptoms, says Dr. Macchia. Biofeedback is one therapy that seems to help. (See chapter 17.) As a last resort, some doctors have tried "surgical approaches in which impulses are fed into the nervous system that supplies feedback to the bladder to block these kinds of discomforts."

If you are one of the many women or the few men who have been sent away frustrated because doctors think there's nothing wrong with you, take heart. Pioneering work with LTI may lead to a definitive cure in the future.

cause frequent urination with cramping," he says. If you're taking Sudafed, try stashing it.

Make water in the water. Some doctors think that painful urination is made slightly less painful if you release the urine in a tub of bathwater.

See also:

- Chapter 26, on medications.

➤ PREVENTION PAIN-RELIEF PROGRAM

Some acute urinary tract problems go away on their own, says Dr. Block. But it's always wise to seek medical help, says Dr. Macchia, if a low-grade infection lasts for a few days or if you suspect your infection is sexually transmitted or caused by vigorous sexual activity—a condition known as cystitis (or more familiarly, the honeymoon disease). And any pregnant woman who experiences a UTI should see her doctor immediately.

UTIs should be treated by physicians with special sensitivity, says Dr. Block. Relationships could be ruined if one partner mistakenly believes the other has gotten a sexually related infection from someone else.

In addition to getting the right doctor, you have to be able to take charge of your own body, says Dr. Macchia.

Take Action, Stop Reactions

To get rid of some acute problems with nonsexual causes, ridding yourself of all possible irritants may clear things up naturally in a few days, says Dr. Block. Take panty hose, for example, which "can cause irritation, burning, and itching because they keep things moist and warm," says Dr. Block. Since some women must wear panty hose on the job, the doctor suggests that these garments be taken off as soon as practicable. "Switching to cotton undies whenever possible helps," he says.

Other common personal items can cause irritation or allergic reaction as well. These include bubble bath, soaps, douches, deodorants, and spermicides, notes Dr. Macchia. If using bubbles leads to UTI troubles, blow them off—the same goes for the other offenders, he says.

Another thing that is absolutely necessary is that a woman practice smart feminine hygiene, notes Dr. Block. Women who wipe improperly may put themselves at risk of infection by literally sweeping bacteria from the anal area into the urethra, he says. "You're supposed to wipe from front to back," he says. "If you're not doing that, by all means make a change."

STOP STDs

It's painful to urinate. You suspect that a love in your life may have left you with a sexually transmitted disease. What do you do?

You *must* see a doctor to get cured. Not only are sexually transmitted diseases (STDs) contagious, but possible complications include such things as infertility, says Richard J. Macchia, M.D., professor and chairman of the Department of Urology at the State University of New York Health Science Center at Brooklyn. You can help ease some of your discomfort while waiting for your appointment by drinking fluids until your urine is colorless, to wash away some of the bad-guy bacteria, he says, but the only cure is drugs.

Common STDs that cause painful urination are genital herpes (see page 386), chlamydia, gonorrhea, and trichomoniasis, says Bruce Block, M.D., medical director of the Shadyside Hospital Family Center in Pittsburgh.

A drug called metronidazole (Flagyl) is used to treat trichomoniasis, says Dr. Macchia. Untreated, the condition commonly causes inflammation of the uterine tubes, he adds.

In many cases gonorrhea can be cleared up by treatment with a simple, inexpensive antibiotic such as ampicillin, says Dr. Macchia. If you have a strain of gonorrhea that is resistant to drugs, a single injection of an antibiotic named Rocephin does the trick, he says.

Urethritis requires the doctor to treat for gonorrhea and chlamydia, says Dr. Block. Tetracycline is the treatment of choice for chlamydia, he says.

To prevent STDs from spreading, make sure that your partner also sees a doctor for treatment, says Dr. Block.

Make Sex Appealing

Repeated bladder infections caused by sexual activity may tempt some women to ponder joining a convent. After all, one study of young nuns found a very low instance of disease-causing bacteria, says Dr. Corriere. But if getting thee to a nunnery ain't your idea of funnery, don't despair. There are ways to make sadder bladders gladder.

Simply reducing the vigor of one's lovemaking by assuming less strenuous positions, such as female superior or lying side-by-side, may prevent bladder infections, says Dr. Block.

But the only way to make these bladder infections go away when they occur is with medication, says Dr. Block. He prescribes an antibiotic such as nitrofurantoin macro-crystals (Macrodantin). The treatment doesn't take long—just three days in many cases.

In complicated cases where the UTI refuses to take a hike, the doctor will probably call for additional tests.

"If this woman keeps getting infections, long-term treatment for three to six months may prevent them," says Dr. Block. "If the infection is due to a sexually transmitted disease, then treating her sexual partner as well sometimes stops the infectious game of tag."

Darn Diaphragm

There are a couple of studies that show women who use diaphragms are a bit more likely to get infections, says Dr. Block. "The diaphragm pushes up against the urethra if the device is too big and can cause some problems," he says.

"The solution is a refitting of the diaphragm or looking at other methods of birth control," says Dr. Block.

What's better than a diaphragm? A cover-up. Women who are sexually active, or who date a partner who is, should demand that their man wear a condom because so many dread infectious diseases can be sexually transmitted, says Dr. Block. "In terms of prevention, someone who's getting frequent genital infections will go a long way toward saving a lot of problems by using condoms," he says.

PROSTATITIS

Pity the poor prostate. When a healthy prostate plays its starring role in reproduction by preserving sperm long enough for conception to occur, no one applauds. But just let it get the least bit puffed up and inflamed, and men start complaining. No less than three million visits a year to urologists are the result of prostatitis.

Prostatitis—inflammation of the prostate gland—is generally diagnosed when a man has painful urination, says Dr. Macchia. (Urinary tract infections are relatively uncommon in men.)

Like the term UTI, prostatitis is really nothing more than a catchall term that applies to both bacterial and nonbacterial conditions affecting the prostate, says Dr. Macchia. In years to come researchers may ferret out and identify all the sub-causes, but because of a general lack of knowledge about this part of a man's anatomy, "we're blaming the prostate for a whole bunch of things," he says.

In many ways, a doctor has to be a sleuth the equal of Perry Mason to make a diagnosis. "The symptoms of bacterial and nonbacterial prostatitis are identical," says Stephen N. Rous, M.D., author of *The Prostate Book: Sound Advice on Symptoms and Treatment* and professor of surgery (urology) at Dartmouth Medical School in Hanover, New Hampshire. "The difference is that as its name suggests, one has bacteria to blame for your miseries and the other does not."

Not everyone who has prostatitis experiences the same symptoms. Many men have a feeling of pressure or discomfort in the area between the scrotum and anus, he says. Others complain that the pain seems to be way up inside the inner part of the penis where it joins the bladder or elsewhere in the pubic region.

Some men report discomfort at the beginning and/or end of urinating, says Dr. Rous. Others report a slight discharge. They may find a brownish stain about the size of a quarter in their underwear, he says.

With an acute bacterial infection in the prostate, a man may also have chills and fever, says Dr. Rous.

If you are diagnosed with prostatitis, be assured that you're not even remotely at risk of getting prostate cancer or an enlarged prostate as a result of your infection, says Dr. Macchia. Moreover, "there are many cases of prostatitis that are not related to sexual activity," he says. "Unless there's a discharge, the possibility of transmitting it to a partner is extremely remote."

On the other hand, "people have to understand that prostatitis can come back," says Dr. Macchia. "Treatment and the body's natural health mechanisms will get rid of the pain, but in a couple of months, it may come back."

Relapse rates even after 12 weeks of therapy can be as high as 40 percent, say doctors.

▶ INSTANT RELIEF

If there were a condition that deserved to be called "male troubles," prostatitis would be it. Here are some ways to ease the discomfort.

Try a hands-on approach. Nonbacterial prostatitis may possibly be caused by a famine-after-feast syndrome, says Dr. Rous. That's a polite way of describing the plight of a man who has suddenly been deprived of regular ejaculation.

"When a doctor takes a very careful history, he finds that the problem came on when their wives had surgery, or they became estranged from their wives," he says.

The simple solution if a partner is unavailable is masturbation, advises Dr. Rous. If religious or moral scruples prevent you from masturbating, see your priest or minister. (Such prohibitions may be set aside for medical reasons.) Alternately, your doctor can massage your prostate when the "ejaculate tends to get engorged," says Dr. Rous. He calls such therapy "chronic remunerative prostatitis" because it takes a load from the patient's wallet as well as his prostate.

Have a hot time tonight. "There's no question about it, heat helps some people," says Dr. Macchia. He recom-

EASING THE PAIN OF PROSTATODYNIA

One common painful condition that involves the prostate defies definition, says Stephen N. Rous, M.D., professor of surgery (urology) at Dartmouth Medical School in Hanover, New Hampshire. Prostatodynia, a term for a prostate condition whose suffix is derived from the Greek word for pain, is a mysterious "ache in the perineal area—the area between the scrotum and the anus," says Dr. Rous, author of *The Prostate Book: Sound Advice on Symptoms and Treatment.*

This is a condition that no one knows much about—except what doesn't cause it, says Dr. Rous. "There's no evidence of bacterial or nonbacterial prostatitis," he says, noting that occasionally prostatodynia is mistaken for these two conditions.

Sitz baths help many people reduce the pain, says Dr. Rous. To take a sitz bath, sit in a tub of hot water with your legs up over the sides of the tub. The idea is to concentrate the heat in the area of the pelvis.

Occasionally, doctors prescribe muscle relaxants to help ease the pain, says Dr. Rous.

mends an old-fashioned hot water bath "where you sit back in a tub and heat the central core of your body, especially the pelvis," he says. "Try to keep your upper body and your legs out of the water."

The main idea "is to bring heat to that area. It stimulates blood flow and has a lot of natural healing properties to it," he says.

▶ PREVENTION PAIN-RELIEF PROGRAM

Once a bout of painful urination causes you to seek medical care, your doctor may take a culture of prostate fluid, says Dr. Corriere. That culture helps the doctor determine what medications are appropriate, he says.

True bacterial prostatitis is much more difficult to clear up than are UTIs in women, says Dr. Rous. But it requires

PROSTATE IN A POOR STATE

Enlarged prostates cause a lot of inconvenience and frustration, but they're not painful—with one exception.

"If you can't urinate and you feel like you've got a lot of urine in you and it hurts like hell, you're probably a middle-aged or older man with an enlarged prostate who can't get the urine out," says Richard J. Macchia, M.D., professor and chairman of the Department of Urology at the State University of New York Health Science Center at Brooklyn. What has happened is that your chestnut-sized prostate has grown to the size of an orange or larger, he says. When the enlarged prostate presses on the tiny opening through which urine must pass on its way out of your body, you've got a painful problem.

This isn't something that happens overnight, says Dr. Macchia. Residual urine builds up over the years so that gradually more and more urine stays behind in your bladder.

Gradually, the bladder gets so distended that it, too, is two or three times its normal size, he says. This is particularly a danger in men who have diabetes because the sensory nerves in the bladder are already damaged, preventing them from feeling the urge to urinate, he notes.

Not being able to empty the bladder properly is a potentially serious condition that often leads to infection and could lead to death if not treated. You must seek immediate medical assistance, says Stephen N. Rous, M.D., author of *The Prostate Book: Sound Advice on Symptoms and Treatment* and professor of surgery (urology) at Dartmouth Medical School in Hanover, New Hampshire. Doctors will use a catheter to drain urine from your bladder and then must operate to reduce the size of the prostate, he says.

the same antibiotics: trimethoprimsulfamethoxazole (Bactrim, Septra) or norfloxacin (Noroxin). The course of treatment, however, is much longer—three to four weeks, says Dr. Corriere.

In extreme cases of bacterial prostatitis—that is, when stones are present in the prostate—your doctor may surgically remove the gland as the last-ditch solution to defeat the recurrent bacteria, say doctors.

There is no known sure-fire drug treatment for nonbacterial prostatitis, but some doctors cross their fingers and try to gain an edge by treating men for a chlamydia infection with tetracycline, says Dr. Corriere. Like chicken soup for a cold, it can't hurt and just might help.

KIDNEY STONES

Kidney stones. The very words can provoke scary shudders in anyone who has had them before. But if you're reading this section because you've got one, we're not telling you anything new.

AAAAARGGGHHHH! There you were having a wonderful time on vacation in the Bahamas when suddenly your side felt as if someone spiked your planter's punch with ground glass. AAAAARGGGHHHH! No matter what you do or what position you assume, the pain remains the same—simply unbear-AAAAHHHH!-ble.

What can you do? Seek medical help quickly, says Dr. Macchia. And consider yourself lucky. Many years ago, people simply had to live—and sometimes die—with these painful stones. Ben Franklin, for example, tolerated them for many, many years and went to his coffin with them.

These nasty little invaders don't always confine themselves to your kidneys. In fact, the term "kidney stone" is a generic term "for any stone in the urinary tract," says Dr. Macchia.

Sometimes kidney stones literally hit you where you live. For instance, so many people in the Carolinas get them for as yet unknown reasons that the area is known as "The Stone Belt," says Dr. Macchia. Similar stone belts are found in other parts of the United States and the rest of the world as well, he says.

➡️ **INSTANT RELIEF**

While you're waiting to see a physician, here is a relief measure to try.

Turn on the heat. Immerse yourself in a hot bath or apply a heating pad "to relieve some of the pain," suggests Thomas C. McNamara, M.D., co-medical director of the Mid-Atlantic Stone Center, Garden State Community Center, in Marlton, New Jersey.

▶ PREVENTION PAIN-RELIEF PROGRAM

If you have a stone, here's one bit of news that ought to bring you some comfort. "Most people who have stones pass them," says Dr. McNamara.

Unless the stone is blocking the ureter (the duct that carries urine from the kidney to the bladder), doctors play it conservatively, monitoring the urine to see if the stone is flushed out naturally, says Simon Saada, M.D., chief of urology and associate director of the Department of Surgery at Victory Memorial Hospital in Brooklyn. "We follow the patient to see if the stone passes," he says.

Treatment consists of increased fluid intake to help the stone pass and the use of a heating pad or immersion in hot water to ease the pain, says Dr. McNamara. "Otherwise, you just go on about your normal business," he says.

In some cases he prescribes nonsteroidal anti-inflammatory drugs. "There is some evidence, although it's not proven, that these may relax the ureter, may open things up, and may allow the stone to pass," says Dr. McNamara.

Solving Calculus Problems

What if you're one of the few, the not-so-proud, whose kidney stone insists on staying put? In almost all cases where a patient is in relatively good health, doctors need to remove the stone, says Dr. Macchia.

"It's a rare patient that you leave the stone in," says Dr. Macchia. "The trouble with stones is that they tend to grow, multiply, and can actually destroy the kidney."

Before a doctor can remove a stone, he or she must first find it.

If you have a kidney stone, quite often your pain gives a doctor all the clues he or she needs to make a diagnosis. The intensity of the pain often gives doctors their first hint as to where the stone is hiding, says Dr. Macchia.

"You get the most pain not when the stone is in the kidney but when it gets stuck in the little tube that connects the kidney to the bladder," he says.

"The stone blocks the outflow of urine and the urine backs up and distends the ureter, causing pain."

The pain is so great for some patients that immediate hospitalization is required, says Dr. McNamara. "Some people need oral analgesics, and some need injectable narcotics," he says.

Your doctor will do tests and x-rays to verify that you indeed do have kidney stones, says Dr. Macchia. Certain back pains, muscular aches, and pain in the ribs and muscles over the kidneys can mimic the pain of kidney stones, he warns. One indication that a stone is present is if the pain spreads all the way to the genitals, he says.

High-Tech Ways to Smash Stones

Fortunately, modern science has found new ways of treating the condition that leave no stone unspurned. Lithotripsy (shock wave treatment) is the treatment of choice for most people whose stubborn stones won't depart on their own, says Dr. McNamara. "It is the treatment of choice in 95 percent of stones in the kidney that need to be treated," he says. In only about 2 percent of cases, where the stone is positioned in an inaccessible or difficult place, must the physician resort to operating on someone, he notes.

What is lithotripsy? Basically, it is a procedure that uses "high-pressure shock waves that are transmitted through water and focused with high energy on the stone," says Dr. McNamara. "The energy of the shock wave is greater than the strength of the stone and therefore it breaks into little pieces."

The devices have electrodes "which we direct with a computer," says Dr. Saada. "We focus the device in the appropriate position for the shock waves to converge on the stone from all directions."

One advantage of shock wave treatment is that it can even destroy stones that are hidden by the person's bones. "If the patient's stone lies on top of or in front of a bone like the pelvis or a vertebra, we reposition the patient and do some maneuvering to free the path of bone so the waves will go to the stone," he says.

As a result of this type of wonderful new antistone device, invasive surgeries with their long, painful healing periods are almost a thing of the past, says Dr. Saada.

If you live in an isolated area that doesn't have a machine, don't despair. "If an institution doesn't have a machine, by law it has to tell the patient that such a machine exists," says Dr. Saada.

One of the nice things about the shock wave procedure is that it's done without anesthesia, says Dr. Saada. "We don't give anesthesia—we give minimum sedation," he says. "The patient lies comfortably on the table, and we fragment the stone."

News from the Stonefront

One of the nice things medical science can do for you is analyze your stone fragments after they vacate your premises to see what they are made of. This information is helpful for those patients whose diet is related to the onset of stone disease, says Dr. Saada. "Depending upon the analysis, you tell the patient what to avoid," he says.

Doctors cannot say with certainty what is causing your stone while it's still embedded in your body, says Dr. McNamara. "You can get some idea initially of what it may be, but you can't tell definitively before they get rid of the stone and you have it analyzed," he says. If your stone is caused by your diet, you can expect your doctor to tell you what foods to avoid, he adds.

Some stones might have a calcium base, leading the doctor to advise you to avoid certain milk products, says Dr. Saada. Also to be avoided is a substance called oxalate, which is found in beans, broccoli, and spinach, he says.

Theoretically, people who take vast quantities of vitamin C supplements also put themselves at risk for stones because the vitamin is converted to oxalates inside you, says Dr. Corriere. "It could cause kidney stones, but very rarely," he says.

Block Those Stones

The best bet against stones is prevention, says Dr. Macchia. People who have had a stone or are at risk because they run in the family are advised to drink between 1 and 1½ quarts of fluids a day, roughly the equivalent of up to eight 8-ounce glasses, says Dr. McNamara. He prefers that people drink water as opposed to certain beverages, "because some fluids (such as fruit juices with ascorbic acid) can contribute to stones," he says.

Rather than spend your hours trying to count the number of glasses you swill, try Dr. Macchia's more practical way of making certain that you don't get dehydrated. He shows his patients a yellow laboratory report. "I say, 'If your urine always looks like this, you're not drinking enough fluids,'" he says. "Your urine should look like water—that's a reasonably good indicator of how much fluid you're taking."

KIDNEY INFECTIONS

If you've got a true kidney infection, you won't have to wonder twice about whether or not you're sick, says Dr. Corriere. The symptoms are as clear as the nose on an anteater's face.

If you've got a true infection in the kidney, most of the time you'll have intense pain in your side, chills, and a fever of 102° or 103°F, says Dr. Corriere. "There's no question that something bad is going on," he says. "You should see a doctor right away."

Failing to see a doctor can lead to serious complications, says Dr. Macchia.

"Kidney infections can lead to destruction of the kidney, hypertension, kidney abscesses, and a whole bunch of other bad things," says Dr. Rous.

Infections in the kidney are more common than many people think, he says. People particularly at risk include those with diabetes, steroid users, anyone with a decreased ability to ward off disease because of a poorly functioning immune system, and those whose urine tends to back up into the bladder.

▶ INSTANT RELIEF

There is no instant relief for kidney infections. "A lot of doctors think you should treat kidney infections for at least two weeks," says Dr. Corriere.

▶ PREVENTION PAIN-RELIEF PROGRAM

A kidney problem is much more complicated than a simple bladder infection, and therefore the period of treatment is much longer, says Dr. Corriere.

Because people with kidney infections tend to be feverish, doctors try to fight dehydration by having the person drink lots of fluids, says Dr. Corriere. In addition, diagnostic tests will determine whether there is some abnormality of the kidney that allows infections to develop, he notes.

But the nuts and bolts of treatment are antibiotics, pure and simple, says Dr. Corriere.

"Fortunately, kidney infections are very effectively treated," says Dr. Macchia. A variety of antibiotics can be prescribed, but two of the most common choices are ciprofloxacin (Cipro) and norfloxacin (Noroxin).

CHAPTER 15

WHOLE BODY

PAIN-FINDER CHART FOR THE WHOLE BODY

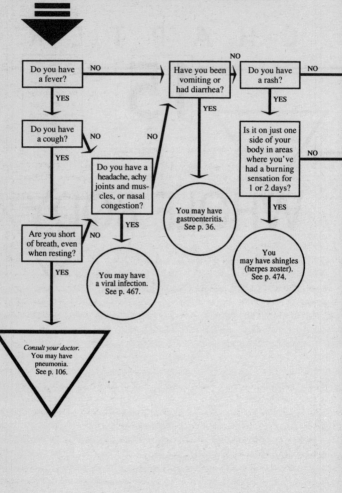

Do you have a fever?

NO →

Have you been vomiting or had diarrhea?

Do you have a rash?

NO →

NO ↑

YES ↓

Do you have a cough?

NO →

YES ↓

Do you have a headache, achy joints and muscles, or nasal congestion?

NO ↑

YES ↓

You may have gastroenteritis. See p. 36.

Is it on just one side of your body in areas where you've had a burning sensation for 1 or 2 days?

NO →

YES ↓

Are you short of breath, even when resting?

NO ↑

YES ↓

You may have a viral infection. See p. 467.

You may have shingles (herpes zoster). See p. 474.

Consult your doctor. You may have pneumonia. See p. 106.

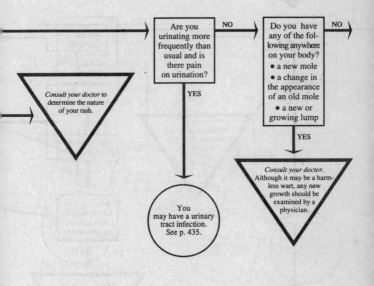

Consult your doctor to determine the nature of your rash.

Are you urinating more frequently than usual and is there pain on urination?

NO

YES

You may have a urinary tract infection. See p. 435.

Do you have any of the following anywhere on your body?
• a new mole
• a change in the appearance of an old mole
• a new or growing lump

NO

YES

Consult your doctor. Although it may be a harmless wart, any new growth should be examined by a physician.

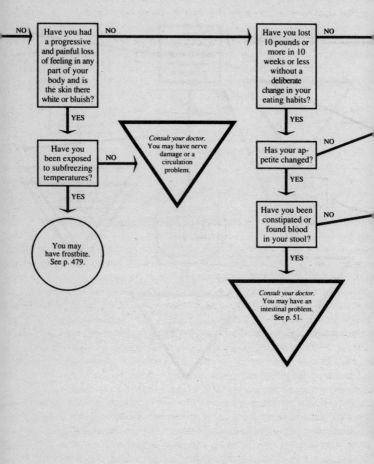

NO →

Have you had a progressive and painful loss of feeling in any part of your body and is the skin there white or bluish?

NO →

Have you lost 10 pounds or more in 10 weeks or less without a deliberate change in your eating habits?

NO →

↓ YES

↓ YES

Have you been exposed to subfreezing temperatures?

NO →

Consult your doctor. You may have nerve damage or a circulation problem.

Has your appetite changed?

NO →

↓ YES

↓ YES

You may have frostbite. See p. 479.

Have you been constipated or found blood in your stool?

NO →

↓ YES

Consult your doctor. You may have an intestinal problem. See p. 51.

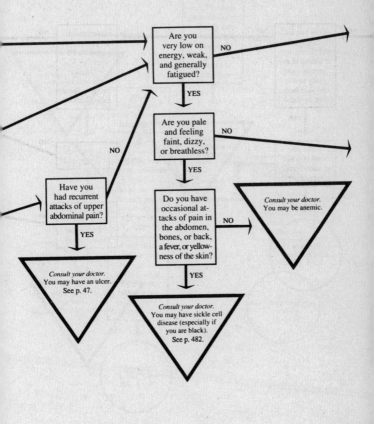

Are you very low on energy, weak, and generally fatigued?

NO

YES

Are you pale and feeling faint, dizzy, or breathless?

NO

YES

NO

Have you had recurrent attacks of upper abdominal pain?

YES

Do you have occasional attacks of pain in the abdomen, bones, or back, a fever, or yellowness of the skin?

NO

YES

Consult your doctor.
You may be anemic.

Consult your doctor.
You may have an ulcer.
See p. 47.

Consult your doctor.
You may have sickle cell disease (especially if you are black).
See p. 482.

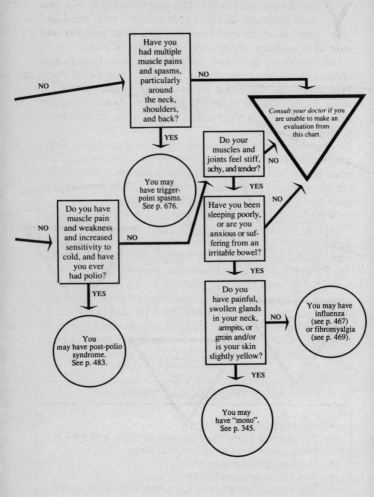

NO →

Have you
had multiple
muscle pains
and spasms,
particularly
around
the neck,
shoulders,
and back?

NO →

Consult your doctor if you
are unable to make an
evaluation from
this chart.

YES ↓

Do your
muscles and
joints feel stiff,
achy, and tender?

NO →

YES ↓

You may
have trigger-
point spasms.
See p. 676.

Do you have
muscle pain
and weakness
and increased
sensitivity to
cold, and have
you ever
had polio?

NO →

Have you been
sleeping poorly,
or are you
anxious or suf-
fering from an
irritable bowel?

NO →

YES ↓

YES ↓

You
may have post-polio
syndrome.
See p. 483.

Do you
have painful,
swollen glands
in your neck,
armpits, or
groin and/or
is your skin
slightly yellow?

NO →

You may have
influenza
(see p. 467)
or fibromyalgia
(see p. 469).

YES ↓

You may
have "mono".
See p. 345.

Your whole body aches. Not just your head. Not just your stomach. Not just your feet. It's your head *and* your stomach *and* your feet *and* your muscles *and* your skin *and* just about every other part of you.

At least that's the way it seems. Sometimes the pain zips around from one place to another like your Great Aunt Tilly when she's transmitting the latest family quarrel: It stops for a chat by your elbow, moves down the street toward your wrist, then slips over to your thumb for a prolonged discussion.

Then again, the pain may seem to be distributed along a network of exquisitely tender points scattered throughout your entire body. You may feel like you're strung with a set of internal Christmas tree lights flashing messages of pain from one dazzling hot spot to another.

What's causing your pain? People always fear, of course, that it's cancer. But pain that travels indiscriminately through your arms—and sometimes your head, back, and legs—could be caused by a fever-inducing virus like the flu. Pain that radiates out from a network of tender spots scattered throughout your body might be due to fibromyalgia, a term that literally means "muscle pain." Pain that comes on explosively in your chest or abdomen can be triggered by sickle cell disease, and pain that lies just at the surface of your body could be the result of sunburn, frostbite, or shingles.

GET PROFESSIONAL HELP IF:

- You have difficulty breathing
- You develop a new mole or lump or notice a change in the appearance of an old mole or lump
- You have blood in your stool
- You have a persistent fever
- Your skin is blistered, blue, hard, and painful after having been exposed to subfreezing temperatures

CANCER

Cancer pain can strike at any time during the disease. It's an early symptom in 40 to 50 percent of those with cancer of the breast, ovary, prostate, colon, or rectum and in approximately 20 percent of those with cancer of the uterus or cervix. It occurs in 70 percent of those whose cancer is terminal.

What triggers the pain? Seventy percent is caused by a tumor's invasion of neighboring nerves and bones, its obstruction of nearby blood vessels and organs, or the swelling and inflammation it triggers in surrounding tissue. Fifteen percent is caused by the chemotherapy, radiation, and surgery that doctors use to fight the disease. And another 15 percent is caused by miscellaneous problems—an underlying arthritis, for example—that vary from person to person.

Fortunately, even when a cancer isn't curable, the pain generally is.

➡ INSTANT RELIEF

Cancer pain can be acute, chronic, or both. When it's chronic (long-term), your doctor will probably suggest a combination of the treatments listed in the "Prevention Pain-Relief Program" on page 462. But when it's acute— when it unexpectedly breaks through the pain relief you've obtained from ongoing treatment—then one or another of the following techniques may bring relief. Keep in mind, however, that these techniques are in addition to—not instead of—any treatment your doctor may have prescribed.

Ask to be touched. Many scientists feel that pain can be decreased or increased as it travels from peripheral nerve fibers through a "gating" mechanism on its way to the spinal cord and brain, says Sally Weinrich, R.N., Ph.D., associate professor of nursing at the University of South Carolina in Columbia. Things like anxiety can apparently open the gate so that pain messages travel up the spine to the brain, while things like relaxation and massage apparently close it.

To see whether or not massage would close the pain gate for people with cancer, Dr. Weinrich arranged for female nurses to give back massages to 14 people who were hospitalized for cancer treatment. Their backs were massaged in a slow, continuous manner for 10 minutes. Their pain was measured on a scale of one to ten before the massage, immediately afterward, an hour later, and an hour after that.

The result? In men, the pain disappeared in some and was significantly reduced in others—an effect that lasted for 2 hours or more. Interestingly, the more pain these men had before the massage, the more likely they were to experience relief afterward.

Women, unfortunately, were not so lucky. The massage did not affect their pain, although, as Dr. Weinrich notes, women had lower levels of pain initially in contrast to the men. She is unsure whether the prior lower level of pain in the women or the gender effect (females giving females back rubs) is the reason for the lack of significant pain reduction in women.

Relax. The anxiety, stress, and physical inactivity that sometimes come with cancer can tense muscles throughout the body and cause them to ache. For this type of pain, doctors say, progressive muscle relaxation can frequently untense the muscles and relieve the pain. (See Chapter 22.)

Try self-hypnosis. Some years ago, researchers at Stanford University studied 86 women who had breast cancer that had spread to other parts of the body, separating them into two groups. Fifty of the women joined a support group and were taught a form of self-hypnosis in which they learned how to evoke images that created competing sensations to pain, such as heat, cold, or numbness. The other 36 women received only routine care.

The result? Women in the support group who used hypnosis had only *half* the pain experienced by women who received routine care. These same patients also felt less anxiety and depression.

See also:

- Chapter 22, on hypnosis, relaxation, and meditation.
- Chapter 30, on support groups.

➡ PREVENTION PAIN-RELIEF PROGRAM

Ninety to 95 percent of those who have cancer can continue to lead an active, comfortable life, says Michael H. Levy, M.D., Ph.D., co-director of the Pain Management Center at Philadelphia's Fox Chase Cancer Center. (The other 5 to 10 percent need not experience pain, but the drugs required to prevent it keep them heavily sedated.)

Unfortunately, despite doctors' ability to keep pain at bay, most studies indicate that between 50 and 70 percent of those who have cancer—including those who are under the care of a physician—experience considerable pain.

Why? Because medical schools often do not teach students even the most basic principles of managing cancer pain, say researchers who review what doctors study. Moreover, of 11 major textbooks on cancer, only two have chapters on controlling pain.

A survey done by the United Nations World Health Organization reveals that doctors habitually underprescribe, underdose, and incorrectly time medication designed to relieve cancer pain.

Narcotics Don't Mean Addiction

Complicating the problem is the unfounded fear among both patients and physicians that people with cancer who take narcotics will become addicts. In fact, for some reason that scientists don't fully understand, people with cancer rarely become addicted.

In a study at Memorial Sloan-Kettering Cancer Center in New York, for example, researchers prescribed narcotics over a four- to seven-year period for 19 patients with chronic pain. The therapy became problematic in only two individuals—both of whom had a history of drug abuse.

In a second, larger study at Sloan-Kettering, researchers prescribed narcotics for 100 people who had cancer pain. A drug problem developed in 6 people who had "significant psychiatric disease." In other words, they possibly couldn't control any other aspect of their lives, either.

Get the Right Kind of Help

The first step in relieving cancer pain should be to find a knowledgeable team of cancer specialists, says Dr. Levy. "No one clinician can really provide total comfort, because even if he or she gets the right prescriptions, cancer pain patients need a tremendous amount of support and education that's primarily done by skilled health professionals called 'pain oncology nurses,' " he says.

These nurses are ten years ahead of other cancer professionals in both education and commitment to relieving cancer pain, says Dr. Levy. Pain team nurses are available in the middle of the night, on weekends, and on holidays. You can call them at any time. Your pain is their first concern, and they know all the tricks to make you feel better. They know whether or not you can take another 20 milligrams of a painkiller, whether or not a walk after dinner will aggravate the pain, whether or not a grandchild's visit will make you feel better or worse.

"They're really the glue that holds cancer treatment together," says Dr. Levy.

Target the Pain

Once you've selected a cancer center, you and your team of cancer specialists can concentrate on getting rid of your pain. And the best way to cure the pain is to cure the disease, says Dr. Levy. Surgery, radiation, chemotherapy, and hormone therapy are all methods used to get rid of a tumor or, failing that, to reduce its size and its effects on surrounding nerves and organs.

The next best way is to figure out exactly what's triggering the pain. Has the tumor invaded a bone? Is it pinching a nerve? Is it causing swelling in an adjacent area? Once this is determined, doctors then can target the specific problem.

In pain caused by cancer spreading to a bone—the most common pain in advancing cancer—the pain itself is triggered by damage to the bone, irritation of the nerves around the bone, and inflammation.

Fortunately, much of this pain can be modified at its source by using the same anti-inflammatory drugs—aspirin and ibuprofen, for example—that are used to treat the inflammatory process in arthritis, says Dr. Levy. These drugs not only subdue inflammation and relieve pain, they also seem to modify the destructive process going on in the bones themselves.

Climbing the Analgesic Ladder

Sometimes anti-inflammatory drugs are given in combination with radiation, which is particularly effective in eliminating bone pain, or in combination with hormones, which are particularly effective in eliminating pain due to breast and prostate cancer, says Dr. Levy.

For other types of cancer, anti-inflammatory drugs are frequently given alone or, as the cancer advances, in combination with gradually increasing strengths of narcotics. Your doctor may begin with a weak narcotic such as codeine, for example, and move very gradually up the analgesic ladder toward a more potent narcotic such as morphine.

Keep in mind, however, that a major consideration in controlling cancer pain is balancing comfort and function, says Dr. Levy. You don't want pain, but you don't want to lie around like a zombie, either. Too much of a narcotic—or the wrong narcotic—can rob you of the ability to think and act clearly. Too little—or the wrong narcotic—can keep you in pain.

A key factor in maintaining your pain/function equilibrium is in taking medication on a regular schedule, rather than on an "as needed" basis. In general, says Dr. Levy, both short- and long-acting narcotics are used to keep you free of pain around the clock.

Breakthrough pain—pain that breaks through the relief provided by a long-acting drug—can be treated with a short-acting supplement that provides an extra measure of relief. Supplements come in pills, suppositories, or liquids. If you find yourself using a supplement more than once or twice a day, cautions Dr. Levy, that's your cue to check with your doctor about changing the long-acting narcotic to a stronger form or dose.

There's absolutely no need for you to "grin and bear it," emphasizes Dr. Levy. Unfortunately, he adds, some people with cancer do, because to admit they have more pain is to admit their cancer is getting worse.

Fighting Nerve Pain

Narcotics and anti-inflammatory drugs are not the only medications used to alleviate cancer pain, says Dr. Levy. Steroids are frequently used to alleviate the swelling that aggravates nerves when they're being crowded by a tumor. Nerve pain characterized by bursts of pain or a "shooting" feeling is frequently treated with anticonvulsants such as Tegretol. Just as an anticonvulsant reduces nerve conduction in seizure disorders such as epilepsy, says Dr. Levy, so does it reduce the conduction of nerve pain in cancer.

Pain that is characterized by a "burning" feeling, however, particularly if it lasts two or three months, is frequently treated with antidepressants, he explains. Antidepressants in this case treat pain, not depression. They are particularly helpful in reducing the pain of nerve damage caused directly by tumors, surgery to remove tumors, or chemotherapy, adds Dr. Levy.

Surgery Can Block Intractable Pain

For the 5 to 10 percent of people in whom pain is not relieved by drug therapy, nerve blocks and other surgical procedures can be a godsend, says Dr. Levy. Drug delivery systems—pumps, for example—deliver morphine directly into the spinal fluid. Nerve fibers carrying pain can be selectively destroyed by chemicals or heat to prevent them from carrying the pain messages to the pain centers in the brain. Such pain-relief measures frequently also allow people who must take heavy doses of narcotics to reduce the amount of medication they use. For some, adds Dr. Levy, this means freedom from the fog of sedation and a new lease on life.

"We have one fellow who's had his pump in for two years," says Dr. Levy. "His big issue was that he had so much pain and needed so much medication that he couldn't function. He wanted to go to the golf course. And now the pump has made that possible."

Altering the Perception of Pain

Although drugs are the mainstay of cancer pain prevention and treatment, relaxation exercises and guided imagery are also used to help patients deal with their reaction to pain, says Dr. Levy. "If someone has deep bone pain that they react to with a muscle spasm that puts more pull on that bone and makes their pain worse, for example, then relaxation exercises can be helpful," he says. (See chapter 22.)

Music therapy has also proved helpful in reducing the perception of pain, says Susan Beck, Ph.D., a research assistant professor at the University of Utah's Oncology Nursing Graduate Program. In a preliminary study of 15 people with cancer, Dr. Beck found that 45 minutes of taped music— whatever kind people like best—could greatly decrease pain in about half the study participants and reduce it at least partially in 75 percent.

"For a small group, that's a good percentage," says Dr. Beck. As one woman said, "When the tape was on, I totally lost myself in the music and couldn't find my pain."

FLU

The minute it hits, you know. Your head starts to throb. Your eyes start to hurt. Your muscles start to ache. Why, oh *why*, didn't you get that flu shot like you meant to? Now you're going to pay the price. The latest version of influenza has hit America's shores and you've inhaled it. It's moved in and set up housekeeping. And it will take your immune system somewhere between seven and ten days to round up all those billions of little viruses and dispatch them.

▶ INSTANT RELIEF

The pain that trudges in and out of your muscles during the flu disappears only when your immune system gets the bug under control.

Take an analgesic. In the meantime, taking a couple of acetaminophen (Tylenol) or some other analgesic will help relieve the pain.

See also:

- Chapter 26, on medications.

▶ PREVENTION PAIN-RELIEF PROGRAM

There are three different forms of influenza—A, B, and C. They all seem to be related at the molecular level, but the one that most of us actually encounter is type A, a microscopic quick-change artist that can alter its appearance every time scientists think they have a good enough description to spot it and shoot it down. They take its measure, develop a new vaccine, and—voilá!—it puts on a new disguise.

This unique ability has made influenza a disease that has plagued the world for centuries. There have been 31 pandemics of respiratory disease attributed to the influenza virus since the year 1510—five of which have occurred in the twentieth century alone.

Fortunately, protection from the latest virus is always only a vaccination away, says Paul Perlman, M.D., associate professor of medicine at East Tennessee State University in Johnson City. Every summer, American scientists study the latest strains of flu, then develop a vaccine that will help your immune system fight them.

New vaccines are usually available in the fall, adds Dr. Perlman. People who should be vaccinated annually include anyone over six months of age who is at risk of getting a severe case or developing complications such as pneumonia, those over age 65, those with certain chronic illnesses, residents of nursing homes and other chronic-care facilities, and those who work in such institutions. People who are allergic to eggs should *not* get the vaccine, since scientists use eggs in making them.

If you *do* forget to get the vaccine and come down with the bug, a prescription for amantadine hydrochloride from your doctor can lessen the length and severity of your illness, says Dr. Perlman. The pain goes away when the fever goes away, so anything that speeds the flu bug on its way hastens pain away as well.

Aspirin or acetaminophen (Tylenol) can also help relieve aches, pain, and fever in an adult. For children under 18, aspirin should be avoided because of its association with a deadly neurological syndrome called Reye's syndrome. Antibiotics should *not* be taken for flu, because they do absolutely no good, adds Dr. Perlman.

If fever or pain lasts for more than seven days, or if you develop wheezing or shortness of breath, see your doctor, says Dr. Perlman. Your flu may be triggering a secondary infection such as pneumonia or bronchitis.

FIBROMYALGIA

The condition has been around for years under various names: generalized tension myalgia, fibrositis, and myofascial pain syndrome are just a sampling. What they all refer to, and what doctors have only recently started calling *fibromyalgia*, is a condition that still has doctors baffled: a network of 11 or more exquisitely tender spots scattered throughout the body from the base of your skull to your knee, with aching, pain, and stiffness scattered right along with them.

What causes all this misery? As doctors like to say when they can't figure out what's going on, "the pathophysiology is uncertain." One theory is that a muscle spasm or tension triggers the pain. Another is that a deficiency in a brain-to-body messenger—serotonin, the neurotransmitter—results in scrambled pain messages.

But the hottest theory right now, says Jeffrey M. Thompson, M.D., a physical medicine specialist at the Mayo Clinic, is based on the knowledge that muscles contain nerves that are activated by pressure. Normally these nerves transmit pain only when they're under heavy pressure, says Dr. Thompson. But if the muscles have been exposed to some sort of microscopic injury—sitting all day at a desk, for example—the muscles release a substance that makes the nerves hypersensitive.

Pull on a shirt and a bundle of nerve fibers in your shoulder muscle will cry out in pain. Button your collar and a bundle of nerve fibers in your neck will swear it's a noose. Take a deep breath and the nerve fibers in your chest muscles will scream that you've been stabbed.

Unfortunately, adds Dr. Thompson, these hypersensitive nerves can get muscles into such a habit of overreacting that they remain in what amounts to an almost constant state of contraction. And—ow!—that hurts.

▶ INSTANT RELIEF

Pain relief in fibromyalgia has two steps, says Dr. Thompson. First, the muscles are gently encouraged to unkink themselves and relax—as in the following instant-relief techniques. Then, as described in the "Prevention Pain-Relief Program," the muscles are retrained so that they stop overreacting.

Use a high-tech washcloth. Pick up a heat pack from your local drugstore, soak it in hot water, wrap it in towels, and put it on the area that hurts, says Dr. Thompson. The heat pack is made of a special material that holds water at an even temperature for an hour.

Follow your fibers. Use your fingertips to trace the path of muscles in the area where you hurt, says Dr. Thompson, then massage them. Press deep into the tissue, but always follow the direction in which the muscle fibers travel. And don't be surprised if you encounter small bumps or nodules. Years ago therapists used to really focus on these spots and try to smooth them out, says Dr. Thompson. Today therapists know that massaging the entire muscle works as well.

See also:

- Chapter 21, on hot and cold therapy.
- Chapter 24, on massage.
- Chapter 29, on physical therapy.
- Chapter 33, on trigger-point therapy.

▶ PREVENTION PAIN-RELIEF PROGRAM

Once you've managed to relax the contracted muscles through a combination of heat and massage, the next step is to retrain those muscles so they remember how to work properly, says Dr. Thompson. The idea is to stretch them out, usually in a kind of diagonal path, so that they won't habitually contract and cause pain.

If your shoulder hurts, for example, try stretching one arm out and across your body until you feel it pull in your back and shoulder blades, says Dr. Thompson. Then stretch

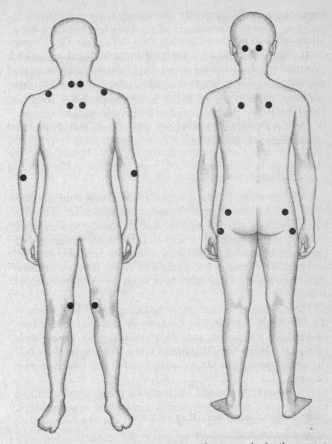

Although you can feel muscle aches throughout your body, there are a number of specific tender points associated with fibromyalgia that can help your doctor make an accurate diagnosis. If your muscle pain seems to concentrate in these areas, let your doctor know.

the other arm. Work gently and slowly from one muscle to another, until you've moved all the muscles that have been affected by pain.

Do these stretches a couple of times a day for a week, says Dr. Thompson; and as your pain lessens, start to move toward an aerobic kind of conditioning program—either walking, swimming, or using a stationary bike. Keep in mind, however, that you need to keep your muscles relaxed. If you find yourself tensing up, pause and stretch the affected muscles, he advises.

Activate Your Natural Painkillers

Exercise provides a repetitive pattern that gets your muscles back into a normal, smooth motion, explains Dr. Thompson. It erases all the painful habits these muscles have learned, and it probably releases endorphins—your body's naturally occurring painkillers—into the area. Eventually, adds Dr. Thompson, you should be doing aerobic exercise three times a week for anywhere from 20 to 60 minutes at a shot.

How effective is exercise in reducing pain? In a study at the University of Western Ontario in Canada, researchers divided 38 volunteers into two groups. One group rode stationary bikes for 50 minutes three times a week, while the other group did simple stretches for the same amount of time.

The result? At the end of 20 weeks, those who had biked their way to fitness reported a significant improvement. Almost 40 percent reported they had cut the intensity of their pain in half.

Listen to Your Body

Biofeedback is another way to both retrain and relax your muscles, says Dr. Thompson. In a study at the University of Parma in Italy, for example, 15 people with fibromyalgia practiced using biofeedback to relax their muscles. They each used progressive muscle relaxation techniques for 20 minutes, twice a week, as the biofeedback machine reported their level of muscular tension.

After seven and a half weeks, 56 percent of the study participants reported a significant reduction in pain. In a follow-up, researchers confirmed the effects of biofeedback and demonstrated that the pain relief engendered by a single biofeedback training course lasted for several months, provided that the people continued using the relaxation techniques at home.

SHINGLES

Like an alien parasite, the chickenpox virus you had as a child hides inside your body, patiently, insidiously waiting for a chance to once again rear its ugly little head. When that chance comes, it erupts as a band of angry blisters. This viral revival is called shingles, herpes zoster, or varicella zoster. This third name comes from the bug causing the condition, the varicella virus, and its likely area of attack—your midsection. (In Greek, *zoster* means "belt.")

Simply getting older is all it takes to be at risk for shingles. The immunity you developed against the virus by having childhood chickenpox drops as you age. People whose immune systems are weakened by steroids, cancer treatments, AIDS, or leukemia help to make up the 300,000 new cases of shingles each year.

Herpes zoster is *not* just a week or two of scratching and crabbiness. If it were, no doubt most of us could survive quite nicely, given a few days of tender loving care. For some, the blisters are the beginning of a bout of constant, burning pain, called postherpetic neuralgia.

"Besides burning, people with shingles often have jabbing, knifelike pain. The pain gives them absolutely no relief," says Marilyn Kassirer, M.D., neurologist at the Veterans Administration Outpatient Clinic in Boston.

There *are* ways to ease the hurting, though. And the best news is that even for most people with long, lingering pain, the condition eventually eases on its own, as nerves heal and return to normal.

▶ INSTANT RELIEF

See a doctor as soon as you realize something's wrong, especially if you suspect shingles on your face. (Shingles can cause blindness if it involves your eye.) Once you're receiving medical care, you can use these remedies to help ease the pain of shingles or, as indicated, postherpetic neuralgia.

Shrivel up and dry. Use a drying solution to make blisters disappear. Drying them up may help relieve pain, since the fluid inside the blisters contains pain-producing hormones known as prostaglandins. When treated in a hospital, shingles blisters are often opened and swabbed with an antibacterial and drying lotion, says Boni Elewski, M.D., assistant professor of dermatology at Case Western Reserve University in Cleveland.

For at-home use, she recommends Domeboro powder or tablets, or similar products that contain aluminum sulfate and calcium acetate. The powder or tablet is used to make a wet compress to lay over the blisters.

Add an antibiotic. In the time between applying compresses, use a topical antibiotic cream to help prevent infections, Dr. Elewski says. Or your doctor can prescribe a cream containing silver sulfadiazine, used to soothe and protect burns.

Since shingles blisters can ooze and become infected, you'll want to avoid anointing yourself with creams containing hydrocortisone, greasy ointments such as petroleum jelly, and powders such as cornstarch, because they can promote bacterial growth.

Add aspirin. Because shingles inflames nerves and skin, anti-inflammatory drugs can ease the pain, Dr. Kassirer says. She suggests oral aspirin or ibuprofen and says her patients have good success easing postherpetic neuralgia using crushed aspirin in a skin lotion (she recommends Vaseline Intensive Care Lotion) applied directly to the painful area. "The analgesic does seem to be absorbed through the skin," she says.

▶ PREVENTION PAIN-RELIEF PROGRAM

Once you've been diagnosed with shingles, your doctor will probably prescribe an antiviral drug (acyclovir is common). If shingles is threatening an eye, you may even get intravenous antivirals. If you begin taking an antiviral drug within 24 hours of the time your blisters erupt, studies show you may heal faster and hurt less, Dr. Kassirer says.

Within ten days of the time your blisters first erupt, if you're in generally good health, your doctor may recommend a course of oral steroids (most commonly prednisone). Several studies suggest that this treatment may help reduce the incidence of postherpetic neuralgia.

Fight Fire with Fire

One increasingly popular treatment for postherpetic neuralgia is over-the-counter cream made with capsaicin—the tongue-searing component of red chili peppers. Several studies suggest that these creams work by depleting a neurochemical that causes pain, called substance P. In some people, the cream works quickly. Most people, though, must use it several times a day for several days and endure a phase when the cream itself causes burning pain.

"People who are warned in advance deal better with this cream," Dr. Elewski says. "It does have a funny burning sensation, but that lasts only a couple of days, and then it's gone. And the pain caused by your condition is totally gone, too, so the discomfort is worth it, if you are willing to put up with it for a couple of days."

Like salsa, capsaicin creams now come in mild and hot versions. The "hot" version, Axsain, contains three times as much capsaicin as Zostrix, the "mild" version. Ask your doctor which version is appropriate for you. Unlike south-of-the-border condiments, these creams carry cautions. Make sure you heed the "Keep out of eyes" advice. That can be a problem if your shingles occurred on your face. Sweat can run down your forehead and into your eyes, carrying capsaicin with it. And the cream can linger on your hands, even with washing. Dr. Kassirer recommends wearing rubber gloves when you apply it.

Other Drugs May Help

If topical creams such as Zostrix or lidocaine fail to quell lingering pain, your doctor may have you take anti-inflammatory analgesics such as aspirin or ibuprofen as well. He or she may instead recommend a course of low-dose antidepressants, not because you're feeling blue but because these drugs help relieve some sorts of nerve pain. And the same kinds of anticonvulsant drugs used to treat epilepsy can also tame tingling nerves. (See chapter 26.)

One nondrug therapy—transcutaneous electrical nerve stimulation (TENS)—is also worth trying, Dr. Kassirer says. "People may use TENS for 30 minutes or so before bedtime, so they can fall asleep," she explains. (See chapter 32.)

Ease Off Stress

For lingering pain, some lifestyle changes may be helpful, experts agree.

"Lots of people say stress can induce these sorts of illnesses, but no studies show stress reduction can prevent shingles," Dr. Kassirer says. "On the other hand, when they get postherpetic neuralgia, many people do turn to stress reduction—biofeedback, meditation, visualization, anything that helps take their mind off the pain. And those things work. They are helpful for any type of chronic pain." (See chapters 17, 22, and 34.)

When all else fails, and postshingles pain remains unrelenting, doctors sometimes prescribe narcotics or nerve blocks. These treatments are considered last resorts, however, and each comes with its own set of problems. (See chapters 26 and 27.)

Vaccine: You'll Have to Wait

Chickenpox is definitely contagious. But shingles is not considered contagious, nor is it thought to be caused by exposure to someone with chickenpox or shingles.

"The only people at risk through such exposure are those who've never had chickenpox," says Myron Levin, M.D., professor of internal medicine and pediatrics at the University of Colorado School of Medicine in Denver. Even so, they wouldn't get shingles; they would come down with chickenpox, which can be a serious illness in adults.

A vaccine that prevents chickenpox in children, Varivax, is under review for licensing by the U.S. Food and Drug Administration. This vaccine has been shown to boost a certain type of infection-fighting ability, called cell-mediated immunity, in adults age 55 or older, says Dr. Levin. These early results lead researchers to speculate that a vaccine may one day be used to prevent shingles, too. That's a prospect most neurologists, and their patients, would undoubtedly welcome.

FROSTBITE

Take temperatures below freezing, add a stiff breeze, bad planning or bad fortune, and perhaps a flask of your favorite peppermint schnapps, and you've set the stage for frostbite.

It doesn't even take all those conditions for frostbite to occur. Simply exposing bare skin to below-zero temperatures for a minute or two can start the process that eventually freezes body parts as solid as a supermarket turkey.

You can even freeze your *eyeballs* if you drive a snowmobile in below-freezing weather without goggles. (And you'll require a corneal transplant to restore your vision, says Murray P. Hamlet, D.V.M., director of the Research Program and Operations Division at the U.S. Army Research Institute of Environmental Medicine, in Natick, Massachusetts.)

Like burns, frostbite develops in degrees. Superficial frostbite, sometimes called frostnip, affects only the top layers of skin. Your skin looks gray and feels thick and numb. As freezing progresses through layers of tissue, the area becomes hard and white. With serious frostbite, your hand really can feel like a frozen lamb chop.

➡ **INSTANT RELIEF**

Superficial frostbite, or frostnip, melts away with gentle warming. You may feel some burning and tingling as the part warms up, and afterward feel a sensation similar to sunburn. Your skin may darken and later peel, just as it would with sunburn.

Put your cold parts in a warm place. If you're stuck outdoors, be creative. Stick your hands in your armpits or waistband. Use your mittened hands to warm your cheeks, nose, or ears. If your feet are frigid, sweet-talk someone into letting you put your feet against their belly for a time. (Tell them you'll be happy to return the favor later.) One of the best ways to get warmed up, Dr. Hamlet says in all seriousness, is for two or more people to get into a sleeping bag together.

Once you're indoors, getting warm is a much less interesting proposition. Simply being in warm air will thaw your parts out. If you wish, a tepid bath will do the same. Avoid strong heat: No hot tubs or roaring fires, experts say. It's too easy to fry the already damaged skin.

Resist rubbing. It's true that friction produces heat. But just as you wouldn't rub a sunburn to make it feel better, you don't want to rub frostbitten hands, feet, or cheeks. You could rub your skin right off, says Ruth Uphold, M.D., medical director of emergency medicine at the Medical Center Hospital of Vermont in Burlington.

Apply aloe vera. Doctors sometimes recommend fresh aloe vera gel or creams containing aloe vera as part of the treatment plan for minor frostbite. The clear, fresh gel from this plant's leaves has long been used as a soothing cover for burns. Researchers say it contains anti-inflammatory and healing compounds. Simply smooth on the gel a few times a day, leaving your skin uncovered.

▶ PREVENTION PAIN-RELIEF PROGRAM

Frostbite most often strikes the feet, hands, or face. It's more likely to afflict people who have been drinking alcohol, people with circulation problems or diabetic neuropathy, or those unaccustomed to the cold. Getting soaked with water or gasoline, handling cold metal—even wearing metal earphones—are sure-fire ways to invite frostbite, even when temperatures are relatively balmy (say, near-freezing rather than below). That's why so many North woods mechanics are minus a fingertip or two.

Dress to Stay Warm and Dry

If you're planning to stay outdoors for an extended time in cold weather, a few simple measures help prevent frostbite. Wear warm, waterproof boots that give your toes plenty of wiggle-room, Dr. Uphold suggests. Wear two pairs of socks—liner socks that draw moisture away from your skin and thick wool socks. And do carry a dry change of socks in case yours get wet. Wear mittens with warm liners and windproof, vapor-permeable shells. Carry gloves if you know you'll need to use your fingers, and carry an extra pair of mittens in case you lose one.

Carry a face mask or balaclava—a knitted hood that can be drawn over your face so all but your eyes are covered. Wear goggles if you're snowmobiling, walking, or skiing in brisk wind. Dress in layers that draw moisture from your body and allow you to open up to cool down if necessary. Purchase outdoor pants and jackets with moisture-releasing vents.

In Case of Emergency

If you get into a situation where frostbite does occur, stay calm, Dr. Uphold says. Rapid thawing is the best way to save tissue. But don't try to thaw out a part unless you can guarantee it won't refreeze, since refreezing causes much more damage.

Frozen feet pose special problems. It is possible to walk a few miles on frozen feet, and you'll do much less harm walking on them frozen than thawed. But unless the temperature is very cold, it's hard to keep feet frozen. Once they thaw out, even partially, they will be too painful to walk on, and walking on them will do serious damage. So unless you have just a bit of frostbite on a toe, arranging to be carried out is your best bet, according to Dr. Uphold.

Thawing a badly frostbitten limb causes intense pain. In a hospital, intravenous narcotics are usually offered. On the trail or road, pain can be temporarily eased with aspirin or ibuprofen and by protecting and immobilizing the limb, Dr. Uphold says.

SICKLE CELL DISEASE

Normal red blood cells are plump disks that can bend around corners, squeeze through tiny capillaries, and then pop back into shape again. In sickle cell disease, red blood cells become rigid, elongated, and sickle shaped. Instead of flowing through tight spots, they get stuck, back up, and create a cell jam that acts like an internal tourniquet, cutting off the flow of blood to tissue, creating a painful lack of oxygen.

A sickle cell jam can occur anywhere in the body—the fingers, arms, ribs, abdomen, and organs such as the spleen and lungs. The swelling, tenderness, and deep throbbing pain can last from several hours to several days, with most attacks easing off in seven to ten days. Severe attacks, though, can be followed by a dull ache that lasts for days or even weeks, says Doris Wethers, M.D., director of the Sickle Cell Clinic at St. Luke's—Roosevelt Hospital in New York City. If cells jam up in the brain, a stroke may occur. That's one of the most serious possible consequences of this disease, Dr. Wethers says.

In the United States, people of African descent are most likely to have inherited the gene that causes sickle cell disease. But Greeks, Italians, or anyone of Mediterranean, Arabian, or East Indian descent can carry the gene. A special blood test can determine if you have one of the various kinds of sickle cell disease (including its most serious form, sickle cell anemia) or if you carry the trait without symptoms.

Children and adults can learn how to manage a sickle cell episode, with medical help if necessary. As painful as these episodes can be, they are seldom life-threatening, Dr. Wethers says. Over the years, though, sickle cell disease can cause tissue damage that shortens a person's life.

INSTANT RELIEF

People who can tune in to the early symptoms of a painful crisis can sometimes do things to minimize the pain, Dr. Wethers says.

POST-POLIO SYNDROME

They endured crutches, heavy metal braces, and claustrophobic iron lungs. Those who lived fought back with a determination that stays with them. They may need that strength, for polio survivors now face a new challenge from the virus that nearly crippled them 30 or more years ago: post-polio syndrome.

Post-polio syndrome can include an array of symptoms: severe fatigue following moderate activity, generalized joint and muscle pain, muscle weakness and loss of muscle use, and breathing problems that can lead to early-morning headaches, insomnia, and increased sensitivity to cold.

The syndrome can show up in sudden, odd ways, says Stanley Yarnell, M.D., director of the Post-Polio Clinic at St. Mary's Hospital in San Francisco and assistant clinical professor of physical medicine and rehabilitation at Stanford University. One man who hauled suitcases around an airport one day discovered the next day that he could not raise his arms to knot his tie. It took him more than a year of rest and gentle exercises to recover the strength in his arms, Dr. Yarnell says. Another man, confined to a wheelchair, had for years relied on his one strong arm for just about everything. One day, Dr. Yarnell says, he dropped his car keys on the ground. He bent over from his wheelchair to pick them up, but when he tried to push himself upright, he found his "good" arm too weak to push.

Symptoms Revisited

The condition is *not* a flare-up of the polio virus, Dr. Yarnell says. The symptoms are thought to be due to overusing the remaining active muscles, changes in body mechanics, and problems in the connections between nerves and muscles, called neuromuscular junctions.

The *pain* associated with post-polio syndrome is often due to years of overuse and altered body mechanics, as surviving muscles try to take on the workload of those that were lost.

Many people using crutches, for instance, may develop tendinitis or bursitis in their shoulders or hips. Both these conditions can be treated with rest, hot or cold therapy, or analgesics.

Most people with polio also have curvature of the spine, or scoliosis, which can cause painful pinched nerves; this can also be treated. Myofascial pain, characterized by sore muscles with tender trigger points that radiate pain, is also common in polio patients and can be treated in a variety of ways. Carpal tunnel syndrome, a form of tendinitis that hits the wrist, is common in crutch users. Arthritis is less common.

Treatment of post-polio syndrome includes pinpointing any condition that can be treated and carefully balancing exercise and rest.

Treatments Revisited
Some people, who thought leg braces part of a distant childhood memory, may require them once again to stabilize their gait. Some are encouraged to use electric scooters.

"Fatigue can be a profound problem," Dr. Yarnell says. "Some people may need to rest about 25 percent of the time." This doesn't mean they need to lie down, he says, but they may need to sit. He asks his patients to rest 5 minutes for every 15 minutes of activity, or to interchange physical activities such as scrubbing a floor with less demanding tasks—making a grocery list, for instance.

Exercise is also important for post-polio patients. If they are inactive, their muscles get flabby, and they end up more tired than ever. Most doctors recommend what they call "nonfatiguing exercise." They'll initially cut activity to well below the point where muscles get rubbery. Then they'll slowly build up again, over months, to a level that is sustainable but not tiring. Swimming is a favorite activity, because it builds stamina with little pounding on joints and muscles, says Paul Peach, M.D., director of the Post-Polio Clinic in Warm Springs, Georgia. Gentle stretching exercises also help relieve aching muscles.

Fighting Back
Some doctors occasionally use a drug to improve communication between nerves and muscles, says Neil Cashman,

M.D., assistant professor of neurology at McGill University School of Medicine in Montreal and director of the Montreal Neurological Institute Post-Polio Clinic. The drug, pyridostigmine (Mestinon), has been used for years in the United States for myasthenia gravis, a neuromuscular disorder with acute muscle fatigue like that sometimes seen in post-polio patients.

In a recent study, Dr. Cashman found that 60 to 70 percent of carefully selected post-polio patients responded to the drug with less muscle fatigue. (The drug did not affect overall weakness.) "Even in a select group of people, not everyone benefits from this drug," Dr. Cashman says. "But it seems to benefit most those whose symptoms are worst." One patient who'd required pressurized air to sleep comfortably at night was able to sleep normally using the drug, Dr. Cashman says.

Some doctors worry that this drug may lead to more muscle damage, especially if people use it to mask their symptoms rather than resting overworked muscles.

"It's true that people don't like being told to rest or to go back to using a leg brace, especially when they worked so hard to overcome polio," Dr. Yarnell admits. But once they discover that a few simple energy-conserving tricks give them more pep for other things, they willingly make the trade-off, he says. And trade-offs may be something they'll have to do the rest of their life.

If you're cold, warm up. Sickle cells are more likely to stack up when your whole body or your hands or feet are cold and blood vessels are constricted. Relaxing in a tub of warm water or warming up painful hands or feet sometimes helps avert a crisis, Dr. Wethers says.

If you're hot, cool down. Becoming overheated can also cause loss of body fluids, which can cause sickle cell jams, Dr. Wethers says. Slow down, get out of the hot sun, and find a cool spot where you can lay low for a while, she suggests.

Hang out at the watering hole. Dehydration can also trigger a painful episode. Drinking plenty of fluids is especially important if it's hot or if you've been exercising or sweating a lot, Dr. Wethers says.

Give yourself a break. Exercising too hard or too long can lead to painful episodes. "We tell people, and especially kids, when you get tired, stop," says Dorothye Boswell, executive director of the National Association for Sickle Cell Disease, in Los Angeles.

Breathe deeply. Some doctors believe that a few minutes of deep, slow breathing done just before you hit the sack can help prevent painful episodes during the night.

Take an analgesic. For children, acetaminophen can help relieve the pain of a sickling episode. In adults, aspirin or ibuprofen is preferred, Dr. Wethers says.

▶ PREVENTION PAIN-RELIEF PROGRAM

What's a prudent diet and lifestyle for someone with sickle cell disease? "We simply tell people to eat a normal, healthy diet and to do all things in moderation," Dr. Wethers says. That means a nutritious diet that goes easy on salt and alcohol. It also means engaging in exercise such as walking or swimming.

Some doctors give their patients with sickle cell disease supplemental folate, a B-complex vitamin. And most give children with sickle cell disease a multivitamin/mineral supplement, since such children are slow growers. But there's little evidence to show that in adults, nutritional supplementation has any impact on sickle cell disease. "About the only thing we do know is that people with sickle cell disease who are poorly nourished do not do well," Dr. Wethers says.

Severe pain, or the threat of side effects, sometimes means a person needs to be admitted to the hospital for intravenous fluids and pain-relieving drugs. People who suffer from frequent painful episodes often try self-hypnosis, relaxation techniques, biofeedback, or TENS, Dr. Wethers says. "We encourage these things, because they do seem to help people reduce their need for pain medication," she says.

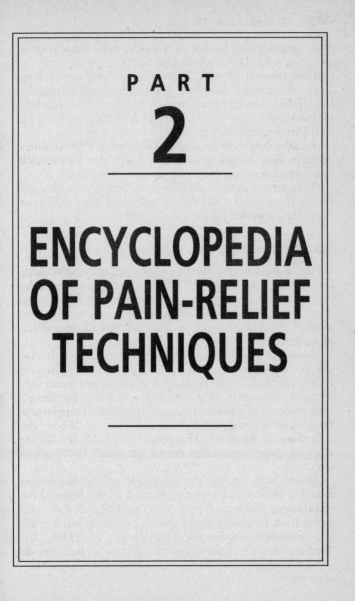

PART
2

ENCYCLOPEDIA OF PAIN-RELIEF TECHNIQUES

CHAPTER
16

ACUPUNCTURE
THE FINE POINTS
OF RECOVERY

Remember the box-office hit *Star Wars*, back in the 1970s? If so, you'll recall old Obi-Wan Kenobi sending Luke Skywalker off to do battle with the enemies of the Empire. As Luke departs, the Jedi Master intones "and may the Force be with you."

The idea of a friendly personal "force" was so appealing to people that T-shirts soon appeared bearing Obi-Wan Kenobi's words. Yet the idea of a "force" being with us isn't really new. In fact, the Chinese have believed for centuries that every living thing contains a life force, or *chi*. They use this belief to explain how acupuncture, the ancient Oriental technique for pain relief and healing, works. Acupuncture—which involves placing tiny, sterile needles into various parts of the body—may be the granddaddy of all healing arts. Archaeologists in China have dug up stone acupuncture needles (ouch!) possibly dating back to 8000 B.C.

It wasn't until 1971, however, that acupuncture came to the Western world in a big way. James Reston, an editor with *The New York Times*, was traveling through China when he experienced a sudden attack of appendicitis. His hosts rushed him to a local hospital, where he underwent emergency surgery. Later, when he complained of severe gastritis—a common complaint following such surgery—his doctors urged him to try acupuncture needles for pain relief. He agreed and was amazed to find the treatment painless. Twenty minutes later, the gastritis pain was gone. Reston's was the first widely reported case of an American being treated with acupuncture.

Reston was so impressed with his experience that on his return to New York, he wrote an article describing it. Americans were fascinated, and a few years later, the first U.S. school of acupuncture opened in New England.

The Case for Needles

Today, an increasing number of physicians in the West are taking a practical look at the benefits acupuncture may offer. There are now enough data to prove that acupuncture is valuable in providing pain relief.

According to the World Health Organization, the many conditions that respond well to acupuncture treatment include trigeminal neuralgia, frozen shoulder, tennis elbow, sciatica, low back pain, osteoarthritis, gastritis, constipation, diarrhea, toothache, postextraction pain, gingivitis, pharyngitis, and conjunctivitis.

Studies have shown acupuncture to be valuable in relieving both migraine and tension headaches, according to Alexander Mauskop, M.D., director of the Downstate Medical Center in New York City.

And 6 to 24 treatments can produce "dramatic" pain relief for many arthritis sufferers, says Robert Sohn, Ph.D., past president of the American Association of Acupuncture and Oriental Medicine. Dr. Sohn, who has worked with acupuncture for more than 29 years, says he's seen people with arthritis "literally get off the table and walk away with pain reduced by 50 percent."

Acupuncture is an important therapeutic technique for a variety of painful conditions, says Lloyd Saberski, M.D., director of the Yale Center of Pain Management. The center already has an acupuncturist on staff and plans over the next five years to actively explore possible uses of acupuncture.

Apparently, a good deal of research remains to be done before Western science gets a handle on everything that acupuncture can do. Or even on *how* it does what it does, for that matter.

How Does Acupuncture Work?

Ask ten health-care professionals who use acupuncture to explain how it works and you'll probably get ten different explanations. There are two primary schools of thought—Western and Oriental—and even these have variations.

Western medicine theorizes that acupuncture stimulates the release of certain naturally occurring brain chemicals, including morphinelike substances known as endorphins. These chemicals flood the body with a sense of well-being and can lessen or eliminate pain.

Other Western researchers believe that acupuncture affects the body's electromagnetic fields. Among them is Daniel Kirsch, Ph.D., former clinical director of the Center for Stress and Pain at Columbia-Presbyterian Medical Center in New York and founding member of the National Institute of Electromedical Information. He accepts the Oriental explanation that acupuncture manipulates the body's energy, but he believes the *chi* force is actually body electricity, a theory many physicists share.

"Everything in the body is electrical, and every cell is like a small battery," he says. Medical studies have proven that electrical fields are at work in the body. Dr. Kirsch markets a pain-relief device, called Alpha-Stim, that works by stimulating cells with electricity. It is available nationwide through medical suppliers. (For information, call 1-800-FOR-PAIN.) The Oriental explanation would be that it taps the *chi*.

The Chinese believe that our body contains a number of meridians, or pathways, along which our life energy flows. Charts dating back to 2600 B.C. illustrate these meridians, and modern versions show the same invisible anatomical road map. Traditional Oriental acupuncturists maintain that as long as all parts of our body receive their supply of life force and our organs remain healthy, things run smoothly. But if the *chi* energy is blocked so that it can't complete its circuit to an organ, pain and illness can result.

Here's where acupuncture comes in. Oriental acupuncture theory maintains that there are hundreds of locations, or *points*, on the body where the meridians can be tapped. By piercing the skin at these points, the theory goes, the normal flow of life energy can be unblocked and good health restored.

For the most part, traditional Western medicine is still uncomfortable with such terms as *life force*. But a growing number of physicians, nurses, and therapists are convinced there's a place for acupuncture as a healing tool. Affirms Dr. Kirsch: "It works, no doubt about it."

Seek and You Will Find

Now what if you're convinced you'd like to try this ancient healing technique that has the modern-day stamp of approval? To begin, ask your physician for a referral. He or she may not be able to recommend anyone, but then again, you might be pleasantly surprised.

"When you're looking for a practitioner, ask your friends how they were treated," says David Molony, an acupuncturist practicing in Emmaus, Pennsylvania. And, he adds, "be sure the therapist has NCCA certification." The NCCA, or National Commission for the Certification of Acupuncturists, is based in Washington, D.C. It has established standards that candidates must meet before they can become certified acupuncturists.

A number of states license acupuncturists or allow them to practice under supervision. For the name and address of your local licensing board, contact the National Commission for the Certification of Acupuncturists, 1424 16th Street NW, Suite 501, Washington, DC 20036.

For additional help in finding a qualified acupuncturist, contact the Traditional Acupuncture Institute, American City Building, Suite 100, Columbia, MD 21044, (301) 997-4888.

Say Ahhh . . .

Once you've found an acupuncturist and made your appointment, you're likely to feel pretty nervous when the big day arrives. If it weren't for that painful condition, you'd probably be a million miles away. Ah . . . the patient ahead of you is coming out, smiling. Maybe there's hope. But then you remember . . . the needles!

Relax. You're in for a fascinating experience, probably far more pleasant than you'd expect. Once inside, you'll be asked a few general questions. If your acupuncturist follows the Western school of thought, you can expect questions similar to those you might hear from your doctor—along the lines of where and why are you in pain. In fact, an increasing number of physicians are either learning to do acupuncture themselves or referring patients to acupuncturists.

If, on the other hand, you are receiving treatment from an acupuncturist who follows the Oriental school, your preliminary examination may be quite different from what you'd expect. It's usually composed of four parts.

- Observation of your eyes, face, skin, tongue, and general appearance
- Questions about your eating habits, medical history, and elimination problems
- Listening to your voice, breathing, and coughing, and noting mouth odor and other signs of illness
- A "reading" of your pulse

Chinese medicine puts a lot of stock in taking the pulse. Traditional practitioners recognize 23 different types of pulse beat, all of which they say can give vital information about your physical condition. As to your tongue, they maintain that its texture, shape, and color can provide clues to where problems may lie.

After your examination, your therapist will discuss what can be done to help you and how many sessions it may take. (This is a good time to ask any questions you may have.) Then you'll be asked to sit, stand, or lie on a table, depending upon where on the body the acupuncturist will be inserting the needles.

Don't Let Those Needles Scare You

Acupuncture needles range from ½ to 5 inches long and are as thin as a hair. Therefore, you'll probably feel little if any pain. "When the point is correctly needled, the sensation can be tingling, soreness, or numbness. It is necessary to experience one of these three sensations or the treatment will not work," says Dr. Kirsch. "Relaxation may or may not occur."

In some cases, the acupuncturist may apply heat, electrical stimulation, or pressure to the needles or may twirl them "to get the energy moving." By now you've probably entered a deeply mellow state. The needles will be left in for 20 minutes or more, but most patients doze off while waiting. The whole procedure—from examination to end of treatment—takes about an hour.

For most people, the aftereffects are positive, say acupuncture experts. Patients report better sleep patterns, more energy, less stress, and a general feeling of well-being after treatment. Sometimes, symptoms will worsen slightly over the next day or so before getting better. Therapists consider this to be a good sign, however; they have observed that these patients seem to benefit even more than others once their body has adjusted to treatment.

Today, with the increasing concern about AIDS and other diseases spread by improper use of needles, acupuncturists are bound by law to use disposable or sterile needles. And, in fact, they do. Acupuncturists have an excellent record for safe practice, according to Dr. Sohn.

Therapists maintain that the best time to visit your acupuncturist is when you're actively experiencing the pain. This enables the therapist to locate the source of the problem quickly and place needles at the appropriate points.

Because each case is different, most practitioners find that the number and frequency of treatments vary, depending on the type of problem and its severity. Acute conditions, such as athletic injuries, may require only one treatment. Chronic cases—problems that people have had for a long time and that are not inflammatory—may or may not improve. (Be sure to ask your acupuncturist during that first session how many visits will be required to treat your condition.)

Drug-Free Surgery

Relieving pain created by a wide variety of conditions is not the only trick that acupuncturists have up their sleeves,

A PRESSING CONCERN

Acupuncture, which must be administered by a professional, may seem like an extreme and exotic treatment to a person who has grown up with Western medical tradition. There is, however, a less daunting way to tap into this powerful Oriental technique, one that involves neither needles nor facing the unknown—acupressure. Both acupressure and acupuncture are based on the Oriental theory of life force and meridians. But acupressure is a "fingers-on" rather than a "needles-in" approach.

By using your thumb or fingers to exert pressure on specific points, you can often get as powerful results from acupressure as you can from acupuncture. Acupressure can be used to relieve discomfort in a variety of conditions, including migraine, arthritis, backache, menstrual pain, eyestrain, facial pain, whiplash, motion sickness, and even sunburn!

Look for specific instructions on relieving a wide variety of pains throughout Part 1 of this book.

however. The ancient needle therapy is also used to deaden pain during surgery.

To date, acupuncture experts maintain, there are 30 types of operations for which acupuncture can be used for anesthesia. It is especially valuable, they say, during operations on patients with high blood pressure or liver, lung, or kidney problems.

Physicians who use acupuncture have found that it offers several other advantages as surgical anesthesia.

- There are no side effects.
- Recuperation is faster.
- The patient, who is conscious, can cooperate during the surgery.
- There is often less bleeding.

Recently, Yale played host to Dr. Xiao-Ding Cao, dean of the faculty of Basic Medical Studies, Shanghai Medical University, and China's leading expert in acupuncture.

According to Dr. Xiao-Ding Cao, physicians in China are using acupuncture as anesthesia during surgeries of the head and neck. These physicians indicate that acupuncture is even more effective when used as anesthesia than it is for removing chronic pain. Acupuncture gives such thorough pain relief, says Dr. Xiao-Ding Cao, that one patient undergoing brain surgery ate an orange during the operation!

So far, however, most American hospitals do not offer surgical acupuncture. You might ask a registered acupuncturist where you could obtain such treatment.

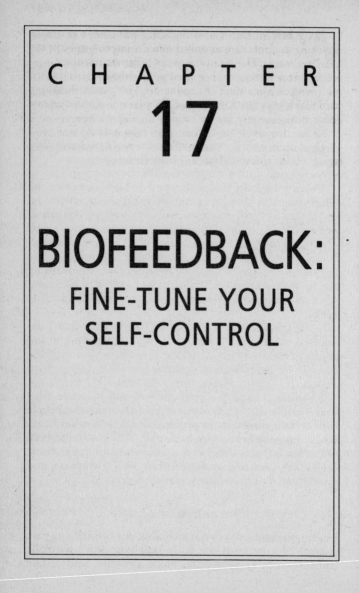

CHAPTER
17

BIOFEEDBACK:
FINE-TUNE YOUR
SELF-CONTROL

When Mohammad R. Sadigh, Ph.D., was a graduate student, he had only a modest interest in biofeedback until he saw it work a minor miracle.

He met a woman who had suffered migraine headaches for 27 years. The future Dr. Sadigh told her about a chapter in one of his textbooks that described how biofeedback can be used to cure migraines.

"Why don't you try this on me?" she asked.

The young man approached the woman's personal physician. "This doesn't seem to be anything dangerous," the physician said with a shrug. "Go ahead and try it."

Twice a week the student hopped on his bike to visit the elderly woman. Using a portable digital thermometer, he taught her biofeedback techniques, as well as relaxation methods that he himself had just learned from his professor.

In just six months, her headaches stopped completely. Today, years later, when she experiences the flashing lights and slightly blurred vision that serve as the early-warning signals that a headache is on its way, she sits back and practices biofeedback—stopping the migraine dead in its tracks.

"After that, I was so excited by biofeedback that I decided to spend a good portion of my life studying it and understanding it better," says Dr. Sadigh, who now is the director of the Gateway Institute, a Pennsylvania pain clinic.

Biofeedback isn't for everyone—as will be made clear later—but Dr. Sadigh says that it can do wonders for people with certain chronic pain problems such as tension headaches, migraine headaches, back pain, and gastrointestinal problems. It is also used to treat temporomandibular disorder (TMD, sometimes referred to as TMJ), whiplash, and a wide variety of neuromuscular disorders.

Choosing Calm Instead of a Storm

Essentially, biofeedback is a technique for helping you gain control of aspects of the body that you don't normally control—such as heart rate, blood pressure, and certain responses to stress. You gain this conscious control in part by working with instruments that provide visual or auditory feedback, says Gerald M. Aronoff, M.D., author of *Evaluation and Treatment of Chronic Pain*. Dr. Aronoff, director of the Boston Pain Center and assistant clinical professor at Tufts University School of Medicine, says that his goal with pain patients is to bring down states of tension, "because a totally relaxed state is felt to be incompatible with suffering from pain."

Dr. Sadigh defines the term by noting that "biofeedback is a process where information is given to the patient about those aspects of his or her nervous system that he or she may not be conscious of. Initially, it may begin to make what is not conscious, conscious, so you can begin to regulate those things."

Even if you are normally tenser than a deposed dictator facing a firing squad, biofeedback can help you bid an unfond farewell to stress and anxiety. And when you do perfect these relaxation methods, chances are your chronic pain will also vanish, says Dr. Sadigh.

Biofeedback is no cure-all, but it is a powerful tool, he says. By itself it doesn't do much good, but when it's used to enhance the body's own pain-control mechanisms, it can do a great deal.

"Pain *management* is the key word I stress—although pain *reduction* is one of my goals," says Dr. Sadigh. "I teach people that they can have control over their pain symptoms after they learn certain simple techniques. They can learn to manage their pain, control their pain, and hopefully reduce or stop it."

Many people suffer long-term pain because they don't know how to handle stress, says Thomas H. Budzynski, Ph.D., director of behavioral medicine at St. Luke Medical Center in Bellevue, Washington. Their muscles frequently are tight.

"Then they injure a part of their body and the muscles tighten up even more," he says. "In that case, sometimes the unconscious part of the brain will maintain pain around the injury even after it heals." Learning how to relax can eliminate those kinds of pains completely.

Who Can Benefit?

To learn how to control your body, there are four conditions that must be met, says Michael G. McKee, Ph.D., in the Department of Psychiatry and Psychology Biofeedback Section at the Cleveland Clinic Foundation. You have to be motivated. You have to have the basic ability to do it. You have to reward yourself for doing it. And you need feedback to know you're doing it right.

Biofeedback isn't right for everyone, says Dr. Sadigh. Some people, for example, seem to tense up more in the presence of machines. They can't let go of that reaction sufficiently to work with the kinds of instruments that are used during biofeedback training. Dr. Sadigh also suggests that those with severe depression or other severe psychological disorders, those with diabetes, or those with drug and alcohol abuse problems may not be suitable candidates.

Tuning Out Tension

How does biofeedback work in practice?

Imagine yourself driving a car. Someone instructs you to drive at precisely 55 mph. It's a simple task to perform if you have a speedometer. All you do is check the speedometer while working the gas pedal and the brake.

But let's say that someone has removed the speedometer. Driving alone on a highway, you might come close to driving 55 mph—or you might earn yourself a speeding ticket.

"That speedometer is the key," says Dr. Sadigh. Biofeedback machinery helps to reduce pain by giving you clues you can see or hear. It can tell you that you are tensing certain muscles or that your heart rate is going up, for example. With the aid of a biofeedback therapist, you use these machines to recognize and respond to the early-warning signs before your body climbs up the wall like the stressed-out Bill the Cat of "Bloom County" cartoon fame.

Imagine, for example, that you have a tension headache—the muscles of your head, neck, and scalp are really tight. "You could take an analgesic to fight the pain, you could take a muscle relaxant to relax the muscles, or you could relax your muscles so that pain isn't being generated," says Dr. McKee.

Dr. Sadigh concurs. He notes that there are some people who would simply prefer to take headache medications every time they have a headache due to stress. Biofeedback is not for them. But for those willing to take the time to practice biofeedback, pain caused by tension can sometimes be controlled without drugs.

Typically, when you go for biofeedback training, you'll have some electronic sensors painlessly taped to your skin to register electrical activity, skin temperature, and muscle tension. The information that the sensors pick up from your body is converted into a signal that you can see or hear— a computer display or audio tone. As you relax, the sound of "beep, beep, beep" becomes more of a "bloo-oo-oopa, bloo-oo-oopa, bloop." The minor adjustments you can make in your body lead to either tension or relaxation, and the signals from the biofeedback machine keep you apprised of how you are doing.

Insight from Machines

There are many forms of biofeedback equipment to assist you in this pain-control venture. One machine, for example, helps people who are in pain because they tend to brace certain muscles, says Dr. Budzynski. This machine displays the muscles of the left and right sides of your back on a computer screen. The right side is outlined in red, the left in green. The trainer asks you to stretch, flex, and rotate your torso. The gizmo can show you that the right side doesn't know that the left is doing all the work or is tensing unnaturally, for example. With a little practice, biofeedback can help you change your groans to grins.

Dr. Aronoff cautions his patients about becoming dependent on machines. He says that the machines are only tools to help people get better by teaching them how to get in touch with their body.

Scaled-Down Models

The high-tech machines that your therapist uses in biofeedback training are costly, but once you've learned the technique, you may wish to purchase inexpensive biofeedback equipment to use at home. Thanks to modern technology, a cure for your pain just might be in the palm of your hand. Many pain centers now sell hand-held, battery-powered biofeedback monitors that tell you whether you're relaxing by measuring the electrical conductivity of your skin.

Also available are inexpensive, disposable thermometers that detect when your fingers and toes have gone cold—a sign that you're under stress. Temperatures vary greatly from individual to individual, Dr. Sadigh cautions. However, in general, temperatures below 80°F are a sign that tension is present. He works with people to help them increase their skin surface temperature to between 85° and 95°.

With biofeedback thermometers and proper training, you can defuse tension that may worsen your pain, says Dr. McKee.

Son of a Gun, You'll Have Great Fun on the Bio

Unlike some medical procedures, biofeedback "is kind of fun to try," says Dr. McKee. "It's enjoyable for most people" to get more in touch with their body, he says.

The wonderful thing about biofeedback is that no one compares your progress to that of any other patient. "You are your own point of reference," says Dr. Sadigh.

When should someone in pain see a specialist for biofeedback? Anyone with chronic pain whose doctors have determined there is no anatomical problem should consider biofeedback therapy, according to Dr. Sadigh.

Even professionals who teach biofeedback are sometimes surprised by just how much certain individuals need the training. Occasionally, on the first handshake, the cold hands of some people are a telling sign of the stress they are feeling, says Dr. McKee. "Sometimes you see a person who looks really relaxed, but when you hook them up to the machine, you're surprised to see that their readings are very high," he says. "Their stress makes it seem like World War III has started in their body."

On one occasion a female lawyer visited Dr. McKee and was hooked up to a biofeedback machine. She happened to mention that a male colleague thought that women shouldn't be allowed to be on a law review because they were meant to be home with children. The surface temperature of her skin dropped 20 degrees, says Dr. McKee. He told her, "Your body's crying out for help."

Practice Makes Perfect

Biofeedback works wonders, not miracles. The most common reason that biofeedback sometimes fails, says Dr. Budzynski, "is that people don't give it a fair chance." He recommends that you practice once or twice daily (roughly 30 minutes per session) for a month before expecting your first positive results. "It takes a little time to get oriented to it."

Dr. McKee says that motivation is very important. "You're learning a new skill, and if you're not committed, then you're not going to benefit," he says. "There's a great emphasis on taking personal responsibility for your own well-being, so if you're not willing to take that responsibility, it won't work."

He also advises people not to expect miracles on one visit. "If your expectations are too high, you may get discouraged after one visit and drop out of treatment," he says. The average patient needs to attend 8 to 12 sessions, although some chronic pain patients must attend indefinitely.

And while much work is done in the office of a therapist

or doctor, it is also essential that you practice what you learn at home. "If you're not willing to do your homework, you're not likely to make much progress," says Dr. McKee.

Learn to Breathe Easier

People who try biofeedback need to concentrate on breathing from the diaphragm or belly during the session, says Dr. Budzynski. Belly breathing helps drop the body out of stressful high gear into a relaxed low gear, he says.

You can learn to breathe this way by lying on the floor with a heavy book just above your navel. "As you breathe in, allow your stomach to push against the book," he recommends. "As you exhale, let the pressure of the book push your stomach in."

You'll probably work on breathing techniques during only a couple sessions until you get the hang of it, says Dr. Sadigh. "Once you become aware, you'll catch yourself" when you're breathing improperly, he says.

Sometimes It's "Buyer Beware"

If biofeedback sounds like something you'd like to try, you need to receive training from a reputable professional. Dr. Sadigh cautions that people should check any individual or institution's credentials very carefully before submitting to treatment. Because biofeedback practitioners as yet do not have to be licensed, a number of untrained and/or disreputable people have started biofeedback clinics, he says.

Anyone who doesn't offer to screen you carefully before admitting you to treatment is highly suspect, he says, noting: "Biofeedback should be done by someone in the medical profession, a psychologist, or someone with a background in this area." Your best bet is to ask your doctor for a referral.

The costs of training vary from $75 to $150 per hour, depending on where you live, says Dr. McKee. One problem you may encounter is reimbursement from your health insurance carrier.

"We feel strongly that we offer a procedure that is helpful in preventing disease as well as treating and alleviating symptoms," he says. "But because we're a relatively new service, we're not included in some reimbursement systems."

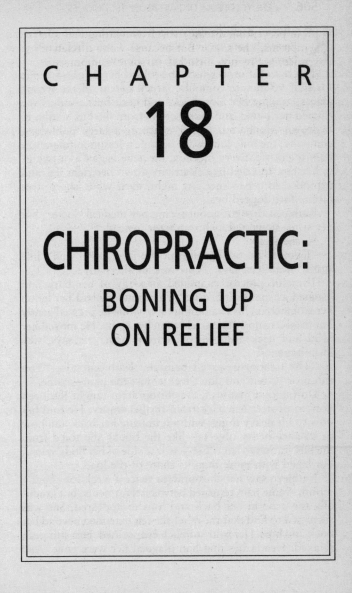

C H A P T E R

18

CHIROPRACTIC:
BONING UP
ON RELIEF

Kathleen Becker's daily trip from her home in eastern Pennsylvania to her New York City office had become, literally, a pain in the fanny.

The bus seat onto which she folded her 5-foot-5 frame for that 90-minute commute struck her in all the wrong places, making her hips, back, and neck hurt. And as she carried her books and manuscripts from the bus station in midtown Manhattan to her office at a large publishing company, the mile-long walk became a lesson in tolerance: pain tolerance. Every morning the ache began as a twinge in her hip, traveled like electricity down her right leg, and exploded into her knee. At night, even while she rested, discomfort dogged her.

Kathleen thought about seeing her medical doctor, but her sister suggested a chiropractor instead.

So she went.

"I don't like taking pills all the time and I don't like shots," Kathleen says. "This was an alternative."

The chiropractor examined an x-ray of her back and listened as she described her symptoms. He had her lie on her stomach on his examining table while he pressed gently but firmly against the vertebrae in her spine. He moved her head and neck around. Relief from pain, she says, was instantaneous.

"The treatment wasn't painful," Kathleen says. "You can hear it, but you don't feel it. Just the pain is gone."

During that first visit, the chiropractor taught Kathleen how to protect her back from further injury. He told her how to lift heavy things without hurting her back and how to balance heavy objects—like the books she toted from the bus station to her office—so one side of her body wasn't burdened with more than its share of the load.

Kathleen saw her chiropractor twice a week for about a month. Some pain returned between treatments, but gradually the ache in her back and hips disappeared. She was surprised to find that the relief she felt extended beyond her back and hips. Her sour stomach evaporated. Her stiff neck relaxed. Headaches that had plagued her were gone. And she discovered that the pills she had been taking for sore knees were no longer necessary.

After a month, her back and neck felt like new. Kathleen was told that she should return for a monthly maintenance program that would keep her skeleton in alignment.

What exactly did the chiropractor do to return this 23-year-old woman's back to its original pain-free condition?

So, What's a Chiropractor?

Chiropractors are health-care professionals who base their treatment on drugless, nonsurgical methods of healing. They follow the premise that subluxations—misaligned vertebrae together with their surrounding ligaments—put pressure on spinal nerves. This pressure contributes to pain as well as to a variety of internal disorders. Manual adjustments put things back into line. In other words, these doctors realign the pieces of your skeletal puzzle properly. They maintain that when things are in their proper order, your body should work the way it was designed to.

The difference between the medical doctor and the chiropractor, says Louis Sportelli, D.C., American Chiropractic Association spokesman, is like the difference between the mechanic who works on your car's engine and the person at the body shop who can straighten a bent frame and align your wheels. The medical doctor is concerned with the internal organs and disease; the chiropractor concentrates on function, structure, and wellness.

"The medical doctor would view the car's engine, looking for dysfunction. We would look at the frame. You can have a bent frame and your car won't function properly," he says.

"We look for the structural imbalance. A limp won't show up on an x-ray, and yet it will throw your gait off and cause abnormal stress and strain to your structure."

In addition to performing physical manipulation, chiropractors encourage proper nutrition and exercise. Unlike medical doctors, they do not prescribe drugs, nor do they do surgery. They are specially trained in treating problems such as back pain and whiplash. If more invasive treatments are necessary—a cortisone injection, for instance, or surgery—they refer you to a medical doctor.

"We don't cure disease," Dr. Sportelli says. "However, some of the functional disturbances of the human body may have a mechanical basis. For example, a cardiologist can look at a cardiogram for the cause of chest wall pain—functional angina—and not find anything wrong with your heart. Yet when your spine is manipulated, the pain goes away. But we didn't actually cure a heart condition."

"The true chiropractic philosopher basically believes in the intrinsic ability of the body to heal itself," says Scott Haldeman, M.D., Ph.D., D.C., adjunct professor at the Los Angeles Chiropractic College and assistant clinical professor in the Department of Neurology at the University of California, Irvine. "It's a naturalist approach to health [that] encourages exercise, stress reduction, and proper nutrition along with chiropractic adjustments. The question is always raised with individuals who say their patients are much healthier than the general population—are they healthier because they live better or are they healthier because of chiropractic adjustment? We just don't know."

Getting Ready

Chiropractors learn their profession by attending many of the same kinds of classes medical doctors attend to acquire their skills.

To enter chiropractic college, the doctor-to-be must first complete two years of undergraduate school, although more than 50 percent earn a bachelor's degree. In chiropractic college, the next four years are spent studying organic chemistry, anatomy, physiology, bacteriology, microbiology, x-rays and physical exams, neurology, orthopedics, cardiology, gynecology, physical therapy, and nutrition. During a fifth year of study, the chiropractic student sees patients in a college-affiliated clinic. Some students may study an additional three years in radiology or orthopedics.

Beyond Body Mechanics

There is no doubt that chiropractic relieves pain—and not just because it promotes proper structure and function of your body, Dr. Sportelli says.

"Some of the latest studies show that the body produces its own opiates, called beta-endorphins, following spinal manipulation," he says. "It creates a good feeling. That's like the runner's high.

"The second reason is, inside each of the spinal joints are little sensitizers called mechano-receptors. Once they are manipulated and the joint is made more mobile, there is an increase in joint play. Once the mobility of the joint is increased, there is an increased range of motion," he says. The person who was stuck in a painful position can now move more easily and in a larger range of motion without pain.

Sorting Through the Claims

Not all chiropractors, however, agree on what they can treat and how often adjustments may be necessary. Some, for instance, believe a monthly adjustment is required. Some don't.

"For a lot of neuromuscular pains, there is no cure, only control," says Kenneth Edington, D.C., president of the National Association of Chiropractic Medicine. "Some doctors will tell you that you need a monthly adjustment to control pain, but that's based on an old theory that there is a bone out of place and the chiropractor needs to keep putting it back in to maintain your health."

Dr. Edington disagrees with that theory. "I think we control muscular and skeletal pain by teaching body mechanics and exercise programs. For instance, if someone has lower back pain, we send them to back [strengthening] school to learn to take care of their back."

Dr. Sportelli maintains that the regular adjustment is necessary to keep joints and bones moving within their proper range.

"By the time someone gets to a chiropractor," Dr. Sportelli says, "the condition is usually degenerative and many times is not correctable. The body won't grow back a new joint. So we treat the symptoms until [the patient] feels better, then we see them on a routine basis for the rest of their life to keep mobility in the framework. It's not unlike having to take insulin daily for the rest of your life if you're diabetic. Insulin isn't a cure, but it keeps diabetes under control."

Choosing an Alternative

Among people who visit chiropractors, three out of four polled in a *Prevention* magazine survey said their chiropractor brings them the pain relief they need. Surveys show that the most commonly treated complaint is back pain, followed by headaches, joint pain, and sports injuries.

"People who believe very strongly promote chiropractic," says Dr. Haldeman. As both a chiropractor and a medical doctor, he is in a unique position to evaluate the claims of chiropractic.

"Chiropractic is beneficial in the management of spine pain syndromes. The research has been carried out and has shown the beneficial effect of chiropractic care for those patients. Low back pain, neck pain, headaches, whiplash, and other injuries account for 80 percent of patient visits to chiropractors," Dr. Haldeman says.

A study reported in the *British Medical Journal* supports the use of chiropractic in treating certain kinds of pain. The study looked at people with low back pain caused by mechanical problems, not by disease.

Following chiropractic treatment, not only did most fare better than people treated in the hospital using traditional therapy, they also maintained their improvement for at least two years.

Picking a Practitioner

If you think a chiropractor is the right choice for you, you just might be able to ask your medical doctor for a referral.

"Although some M.D.'s are still leery of us, acceptance is better," Dr. Edington says. "We're getting more referrals as soon as they see we're talking the same language."

"There's been an explosion in the last couple of years of medical doctors and chiropractors joining forces as a cooperative health-care team," says Dr. Sportelli. "More than 80 hospitals now have chiropractors on their staff."

Your First Visit

Your first visit to the chiropractor will be much like your first visit to your medical doctor.

It will take about an hour. A staff member will record your medical history, including information on other treatments you have had. The doctor will do a physical examination and ask lifestyle questions, such as "Do you do repetitive work?" (looking for joint or muscle strain) and "Are you happy at home?" (looking for potential posture problems caused by depression). Finally, the doctor will test the range of motion and the strength of your muscles and joints.

Then the chiropractor will probably have x-rays taken of your spine. The doctor wants to know the condition of your skeletal system before attempting to manipulate your spine, says Dr. Sportelli.

After examining the x-rays, the doctor will do whatever adjustments seem to be necessary. The adjustments may sound loud, but the cracking and popping is comparable to the noises your knuckles make when they are popped. The adjustment shouldn't hurt, says Dr. Sportelli.

You may feel some soreness or aching in your spinal joints and muscles afterward, but that's a natural reaction and will pass in a couple of days, notes Dr. Sportelli.

Your health insurance will probably pay for your chiropractic visit if you are having a specific complaint treated. Routine, "preventive" treatments are usually not covered.

Going Back for More

If you've gone to the chiropractor for a specific complaint, you'll probably have to return for a 5- to 30-minute appointment within a week.

"You should get *some* relief right away," says Dr. Edington. A normal treatment program that gives significant relief from pain will include from five to eight visits over a three-week period, he says.

Typically, a person with low back pain who doesn't have a long history of the problem or some underlying cause, such as osteoarthritis, will see the doctor two or three times a week for about three weeks. Many chiropractors continue to treat their patients after the pain is gone to prevent a relapse.

It may take a while to find complete relief from pain. Neither a medical doctor nor a chiropractor can cure everything with a single office visit.

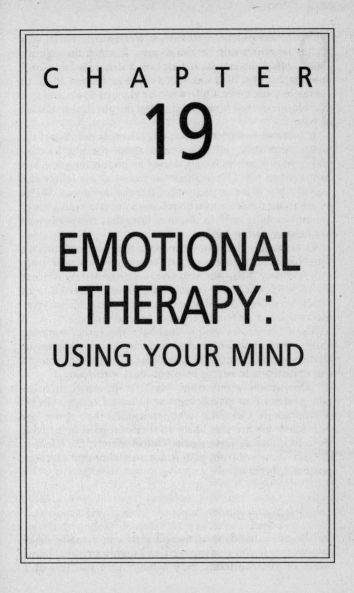

CHAPTER
19

EMOTIONAL THERAPY:
USING YOUR MIND

One day psychologist Patrick W. Edwards, Ph.D., was late for a talk he had to give. Rushing through his office, he caught his arm on a metal basket. For 5 minutes, his arm bled unnoticed while he rushed about to complete some tasks. Only when he glanced down and saw that blood covered his arm did he feel the physical sensation of pain.

It's not so remarkable that Dr. Edwards didn't feel the minor cut. We've all heard tales about the pro football player who fractures his leg during an important game and continues to play. He realizes the extent of his injury and feels the hot blaze of pain only after the last down. We've heard about the woman who rescues someone from a burning automobile, only to discover later that she performed her heroics with a broken arm.

Occasionally the pain we manage to ignore *can* hurt us. Jim Noble, a laborer and part-time country singer from Independence, Missouri, was certain he had merely strained his back. He managed to ignore the brutal pains of a heart attack for more than a day before seeking help. He survived the attack but suffered extensive heart damage.

These anecdotes simply highlight the rather amazing ability of the human mind to focus on a task by ignoring all distractions—including pain. It's an ability that you can call upon consciously to help you deal with pain.

"Distraction is important," says Dr. Edwards, an assistant professor of psychology at Lander College, Greenwood, South Carolina, who concludes that if we are distracted, we are less likely to focus on pain or to label the sensations we feel as pain. Unfortunately, the talent to distract ourselves from pain is not an ability that everyone possesses, he says.

Changing the Channel

On the other hand, your mental state can actually make pain worse. If you're depressed and highly stressed, being aware of your suffering may actually give you less of a threshold for withstanding pain, says Steve Allen, Jr., M.D., assistant professor of family medicine at State University of New York Health Science Center at Syracuse and son of the famous comedian. "There's evidence that you will probably be out of the hospital sooner and require less pain medication when you're not depressed," he says.

Many times the way we view a physical problem causes an "emotional fallout" that has a lot to do with how much pain the problem causes us, says Neal Olshan, Ph.D., author of *The Scottsdale Pain Relief Program.*

But just because your pain may be heightened by your emotional state doesn't mean that you're not playing with a full deck.

"When you get depressed, your biochemistry changes, and any given amount of pain hurts more than it would otherwise," notes Michael G. McKee, Ph.D., of the Department of Psychiatry and Psychology Biofeedback Section at the Cleveland Clinic Foundation. "When you get depressed, it's hard to get out of bed. You go round and round in a vicious circle." What happens when you focus on your pain is that it gets worse until it dominates your life, he says.

That's why skipping work when you're in pain is hardly the best answer to your problems, according to Dr. McKee. In fact, once your mind is on the tasks in front of you, this morning's pain may rapidly fade into only a memory.

Doctors and psychologists have come to realize that pain originates in the body *and* mind—and that *both* must receive attention if treatment is to succeed. They've developed a number of strategies for bringing the healing powers of the mind and emotions into full play.

Reward Yourself for Good Behavior

You actually may help your pain fade into the woodwork by bribing yourself to ignore your pain, says Dr. McKee. The reward you give yourself depends on you. Only you know what truly appeals to you. Using rewards and punishments to shape and change behavior is at the heart of a pain-relieving strategy known as behavioral therapy.

"A reward could be things like going to a movie, just watching television, having a special meal, buying a record," says Dr. McKee. What you are doing, he says, is metaphorically giving yourself a gold star.

One caution: Dr. McKee warns that you should not give yourself a reward that may serve to make pain worse. For example, you should not treat yourself to a game of tennis if you have tennis elbow.

Erase Pain Behavior

The body and mind try to work together to adjust to chronic pain. If the suffering goes on long enough, a pain lifestyle—the most difficult aspect of chronic pain to break—is the result, says Dr. Olshan.

He cites the example of a male patient of his who is a surgical nurse. The young man hurt his back lifting a patient and had three back surgeries. Two weeks after he returned to work, his supervisor told him she'd have to let him go.

"Why? I'm doing my job," he said.

"Yes, but I have to let you go because of your pain behaviors," she told him. He was unconsciously doing such things as grimacing, moaning, and leaning on counters as he went about his work. He was making his fellow employees, not to mention the hospital patients, uncomfortable.

Dr. Olshan uses mirrors to show people in pain how they look to others. Gradually, even if the pain is still there, they learn to suppress their pain behaviors in front of other people.

He also advises people in pain to pay close attention to what happens during conversation. "If you're in a conversation, and the conversation switches to somebody else, spend a few seconds and think: What did I just say? Was I talking about my pain again? Was I rubbing my temples or otherwise acting as though I were in pain?" says Dr. Olshan. "One of the things I've noticed is that if you, with enough consistency, physically act as though you're in pain and verbalize pain, you sabotage yourself." In other words, if you would be pain-free, act as if you're pain-free.

Dr. Olshan recommends that you ask loved ones or friends to help you end your pain lifestyle. He advises you to tell them, "If I start moaning and groaning, if I grab my back, if I show any pain behavior, tell me or give me a signal somehow." Children are often the best observers of behavior, he says. Don't be afraid to ask them to participate in this helpful exercise.

Never Give Up, Never Give In

Just as rewarding yourself is important, it's equally important not to punish yourself when you're in pain. A group of your friends wants to go out after work to play volleyball. You can't play because you've got a bad shoulder, arthritis in the knee, whatever.

"You have a choice," says Dr. Olshan. You can say, "Poor me," or make up an excuse that may be readily seen by everyone, or pout and try to get people to feel sorry for you, or play and reinjure yourself. "Or," he says, "you can keep score and become an active participant without having to play."

Dr. Olshan recommends that you seek other solutions before giving up a favorite activity because of pain. "Take the time to look at alternatives," he says.

Learn to Breathe

People in pain must learn to know their own body, says Dr. Olshan. You have to learn what you're doing that enhances your body's well-being and what detracts from it. "We have to be stimulus creators," says Dr. Olshan. "We have to create the stimuli in our environment that are conducive to controlling pain."

This kind of pain control is not magical. It involves learning a set of skills that you incorporate into your lifestyle.

People in pain tend to breathe high in the chest—a type of breathing done by our ancestors when it was time to fight or take flight, says Dr. Olshan. While breathing is a physical activity, it has an immediate impact on your emotions—and perception of pain. Many times if you're in a lot of pain, you'll be "doing a lot of gasping," says Dr. Olshan. This gasping triggers nerve endings, sending a message to the brain that you're having a reaction to trauma. In turn, this sets in motion certain reactions in your body that increase pain.

"Pain is like quicksand," he says. "The harder you struggle, the more you sink." You can learn how to do a form of abdominal breathing, however, that is completely counter to the anxiety reaction you have when your pain is increased, he says.

"Learning how to regulate your breathing and to do abdominal breathing is very important," he says, noting that such a technique is taught by Lamaze experts to lessen the pain during childbirth. "What's great about it is that you can do it anytime, anywhere. You can do it at the office or while driving a car."

Explaining how to do deep breathing is easy. Actually doing it takes considerable practice—especially if your breathing has been shallow and rapid because you've been stressed out and pain-ridden for a long time. "Put one hand on your abdomen and one on your chest and watch which one moves," says David E. Bresler, Ph.D., former director of the UCLA Pain Control Unit and executive director of the Bresler Center in Pacific Palisades, California. "Practice until you succeed in having the one on your chest relatively stationary and the one on your abdomen moving in and out as you breathe."

Dear Diary

Getting a handle on what aspects of your behavior lead to increased pain levels is not always easy. One of the most beneficial things you can do in this regard is to keep a written diary, says Dr. McKee.

"We ask people to keep a pain diary hour by hour," he says. In the diary they rate both pain and suffering. Sometimes the frequency, intensity, and duration of the pain do not change, but the suffering it causes is less or greater at certain times.

A pain diary is often revealing. It helps you pinpoint what events, people, or activities cause *you* to vibrate in pain like phone lines during an earthquake. What causes you pain can cause another joy, and vice versa. Just as one person's meat is another's poison, so too do different things cause tension, anxiety, and pain in all of us.

Miss Grundy hates teaching. Walking into a classroom, to her, is about as appealing as tap dancing in a minefield. Those who love teaching, of course, are never more joyful than when addressing a class of eager pupils.

Depending on your mindset, a major purchase, the birth of a child, even the arrival of your mother-in-law for a three-week stay may be joyful occasions or anxiety-causing events. If you are a person in pain, how you view these events determines whether your pain is increased or lessened.

And knowing your personal pain triggers may help you avoid them, notes Dr. McKee.

Learn to Bear Up

The people who stream into Dr. Bresler's pain clinic often demand that he kill their pain. "Give me a pill, cut it out, get rid of it," they beg. This insistence on "killing" pain is a uniquely Western concept, says Dr. Bresler. "That term is not translatable into any other language," he says.

Dr. Bresler teaches patients that killing their pain may not be possible in every case but that everyone has a reasonable expectation of learning to tolerate it. There may be times when your pain flares up but your tolerance is so high that it hardly bothers you, says Dr. Bresler. Maybe you're enjoying a friend's company, reading a good book, or enjoying an absorbing movie.

Increasing tolerance to pain is a critical part of care, says Dr. Bresler. When you come into a pain clinic with arthritis, the doctor can inject cortisone into the joint to reduce pain and inflammation, although what's left may still be intolerable. Or the doctor can teach self-management skills that do not directly affect the joint but may elevate your tolerance to the point where that joint pain doesn't bother you any more. The wise patients choose Plan B, says Dr. Bresler.

Most of the pain-management skills that Dr. Bresler teaches his patients involve guided imagery that is designed to produce endorphins—the body's own naturally produced healing chemicals. (For more on this technique, see chapter 34.) He also offers commonsense advice: They should make sure to get a decent night's sleep, stick to a diet that is compatible with the lifestyle they're trying to achieve, and learn to handle their emotions and everyday stressful situations with a minimum of wear and tear on the immune system. "The other self-management strategy we want people to have is a good exercise program that is self-reinforcing and self-maintaining," says Dr. Bresler.

Dr. Bresler says that his aim is similar to a tried-and-true bromide. If you give a man a fish, he is content for only one meal; but if you teach him to fish, you've made him self-sufficient for the rest of his life. "That's the premise of our program," he says. "We teach patients to manage pain on their own."

Switching Focus

If you are in chronic pain, it's sometimes hard to gain relief unless you can focus your mind on things that are desirable to think about, says Carl Simonton, M.D., coauthor of *Getting Well Again*. It's important to concentrate on things that bring joy or at least a calm feeling of well-being into our life, he says.

If we think about pain every waking moment, naturally we are going to feel the pain intensely all the time, he points out. "We create our emotions with our thoughts and beliefs," says Dr. Simonton. "If I change the way I think, then my emotions will automatically change."

Dr. Simonton, who runs the Simonton Cancer Center in Pacific Palisades, California, is no more immune from pain than the rest of us. He believes that chronic pain often represents the body's attempt to protect us from something else. If you're worried that a child or grandchild may be on drugs, your body may manufacture a nagging migraine headache. The pain might be bad enough to prevent you from concentrating on the family crisis. Dr. Simonton speaks from experience. Twenty years ago he had great difficulty in his work. No matter how hard he tried, his expertise was not enough to solve his problems. In the midst of agonizing over his work-related difficulties, his back went out, leaving him in excruciating pain.

While in pain he asked himself what he would be thinking about if he were suddenly pain-free. He realized that he would be worrying about his problems at work and that his pain was helping him avoid doing so.

Because he was motivated to heal his back, he began to develop safe topics that he could think about. He could think about his family, music, and sailing—three topics that he loved and that brightened his life whenever he thought about them.

In two words, his solution was "stop worrying." He began to think desirable thoughts or at least neutral thoughts. His back didn't get better at once, and whenever it did hurt, he realized that he'd somehow slipped into the bad habit of thinking negative thoughts about his work.

Dr. Simonton insists that there is a process central to healing: "Dr. Albert Schweitzer said it as well as anyone when he said that within each person exists a wise physician. I believe that we have within us the answers to what we need to do to come into harmony with ourselves. Pain is an indication of disharmony. We can do a lot about the mental aspects to impact the physical, and then begin to do physical things to also impact the mental aspects."

Pain as a Family Matter

You may think the way you react to pain is uniquely and personally your own. Actually, the way you react to pain may well be something you learned from your mother or father, according to Dr. Edwards. If both parents showed strong responses to pain—say, grimacing, taking to bed, or complaining—you are likely to respond today in a similar fashion. "If you had parents experiencing a lot of pain, then you would find that their offspring would tend to have pain problems," he says. Headaches, for example, might run in your family.

In the Edwards household, his mother was the one who most frequently showed pain, he recalls.

Dr. Edwards thinks that he and his siblings reinforced his mother's pain responses by paying more attention to her when she was suffering. In fact, whenever they saw their mom lying down on the couch, one of the children was sure to pipe up, "She's going to want us to cook supper." Ignoring her didn't work. "She'd just do it more until she got the desired effect," he recalls.

Dr. Edwards's mother is hardly an isolated case. If you're experiencing pain, it might surprise you to realize that you may have a hidden agenda that rewards your display of pain, says Dr. Edwards. These rewards include getting attention from loved ones or co-workers, missing work, and receiving financial gain from an insurance company or workers' compensation.

Quite often, people are unaware that they are reacting in an extreme fashion to pain because they have something to gain, says Dr. Edwards. Pain is something we experience, but also "it's something we create to a degree," he says.

Whether we hide our pain, flaunt it, or do something in between, we all have a similar process to follow when we're hurt, says Dr. Edwards. After we perceive pain, we label it and decide what we're going to do about it. "The important point," he says, "is that when people have an ache or pain, they need to ask themselves, Am I making my suffering worse?"

Dr. Edwards stresses that pain is not imaginary even when people unconsciously rev it up. "There is some physical stimulation coming from the body—such as a pinched nerve or a cut—that causes the pain in the first place. However, people need to question the way they are reacting to this physical stimulation. Ask yourself, Am I magnifying or underplaying it? What kind of body language am I sending out?"

You need to be aware of whether you are using your pain symptoms to get love, affection, and attention from family members, says Dr. Bresler. If you're getting massaged, patted on the back, and cooed over when you express pain, this gets reinforced to such a point that you could be feeling rewarded for being in pain.

Dr. Bresler asks overly supportive family members to leave the person in pain alone. Instead, when he or she feels better, the person then can get gobs of love and support from family members. In most cases, says Dr. Bresler, the whole family is his patient—even if only one member shows pain symptoms. It's essential to involve the entire family in pain therapy for one family member, he says, because all family members are affected.

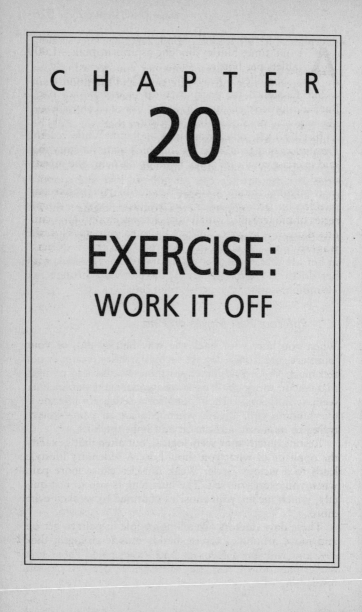

CHAPTER
20

EXERCISE:
WORK IT OFF

At one time, Shirley bought aspirin in bulk—1,000 tablets per bottle.

She filled hot water bottles by the gallon.

She fashioned ice pack after ice pack after ice pack. But nothing relieved the pain in her neck and shoulders—mementos of an automobile accident.

Just by luck, relief was right at hand. While reading *Prevention* magazine, Shirley stumbled across a story that said exercise might be a key to stopping pain. She investigated.

A physical therapist taught her to do exercises recommended by her orthopedic doctor. And today, a simple series of movements, which takes her no more than 5 minutes daily, has become Shirley's panacea for pain. Plus, she was so pleased with the positive effects of exercise in her life that she bought a stationary bicycle and, with her doctor's approval, now spins her way through her 30-minute newspaper break each day.

Put Your Best Moves on Pain

When you hurt your back the way Shirley did, or your joints are sore from a disease such as arthritis, you may not feel much like exercising. Even those tweaks and twinges that tend to sneak up on us as we age can make the sidelines seem awfully appealing. Opting for a sedentary lifestyle is like holding your breath when you are in pain—you're trying to minimize movement and limit the hurt.

Resting quietly may seem logical, but often that's exactly the opposite of what you should do. A sedentary lifestyle leads to a vicious circle: Weak muscles cause more pain when you exert yourself. The hurt tempts you to rest quietly, which means your muscles continue to weaken even more.

These days doctors are telling people in pain to get up and move around. Exercise builds muscle strength, they say, and will speed recovery and lessen pain. Those first moves may not be easy, but sensible exercise will pay off in the long run.

"I think that everybody should try to do some type of aerobic exercise. You might not be able to jog, but you might swim. Or walk," says Kenneth Edington, D.C., a chiropractor and exercise physiologist in Milwaukee.

What it comes down to is this: It's worth the effort because the payback is in the form of faster healing and pain relief.

Hippocrates put it this way 2,400 years ago: "All parts of the body which have a function, if used in moderation and exercised in labors to which each is accustomed, become thereby healthy and well developed, and age slowly; but if unused and left idle, they become liable to disease, defective in growth, and age quickly."

Dr. Edington rephrases it a bit, saying, "Even though you may be a little sore when you move, you will rehabilitate faster."

So, how do you get started?

Easy Does It

The first rule of exercising to help banish pain is this: See your doctor and find out what is causing the pain. If it's a disease such as arthritis that's behind those twinges and pings, you'll want to enlist your doctor's help in starting an exercise program appropriate for your condition. For instance, your family doctor may be able to prescribe stretches for a stiff, aching back or steer you to a program exactly tailored to your needs, such as water-exercise classes. Sponsored by the YMCA or YWCA throughout the United States, these classes cater to people with arthritis, allowing them the benefits of exercise while the water supports their weight, taking the pull of gravity off their inflamed joints.

Even if you know what is causing your pain, make sure you see your doctor before starting any exercise plan. Some painful conditions, such as back pain, could be worsened by the wrong moves.

Taking Mother Nature's Prescription

Exercise is probably one of Mother Nature's best and easiest prescriptions to fill, say the experts.

"Exercise gets the body started doing what it's built to do," says D. W. Edington, Ph.D., director of the University of Michigan's Fitness Research Center in Ann Arbor. "It's in a more natural state when it's moving."

Exercise won't work as quickly to relieve pain as some other types of pain relief—downing two aspirin, for instance—but getting your body moving on a regular basis produces long-term benefits, says Kathleen Haralson, physical therapist and associate director of the Regional Arthritis Center at Washington University School of Medicine in St. Louis.

"Vigorous exercise has been shown to lead to significant alterations in the body's intrinsic pain-regulatory system. It can lead to increased serum levels of beta-endorphins, which are hundreds of times more powerful than the equivalent dose of morphine," she says.

Beta-endorphins are naturally occurring, morphinelike chemicals in the brain that act just like the painkilling drug morphine. Endorphin, by the way, is short for endogenous morphine. *Endogenous* means that it's manufactured by your body. Just like morphine taken as a pain-relieving medication, your body's own endorphins raise your pain threshold. This means your body can tolerate more pain before your nerves scream.

While endorphins reduce your level of pain, they improve your overall sense of health and well-being, too. If you have pain—back pain, for instance—you may feel better during and after exercise because your beta-endorphin level rises with exertion.

"You don't have to do something strenuous to do some good," Dr. D. W. Edington says. "Even moderate exercise increases the circulation: Wounds heal quicker, pain goes away faster."

Mind/Body Benefits

Exercise also produces psychological benefits that can help you cope with pain. It draws attention away from pain, and it promotes healing and soothing sleep, Haralson says.

"When you are sitting there in pain, it's a pretty small world you're concentrating on. If you get out and expand your world, then the pain becomes a smaller, lesser part of your world," Dr. D. W. Edington says. Experts say that exercise also acts as a stress reliever. It promotes your self-confidence. It seems that the right kind of movement can turn down your pain amplifier while boosting your natural good feelings.

When you exercise you begin to see yourself a little differently—a little more positively. Instead of seeing yourself as an invalid or someone who is prevented by pain from doing things, you become more self-confident. "You get a sense of accomplishment, especially when you are doing something you didn't think you could," says Dr. Kenneth Edington. Other people begin to see you in this new light, too—an additional ego boost. Not only that, researchers say exercise provides a good outlet for anger and tension—two by-products of pain.

Banishing Extra Pounds

Exercise has one additional benefit that is very important to pain relief—it can give your weight-loss program a power boost. A number of painful conditions are relieved when you drop those extra pounds, and your doctor may well tell you to cut back on calories. (See chapter 35 for the dietary side of the weight-loss picture.) You'll find that a successful weight-loss program is easier to maintain if you're exercising regularly. And you might even be able to indulge in an extra snack or two.

Even a 130-pound woman who is totally sedentary uses up 1,690 calories a day. That means on a 1,200-calorie diet she can lose 490 calories a day, or about 1 pound a week. It takes approximately 3,500 calories to create a pound of fat.

Taking in so few calories, though, often leaves people prowling the kitchen for food. If this same woman were to add two 15-minute sessions of easy walking (at 2 miles an hour) a day, she'd burn an extra 120 calories. That's enough to eat an extra piece of fruit, a slice of cheese, or three cookies each day and still lose a pound a week. If she also threw in a 20-minute gentle swim session a week, she'd burn an additional 200 calories, enough to indulge in a slice of pizza or a beer (or both, if she swam 40 minutes!) every Friday night and still lose her pound a week. It's those caloric extras, along with body toning and just plain feeling good, that make nutritionists consider exercise an essential part of any successful diet. (See chapter 29 for more on incorporating exercise into your pain-relief program.)

The Right Moves

In the past, if you had chronic pain, you may have thought that you couldn't exercise or that your doctor wouldn't allow you to exercise. Even patients at chronic pain clinics are now sweating their way through regular workouts.

Doctors recommend stationary bicycles, swimming, walking, and low-impact aerobic dance to build muscle strength, endurance, and flexibility.

If your doctor doesn't recommend an individualized program to suit your particular condition, you have a wide variety of suitable activities to choose from. Rhythmic activities for strengthening large muscles, for weight control, and for stress reduction include walking, hiking, jogging, bicycling, swimming, and dancing.

Your doctor may even recommend weight training to help you strengthen muscles. You would begin by lifting light weights and then use progressively heavier weights as you gain strength.

Flexibility—a quality often missing in someone with pain—can be gained through stretching.

You might sneak a little extra exercise into your pain-relief program by encouraging yourself to remain active, doing such things as climbing stairs, light housekeeping, and gardening.

Pain specialists say that almost any exercise can be safe and effective if you start slowly and build gradually.

Walk Away from Pain

"If I had to choose one exercise, regardless of the pain, I would choose walking," says Dr. D. W. Edington. "Swimming is also good because your natural buoyancy eliminates gravity, but you have to know how to swim."

Besides not requiring any kind of special skill or equipment, walking is one of the easiest forms of exercise around. "It improves almost every system of the body and makes a major contribution to the quality and duration of a person's life," according to James M. Rippe, M.D., director of the Exercise Physiology and Nutrition Laboratory at the University of Massachusetts Medical School and author of *Dr. James M. Rippe's Complete Book of Fitness Walking.* Walking can lop off the extra pounds that add stress to an already stressed-out skeleton. It can increase your stamina, flexibility, and balance.

A Beginning Walker's Program

Walking is super exercise, but if the farthest you usually walk is from your back door to your car door, your walking program should begin with a few steps.

Think of walking in the way you would think of moving a giant rock. You don't just pick up the rock and walk away, you lean into it, hoping to roll it along. You work a little. You rest a little. You take your time. If you go too fast or too far in the beginning, you will get stiff and sore and you'll take longer to reach your goal of regular, pain-free walking. You may also get frustrated and quit. So go slowly.

Plan a walking routine that you can do at least three days a week but not more than six. You need to walk a minimum of three days each week to begin to get your body into condition. If you let too many days go by without walking, your body will always be at the starting point.

Your walks should make you feel invigorated and relaxed, not fatigued. For some people, that will mean a half hour on the road. For others it may be 15 minutes. And if you can walk only to the end of your driveway and back comfortably, that's all right, too. Stop when you feel winded or out of breath—you'll go farther next week.

Take your first walk in your neighborhood. Walk to the end of the street and back. Walk around the block. If you aren't sure how far you can go comfortably, stay close to home.

Begin to exercise "gingerly," says exercise scientist Michael Wolf, Ph.D., president of Fit-Tech in New York City. "Build gradually as you feel your capacity increasing. Each time go a little farther and push a little harder, but just until it doesn't feel good. Walking is a great lifetime exercise, but you don't start walking four miles on Day One. You walk until you are tired, then you sit down on a bench."

While you walk, zero in on how your body is feeling, Dr. Wolf says. "Any sign that you are doing too much—whether it shows up right away, that evening, or the next day—means you should pay attention."

Signals that alert you that you may be pushing yourself too hard include a feeling of malaise, injuries, and general aches and pains in the joints. If it's a strong signal, see a doctor. If it's just soreness, it's probably your body's way of saying you haven't done this in 20 years, so lighten up, Dr. Wolf says.

Take the Next Step

After three to five days of walking at a comfortable pace, add 5 minutes to your walk. If that feels good, stick with it for a week or so. If it doesn't, drop back to your original walk for another week.

Add a few minutes to your walk every week or so until you are walking for a half hour three days a week. When you've reached that goal, speed your pace just a little.

Let comfort dictate your pace. You should always be able to carry on a conversation without gasping for breath.

"The only rule is just do it," says Dr. Wolf. "It's much more important that you get out and go 15 minutes if that's all you feel like doing today. Then, go ahead and sit down and watch the birds a while."

C H A P T E R
21

HOT AND COLD THERAPY:
TURN ON INSTANT RELIEF

Y ou've spent a long day planting the garden. Now, as you slap the dirt off your jeans, you realize that your back and legs are starting to ache.

You climb into the shower and adjust the water flow to a delightfully hot barrage. You turn around. The stinging jets beat a rhythm against your aching leg and back muscles. You close your eyes—and savor the healing power of a hot water massage.

You've discovered a magic potion that many people routinely use to stop or prevent pain. Heat is one of the oldest natural pain relievers around. However, water is not the only way to apply heat. A heating pad is often the first thing people reach for when they are in pain. Doctors sometimes prescribe radiant heat—like that from a light bulb—for pain relief. And you can generate your own soothing heat with a plastic body wrap.

Cold is an excellent pain reliever, too. Ice packs, ice massage, frozen gel, and cold compresses are good options for stopping sudden pain.

The beauty of using heat or cold to soothe pain—called hot or cold therapy—is that both are so readily available and so easy to use. They are as close as the bathroom or refrigerator and as simple as grabbing a bag of frozen peas.

When Hot Is Not Cool

Doctors and physical therapists recommend the painkilling power of both of these natural analgesics. But which is the better choice?

Cold stops pain short by dulling the sensory nerves. It helps to prevent both inflammation and joint stiffness. It also slows blood flow to an injured area—helping to prevent soreness and bruising. Heat, on the other hand, encourages blood flow. Increased circulation flushes away the natural body wastes that can cause soreness. Warmth also relaxes muscles, allowing them to uncramp and helping you to regain mobility—a first step in getting your aching joints or muscles back to normal.

While both heat and cold can relieve pain, the treatments

are not interchangeable. Using heat when you need cold—
as in the case of a twisted ankle—can increase swelling and
delay healing. Using ice when heat would do the trick—on
an arthritic joint, for example—may make you just plain
uncomfortable.

Simply because your choice feels good doesn't make it
right. Many people who experience sudden, sharp back
pain enjoy the soothing sensation of a heating pad when
their muscles scream. But an ice bag would be the better
choice initially.

"You'll walk with a stiffer sensation in your back if you
use heat in the early stages because it will leave your tissues
congested," says Joseph Estwanik, M.D., an orthopedic
surgeon in Charlotte, North Carolina. Dr. Estwanik consults and travels with the U.S. Olympic boxing team.

"If you numb the muscle while it's still trying to spasm,
there's less pain and less stiffness," he says. Once the spasm
is gone, it's okay to reach for the heat. It'll help your mobility in the affected area, says Dr. Estwanik.

So the first rule of hot and cold pain relief is: When
there's any doubt, choose cold first.

"Ice accomplishes many things that heat would do, but
with half the potential drawbacks," Dr. Estwanik says.

Cool It Off, Heat It Up

Cold water and ice, experts say, work best for injuries
and acute (sudden) pain. Cold is an excellent antidote for
headache, as well as back, knee, and shoulder pain. Cold
is a good choice for alleviating pain from surgery, minor
burns, itching, bursitis, and back labor during childbirth.

Moist heat and dry heat alleviate pain caused by some
types of disease—including joint stiffness from arthritis.
Heat is also excellent for relieving the pain from pressure
sores, boils, and gastrointestinal upset. Look to warmth to
stop pain in the rectal area and pain from menstrual cramps.

Sometimes the distinctions aren't clear-cut, and you may
have to experiment to find out which works best for you.
Either heat or cold will take the twinge out of overused

muscles—the soreness you feel after a full day in the garden. Either is a good choice for muscle spasms, joint stiffness, low back pain, and jaw pain. The effect of cooling, however, lasts longer than that of a heat treatment. After heat is removed, the increased blood flow brings muscles rapidly back to their normal temperature. After cold is discontinued, blood vessels remain constricted for a while, so rewarming takes longer. The choice is yours.

However, heat and cold aren't the right pain relievers for everyone. People with fragile skin, areas of numbness, or circulatory problems (caused by diabetes, Raynaud's syndrome, or other illness) should check with their doctor before experimenting with these treatments.

Putting the Freeze on Pain

Suppose, as you're returning your hoe to the garden shed, you trip over a stone and turn your ankle. If you find yourself reaching for an ice pack, that would be the right choice.

Ice is not just nice—it's the main ingredient in RICE, a catchy little formula doctors use to describe a common first-aid technique. RICE stands for rest, ice, compression, and elevation.

To treat that sprain using RICE, you would wrap an elastic bandage around your throbbing ankle, set it on a stool so it's slightly elevated, and not walk for a while, allowing your ankle to rest. And you'd apply ice, which does double duty. It will stop any bleeding, bruising, and swelling that can cause long-term soreness, and it becomes your on-the-spot analgesic.

"If you get hurt—a burn or a sprain or a fracture—the area looks red and feels warm to the touch. Inflammation is the body's response to an injury. What we want to do is stop the inflammation that's causing the 'heat.' We do that with ice," Dr. Estwanik says. "In addition to physiologically improving the injury, ice numbs the sensory nerves and helps with the pain. We win two ways."

How to Chill Out

Do you have an ice bag handy for that ankle?

Sure you do. Just drop some cubes into a resealable plastic bag. *Voilà!* A low-cost ice bag.

There are many ways you put the chill on pain: an ice pack, an ice towel, an ice massage, a contrast bath, vapo-coolant (an ethyl chloride spray), or frozen gel. But using ice for pain relief can be as simple as opening your refrigerator door.

Try a gel-filled plastic bag that can be frozen and refrozen. Make a do-it-yourself gel pack by filling a resealable plastic bag with one-third alcohol and two-thirds water. Seal tightly and place in the freezer for a flexible, unfrozen slush. Or you can make a flexible cold pack by placing a cold, damp cloth or towel inside a sealed plastic bag. In a pinch, you can press a bag of frozen peas or corn against your aching head—it works just as well as a bag of ice, says Kathleen Haralson, physical therapist and associate director of the Regional Arthritis Center at Washington University School of Medicine in St. Louis.

"I prefer old-fashioned ice to the chemical ices," Dr. Estwanik says. "With the chemical ices, you run the risk of freezing the skin. You're somewhat protected using ice because as it touches the skin, it melts, and that water provides a natural layer of insulation between the ice and the skin."

You can get fancy with a Thermosport Wrap—a vinyl bladder that you fill with ice (or cold water or hot water, depending on the relief method you prefer). You insert the bladder into its sleeve and secure the whole thing against your injury with adjustable Velcro straps.

You can sometimes use cold to *prevent* pain, too. When you feel the tension that precedes some kinds of pain (back pain, for example), slip an ice pack onto the area.

Never use any kind of ice for more than 20 minutes at a time because your skin may freeze, blistering just as it would if you used a wrap that was too hot. And be sure to wait about an hour between applications so that your skin has a chance to rewarm itself. You may want to use a thin towel or sheet between the ice bag and your skin to help protect against supercooling.

Give Yourself an Icy Massage

If you don't like the intensity of holding an ice pack against your skin, try an ice massage. Freeze paper cups filled with water to make convenient ice applicators. When you need to massage an area that smarts, tear the paper away from the sides of the cup, leaving yourself a "handle" portion at the bottom. Massage the sore area slowly with short, circular, overlapping strokes two to three times daily.

A towel or cloth soaked in water, called a compress, delivers comfort, too. For years, migraine sufferers have applied cold, damp washcloths to their head. Cold decreases the blood flow and helps reduce migraine pain. In one study, a cold pack in an elastic bandage was applied at the beginning of a migraine and left in place for 30 minutes. Pain was reduced in more than half of those with headaches.

Cooking Up Relief

Warmth has always been a comforting sensation and a great pain reliever. Even in ancient Rome, people flocked to bathhouses for comfort and warmth. Even as Roman legions fought to conquer foreign lands, they found time to build and luxuriate in hot mineral baths. The most famous, perhaps, was in Bath, England, where the 120°F water temperature certainly helped to ward off the damp British climate.

If you have arthritis, you already know how good a warm bath feels when you need to be refreshed. It's an equally good choice for an athlete with a charley horse. But did you know there are several ways you can take that bath?

Rub-a-Dub in More Than a Tub

The sitz bath is a traditional remedy for pain following rectal or vaginal surgery or for treating pelvic infections.

This hip-deep bath, which you can duplicate at home in your own bathtub, is simply a shallow tub of water heated to approximately 105°F—just slightly over body temperature. You sit with your feet up, or kneel so your buttocks, upper thighs, and lower abdomen are in the water, and let the water lap against your wounds. Sometimes your doctor will have you add medication to the water. The sitz bath was the forerunner of the whirlpool, says Dennis Mittleider, director of physical therapy at Hinsdale Hospital in Hinsdale, Illinois.

Like a bubbling mineral spring, the whirlpool, another hip-deep bath, can be cool or warm. The whirlpool adds a soothing turbulence to the water, which serves as a counterirritant. That means the whirling bubbles stimulate large sensory areas on your body and distract your jangled nerves from pain. Also, the water reduces the force of gravity, taking pressure and discomfort away from joints, Haralson says.

You can use a whirlpool at your local gym or buy a small one for your bathroom. And while you are heating up in the tub, you can call on the power of cold at the same time. A cool compress against the forehead while the rest of your body is toasting adds to your comfort and relaxation.

How to Get Out of Hot Water

Spend no more than 15 to 20 minutes at a time immersed in a whirlpool or hot bath, warns Haralson. Your body adjusts to the heat, so it won't get as much benefit after that time. Also, you may become faint from the heat.

For someone who doesn't want to use a heated pool or bath, a hand-held shower with a massage unit offers a comforting tingle to soothe jangled nerves. Direct the stream from the showerhead against sore muscles.

Heat is especially good when used *before* exercising with a sore muscle or joint, says Willibald Nagler, M.D., the physiatrist-in-chief at New York Hospital—Cornell Medical Center. He is the author of *Dr. Nagler's Body Maintenance and Repair Book*. "Heat can make the skeletal muscles 10 percent more elastic," making subsequent range-of-motion exercises easier and more comfortable, he says.

If It Hurts, Get It Hot

Even when the muscles aren't already sore, a day of painting the walls or ceiling can make your arms feel as if you've been reaching for the stars. That's a good time to refresh those tired limbs with a little heat.

Because water is an excellent conductor of heat, the effects of moist heat are likely to be greater than the effects of dry heat. However, you have to be careful about using too much of a good thing. Moisture's excellent transport of heat can lead to burns. If you need to lower the intensity of the heat, cover your skin with a dry towel.

Warmth is a soother no matter how you apply it—in forms ranging from hot towels to heating pads, from steamy baths to the heat from a 40-watt light bulb, from plastic wrap that retains body heat and bubbling whirlpools to heat-producing creams that are rubbed into the skin. Warmth can be applied to any sore joint or muscle for soothing relief.

Experts advise applying heat for 20 to 30 minutes at a time and waiting a couple of hours between applications.

A plain heating pad held over a sore elbow or against an aching knee is sometimes enough to offer comfort. An electric blanket works just as well, Haralson says. And don't forget to try an old-fashioned hot water bottle!

If the twinge is in your neck, simply wrap a fluffy towel around the area. Your body will generate the necessary heat. You can rely on body heat, too, by wrapping plastic food wrap or a plastic dry cleaner bag over an injured area and taping it in place. (It goes without saying that you should never put a plastic bag over your head or face.)

Or you can expose an injured limb to the radiant heat generated by a household light bulb. Simply hold a 40-watt light bulb about 18 inches from the painful area.

For moist heat, a towel dipped in hot water or dampened and then heated in a microwave oven will soothe legs still throbbing from a Saturday touch football game. Towels lose heat quickly, though, and need to be replaced or re-heated about every 5 minutes.

For moist heat that heats longer, try a hydrocollator

pack—a canvas bag that contains silicone gel. You heat the silicone layers in boiling water and wrap the pack in one to two layers of towel to protect your skin from burns. Then place the pack on the sore area and let the heat go to work. You can find this aid in pharmacies and medical supply stores.

Never use heat on areas that already are hot, swollen, or red or on a fresh injury. And never use more than one form of heat at the same time. For example, using a heating pad over a topical heat cream such as Ben-Gay can produce dangerous burns and blisters.

Rubbing Out Your Woes

Another way to apply spot heat is from a tube. A rub-on analgesic such as Ben-Gay, Icy Hot, or Deep-Down can provide comfort and relief.

You massage the over-the-counter cream, which contains menthol, into your sore muscles. The cream works by opening capillaries to your skin, increasing the blood flow so that you feel a soothing warmth. Some say it is a counterirritant that may relieve pain by distraction or by decreasing the perception of pain.

Rub-on heat is appropriate for arthritis, muscle, joint, and tendon pain, low back pain, tension headache, neck pain, sore throat, menstrual cramps, gas pain, itching, and sports injuries. Do not use it on open wounds or irritated skin. Also, do not use this kind of heat if it increases your pain.

So what do athletes really use?

"The one we really like in the National Basketball Association is Flex-all 454," says Terry Kofler, trainer for the Charlotte Hornets basketball team. "We use it to reduce pain."

Finding Relief in Contrasts

Some people like their pain relief both ways: hot and cold. In Finland, it's called a sauna. First, bathers sit in a room where water is poured over hot stones. The bathers are enveloped in the hot, soothing steam. Then they plunge into a cold pool.

While Scandinavians may take saunas for fun and fitness—and you can, too, with an okay from your doctor—physical therapists employ a similar technique to ease pain. Called *contrast therapy*, the treatment uses alternating heat and cold on a pained body part. It can be used whenever heat or cold would be useful. You can use alternate hot and cold baths, or hot and cold packs, for 10 minutes each. This kind of therapy is usually reserved for severe pain.

Since it's hard for someone to set up two full bathtubs at home and keep both at the right temperature, large-scale jobs are best left to a physical therapist. But you can make a contrast bath easily for a sore hand or foot by using two bowls—one with hot water, the other with icy water.

Or alternate a steaming towel with ice applications, leaving each on the affected area for 5 to 8 minutes. This therapy has also been shown to be effective for relieving the muscle pain of temporomandibular disorder (TMD, sometimes referred to as TMJ) or a direct blow to the jaw.

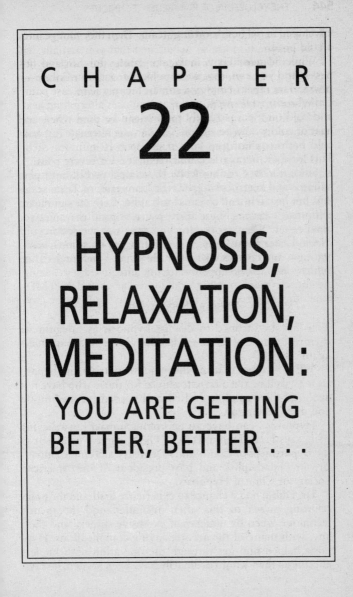

CHAPTER
22

HYPNOSIS, RELAXATION, MEDITATION:
YOU ARE GETTING BETTER, BETTER . . .

n your mind, you're skiing. Under hypnosis your powers of imagination are so heightened that you actually feel the cold wind on your face and hear the swish of skis spewing a jet of white powder behind you. You're vibrating to the fast thrill of the descent, feeling no pain.

Whoa . . . feeling no pain?

The mind is a powerful instrument for pain relief, and certain tools—hypnosis, relaxation, meditation—can help you tap into that deep font of soothing relief.

Hypnosis, relaxation, and meditation are first cousins, says Harold B. Crasilneck, Ph.D., clinical professor of psychiatry and anesthesiology at the University of Texas, Dallas. But just as not all cousins look alike, there are significant differences among these three psychological therapies for pain relief. What works for you may not work for your Uncle Lester from Odessa. You'll have to do some investigating—and consult with your physician—before deciding which one may be appropriate for you.

Hypnosis: Open to Suggestion

You may be inclined to dismiss hypnosis as a legitimate therapy because of its somewhat dubious reputation. Guess again.

When it comes to using the mind to control pain, hypnosis may well be the alternate choice for those who have not acquired the discipline and control needed for meditation and deep relaxation.

Hypnosis "can have an enormous impact" in relieving pain, says Louis Dubin, D.D.S., Ph.D., clinical professor in the Department of Community Dentistry at Temple University in Philadelphia and past president of the American Society of Clinical Hypnosis.

Dr. Dubin had a chance to experience firsthand the pain-relieving power of this often misunderstood therapeutic technique when he underwent extensive surgery and therapy, with many of the accompanying complications. Hypnosis helped him get through the operation with far less anesthesia than would ordinarily have been needed, he says.

It also helped reduce postoperative discomfort and put him back on his feet sooner.

Don't Labor under Mythconceptions

Hypnosis has a long, honorable history as a pain-relief technique. Before chloroform and ether became the fashionable forms of anesthesia, hypnosis was a standard method of reducing pain during surgery, notes Dr. Dubin. He cites the example of one English surgeon who performed 3,000 operations on British soldiers during a single campaign in India in 1845. Another nineteenth-century physician used it to anesthetize patients before amputating limbs and removing tumors.

Hollywood has created the unfortunate image of hypnotists as charlatans and quacks, laments Dr. Dubin. Except for a few unscrupulous people, nothing could be further from the truth.

"We're very careful of our image," he says. "We've spent years getting rid of the Rasputin nonsense that TV, movies, and some of the media put out."

Don't be misled by some slapstick comedy film you once saw. Under hypnosis you can't be made to rob a bank, assassinate a dictator, or commit some wacko crime (unless you secretly harbor a desire to do any of these things).

"Generally, if you wouldn't do something in the awakened state, you won't do it in the hypnotic state," says Dr. Dubin. "You won't give away any secrets or anything."

Not for Everyone

Professionals are aware that not everyone is a good candidate for hypnosis, notes Dr. Dubin. All who come to him undergo a rigid medical and psychological workup to determine that pain caused by serious illnesses—such as cancer and heart disease—receive proper medical attention beyond pain control. People with certain psychological problems may also be excluded from treatment.

For most of us, however, hypnosis may prove beneficial in relieving a number of problems and painful symptoms.

"I have found in the past 25 years of practice that the

more pain someone is in, the better their response to hypnosis," says Dr. Crasilneck. "What I look for in a patient is the desire to get well, the desire to cooperate, and the desire to escape from pain." It also helps for the patient to trust the hypnotherapist, he adds.

Hypnosis is not a panacea for all that pains you, however, says Dr. Dubin. It can be used as a pain reliever for only 30 to 40 percent of the populace. "It's unique with every individual," he says.

The ability of hypnosis to relieve pain apparently also depends on the type of pain being relieved. Experts say it can, for example, help 90 percent of dental patients.

How It Works

Why does hypnosis often work so well to block pain? One theory has it that hypnosis is successful because it relieves anxiety. Another is that it has an effect on both the immune and nervous systems.

Hypnosis is an altered state of consciousness in which your mind disassociates from the environment your body is in, according to Dr. Dubin. He likens it to the experience of being so engrossed in a novel that you no longer are aware you're on your own couch.

With hypnosis, says Dr. Dubin, you become so engrossed that you block out your awareness of things happening in the present—including anxiety and tension, which often worsen pain. Similarly, he says, you can disassociate yourself from the pain you ordinarily might feel during a surgical procedure by taking yourself somewhere else—to your favorite ski resort or a secluded beach, for example—in your imagination.

People under hypnosis frequently lose all perspective on time, says Dr. Dubin. One patient who underwent a 6-hour operation estimated when he awoke that he'd been under only 10 minutes, he says.

Snapping Out of Pain

The list of aches and pains that can be lessened or cured by hypnosis is impressive. Dr. Crasilneck says people from as far away as Europe seek him out for treatment for such conditions as tension and migraine headaches, back pain, arthritis, cancer, childbirth, ulcerative colitis, tic douloureux (a facial disorder marked by severe pain), shingles, and muscular dystrophy. He has also worked with people who have suffered severe burns.

Hypnosis can be used in two ways, notes Dr. Crasilneck—as the sole treatment to fight pain or as an adjunct to other treatments.

Hypnosis also works with chronic pain. If it can't eliminate pain, it can alter your tolerance level, explains Dr. Dubin. "If on a 1-to-10 scale your pain is an 8 or 9, you can lower that figure to a tolerance level you can live with," he says.

Taming the Mouth That Roared

Even pain during a lengthy dental procedure can be eliminated or reduced, says Dr. Dubin. "Hypnosis can help you where ordinarily your jaw would start to get tight and your muscles fatigued," he says. "It doesn't mean that fatigue hasn't bothered your muscles, only that you don't feel it on a conscious level."

Hypnosis can help with a wide variety of mouth pain. One study shows that it may be useful in treating root sensitivity—an often-chronic pain response centered in the root of the tooth. Up to 10 percent of the population has this affliction, which turns gulping a cold beer or a bowl of hot soup into a painful experience. Root sensitivity also makes toothbrushing unpleasant and dental work agonizing.

Hypnosis can also help fight the pain of certain painful mouth disorders, such as temporomandibular disorder (TMD, sometimes referred to as TMJ), when they have a physical or psychological cause, notes Dr. Dubin.

A skilled therapist, he says, may help root out the causes of bruxism—a condition in which patients grind their teeth at night. Bruxism can put painful pressure on the jaws, pressure that radiates to the shoulders and back. Bruxism might be traced back to fear of a dominating parent, a sexual disorder, "or any one of a million things," says Dr. Dubin.

Hypnosis can also be used to attack the pain of bruxism directly, he says. Dr. Dubin teaches people with bruxism to mentally gather all the tension from their body and put it on just two spots located on either shoulder. With the help of hypnosis, they then open an imaginary valve and allow the tension and stress to flow right out, he says. The valve is imaginary, but the tension relief is real.

For people who fear seeing a dentist because of some painful, traumatic remembrance of times past, hypnosis can save the day. A therapist can take you back to your childhood and can help you replace your bad memory with a good one to mitigate your terror.

"We'll superimpose a wonderful chap who holds your hand in place of the gruff old rascal who hurt you," says Dr. Dubin. "You'll walk out saying, 'This is the best dental experience I've ever had.'"

Saying No to Drugs

In many cases, hypnosis is capable of blocking your perception of pain to such a degree that you don't need to resort to drugs, says Dr. Crasilneck. With hypnosis, many people are able to toss out the narcotics they had been taking to induce sleep, he notes.

"Some of my colleagues have performed cesarean sections using hypnosis," says Dr. Crasilneck. "They have done neurosurgery with hypnosis and a local anesthetic. I have personally used hypnosis and nothing else in the delivery room when a woman couldn't take an anesthetic."

Lasting Results

Fine, you may say—as long as you're under hypnosis, you're feeling no pain. But who wants to have to trot on over to a therapist's office for every little twinge? Another nifty feature of hypnosis is that you don't need to make an appointment once or twice a week to get help. While you are receiving treatment, you can be given what is called a posthypnotic suggestion, which can help blot out future pain.

"A therapist can give people a suggestion that they'll be pain-free for a long period of time, or that they will not be nauseous during chemotherapy if they are being treated for cancer," says Dr. Crasilneck. "It's an excellent tool."

Dr. Crasilneck also teaches self-hypnosis to people who cannot easily visit his office. Sometimes he supplements office visits with a tape recording of his voice to help his patients over the rough spots.

Finding a Hypnotherapist

If you'd like to see if hypnosis can work for you, remember rule number one: Exercise caution when selecting a therapist. Never, ever, allow anyone to hypnotize you unless that person is qualified to do so, warns Dr. Crasilneck. He cites an instance in which someone with only two weeks of training opened up a clinic in Texas and referred to himself as a doctor. "In my opinion, no one but a physician, psychologist, or dentist should use hypnosis for pain relief," he says. "We're trying to get state legislation passed to prevent just anybody from using it."

Ask your physician for a referral to a reputable hypnotherapist. You might call a medical college and ask if there are any therapists in your area trained in using hypnosis for pain relief.

You can also contact the Society for Clinical Experimental Hypnosis, 128 Kings Park Drive, Liverpool, New York, 13090, (315) 652-7299, for a referral; or send a self-addressed, stamped envelope to the American Society of Clinical Hypnosis, 2200 East Devon Avenue, Suite 291, Des Plaines, IL 60018.

Don't hesitate to ask your hypnotherapist for credentials, says Dr. Crasilneck. Someone who is truly qualified won't hedge or object. "When people say 'Where did you get your degree?' I'm delighted to tell them," he says.

What to Expect

Typically, the first session with a hypnotherapist is for the purpose of establishing rapport and answering questions. You and the therapist need to establish a solid working relationship in order for hypnotic suggestions for pain relief to really work, says Dr. Crasilneck.

Once you are comfortable, hypnosis begins with a process known as induction. The therapist holds a coin or some other small object above the level of your eyes and asks you to block out all sounds, says Dr. Crasilneck. In time, if all goes well, you relax and your eyelids begin to droop, freeing your body from tension and stress.

The heavier your lids get, the more you blink. At this point the therapist gives you a suggestion—telling you, for example, that your eyelids are so heavy that you are unable to open them. You'll then be led into a state of very deep relaxation.

Before trying to control your pain, the hypnotherapist may give you additional suggestions. He may, for example, tell you that your middle finger has become cold and numb—incapable of feeling a fingernail file thumped against it.

Once you accept a suggestion or two, the therapist will tell you that your unconscious mind has the power to do all things. And he will tell your subconscious mind to block much of your pain sensations, just as you blocked all sensations in your finger moments earlier.

Another technique that practitioners successfully employ is to remind you about how it feels when you plunge your hand into snow or frigid water, says Dr. Dubin. Cold makes your body numb.

"If I stick a needle into that hand, and it's numb from cold, you won't feel it," he says.

Suggesting that the area feeling pain has grown numb with cold is a technique often used in dentistry, says Dr. Dubin. It can make your gums numb. Not only that, hypnosis can make your gums numb without them *feeling* numb, he notes. There's no need to leave the dentist's office feeling like someone's bartered your lips for two slabs of blubber from an Eskimo.

Results Take Time

Of course, if you're undergoing hypnosis for pain relief during dental work, childbirth, or surgery, you need to experience definite and immediate results. (Your physician or dentist should be able to tell you whether this type of anesthesia is right for you.)

Relief for chronic pain may take longer. You should not put pressure on either yourself or the therapist to expect overnight success, warns Dr. Crasilneck.

"Unfortunately, some people in pain expect immediate results," he says. "And sometimes we *do* get immediate results, but it is more likely to occur after several sessions."

Sessions last from 30 to 60 minutes, he says. The number of sessions varies, depending on the pain problem and the patient. "Sometimes it's 6 sessions and sometimes it's 16 sessions," he says. "You don't know until you put it to the test."

Relaxation Brings Relief

Even if you're not a candidate for hypnosis, you may find a related technique helpful. Almost anyone can find some pain relief through relaxation, but health-care professionals carry it a step further and teach deep relaxation as a therapy.

Relaxation is "a state in which your autonomic nervous system is at a level of reduced stimulation," says Jon Kabat-Zinn, Ph.D., director of the Stress Reduction Clinic and associate professor of medicine at the University of Massachusetts Medical Center, in Worcester, and author of *Full Catastrophe Living: Using the Wisdom of Your Body and Mind to Face Stress, Pain, and Illness*.

"The way individuals respond to relaxation certainly varies greatly," says Kenneth L. Lichstein, Ph.D., professor of psychology at Memphis State University in Tennessee and author of *Clinical Relaxation Strategies*.

A number of studies have shown relaxation to be effective against a wide variety of pains. It can relieve breast pain associated with the menstrual cycle as well as some forms of breast pain caused by injury.

"Relaxation is also useful in relieving muscular pain, such as some forms of back pain," says Dr. Lichstein.

What's more, the benefits of relaxation therapy can last for years, according to one study. The State University of New York at Albany's Center for Stress and Anxiety Disorders kept tabs on a group of people who were treated for migraine and tension headaches with biofeedback and/or relaxation techniques. Nearly eight out of ten people with tension headaches reported improvement, as did nine out of ten people with migraines.

Putting Out the Flames of Colitis

Even some chronic pains that are fairly recalcitrant may respond to relaxation therapy. New evidence indicates that relaxation techniques may ease the pain of a bowel ailment known as ulcerative colitis. California psychologist Larry Shaw, Ph.D., became interested in conducting a study on how relaxation affects ulcerative colitis because his wife had a closely related bowel disease.

Dr. Shaw found that the relaxation techniques he used didn't involve the bowel itself. Instead, the techniques addressed the psychological component of the disease.

"The disease gives people a sense of hopelessness, of being out of control," says Dr. Shaw. But relaxation techniques gave these people something positive they could do on their own, thereby making them feel "less helpless," he says.

Even though the people in his study still had the long-term chronic illness, once they learned deep relaxation they were able to reduce the intensity of their pain, notes Dr. Shaw. As a result, he says, "they were able to reduce the medication needed to alleviate that pain." Relaxation is best used as an adjunct to conventional therapy for ulcerative colitis, he says.

Granddaddy of Relaxation Techniques

Deep relaxation therapy involves more than grabbing the *TV Guide* and heading for the sofa (although who's to say that that doesn't bring its own form of pain relief?). The kind of relaxation that sometimes leads to dramatic pain relief must be learned.

There are literally dozens of relaxation techniques, but progressive relaxation is the most established, says Stephen T. Wegener, Ph.D., clinical assistant professor in the Department of Behavioral and Medical Psychology at the University of Virginia. "It's also the one that's usually taught first," he notes.

Basically, you perform progressive relaxation by tensing and then relaxing muscles throughout your body, says Dr. Wegener. It's called "progressive" because the tension and relaxation proceed from one part of the body to another in a set order. A therapist might ask a person to tense a set of muscles for 7 seconds, then release the tension, notes Dr. Lichstein.

"This technique allows people to be aware of what tension and relaxation feel like," says Dr. Wegener.

Ideally, you should have someone work with you to learn progressive relaxation. Each session should take 20 to 25 minutes, and it takes a good deal of practice to become proficient. Ask your physician for a referral if you'd like to learn this technique.

Quick Release

There are shorter, easier forms of relaxation therapy that you can practice yourself, says Robert H. Phillips, Ph.D., a psychologist who directs the Center for Coping, on Long Island. He has developed a modified "quick-release" procedure designed to reduce "different types of discomfort or pain affecting any part of the body, whether it's muscular, intestinal, or headache pain."

Here is the five-step procedure for the technique.

1. Assume a comfortable position and close your eyes.
2. Take a deep breath. Hold it for 6 seconds while tensing all your muscles.
3. Breathe out and let your body go limp. Breathe deeply for approximately 20 seconds.
4. Repeat steps 2 and 3 twice.

5.   After the third repetition, let your body go limp and breathe deeply for 1 minute.

One caution. If you have a condition that may be made worse by tensing your muscles—arthritis, for example—or a condition that prevents tensing—cerebral palsy or paralysis, for example—talk to a professional about modifying the technique, advises Dr. Wegener.

Meditation: Turning Within

Relaxation techniques are relatively easy to learn. Meditation, on the other hand, requires a long-term commitment, says Dr. Kabat-Zinn. It becomes as much a part of a person's lifestyle as eating right and exercising daily.

Dr. Kabat-Zinn uses the term "mindfulness" to describe the kind of meditative techniques that can help people cope more effectively with pain and stress. Mindfulness implies greater moment-to-moment awareness and means that people open up more to joys and problems alike by "owning," in effect, every minute of their life, he says.

Although he uses mindfulness in a nonreligious context, Dr. Kabat-Zinn says that the method has its roots in ancient Buddhist teachings. You don't have to belong to any particular religion to practice mindfulness. "Anyone can use it effectively," he says.

Get Nowhere Fast

Meditation, unlike relaxation, is not directed toward any single goal, says Dr. Kabat-Zinn.

"Its perspective is that you don't have to get anywhere in particular—what you're feeling is what you're feeling," he says. "You don't have to escape from your pain. In fact, it is possible to open up to it and penetrate into it and through it until, ultimately, you learn to transcend it."

Transcending pain entails acceptance of your pain, not denial, says Dr. Kabat-Zinn. Tormenting yourself by lamenting that you no longer can do what you did 10 or 20 years ago just robs you of energy that you could be putting to positive use to help yourself cope better.

"How you feel about your body and your pain can exacerbate or reduce the actual sensations of pain itself," he says. "You can learn to live with pain without having it erode the quality of your life. If the pain is reduced to 50 percent or 75 percent in severity and its frequency is reduced, say, from 10 to 40 percent, you've made major strides."

Begin with the Body Scan

Here is a meditation technique that Dr. Kabat-Zinn recommends to "reestablish contact" with your body.

Begin by lying on your back with your eyes closed and relaxing as much as you can. Take your mind on a mental journey through your body, just one section at a time.

Focus your attention on your breathing, noting how it feels as it flows in and out of your nostrils. Start with the toes of your left foot; then slowly work your way up the foot and leg. Breathe deeply, and simply note how each region feels.

Your mental tour bus next goes to your pelvis, down to the toes of your right foot, and slowly back to the pelvis again, notes Dr. Kabat-Zinn. Then scan your torso, your lower back and abdomen, your upper back and chest, and your shoulders.

Shift to your fingers, he says, much the way you did with your toes, and work your way up your arms to the shoulders. Scan your neck, throat, face, back of the head, and top of the head.

At the end of the exercise, when you're ready, he says you should return movement to your body slowly. Shuffle your feet, wring your hands, and massage your face before going back to your day's routine.

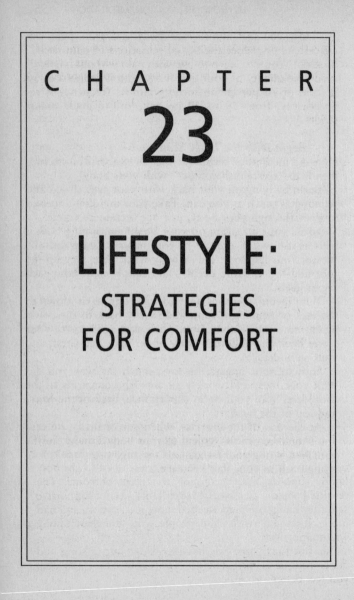

C H A P T E R

23

LIFESTYLE:
STRATEGIES
FOR COMFORT

P icture poor Fred in Room 13B. He's been hospitalized for three weeks. What brings him cheer are nurses and attendants, for he has no family to brighten his day with fresh pajamas or a newspaper with the latest baseball scores. Sometimes the scraggly ivy in the corner, left over from a patient gone home, is his only companion. That, and his pain.

Fred occasionally hears laughter and warm voices and chairs being moved about in the room next door. Yep, he tells himself, that guy next door has visitors again. Maybe it's his twin grandsons, the ones the nurses gush over. Or maybe it's his oldest son, the college professor, who drops by every day after work.

It's too bad Fred doesn't have a son or daughter to talk football with, a niece to bake him chocolate chip cookies, a wife to nag him about his hair.

Living alone is part of Fred's lifestyle, and it may well be a factor in his pain. Researchers have found a host of lifestyle factors that can and do have an impact on pain: smoking, alcohol, caffeine, sleep, pets, leisure activities, vacations. We'll look at all these areas. But first, let's get back to Fred and his solitary lifestyle.

Family Feels Good

If he had a supportive family nearby, Fred might be faring better.

Researchers at the Vanderbilt University Medical Center in Nashville, Tennessee, looked into the impact that family has on people in pain. One year after completing an outpatient pain program, 181 patients were studied to see how family support influenced their treatment outcome. The results? People who described their family as not supportive said they had more pain, needed more medication, and had more emotional stress than people who said their family was supportive.

It's not that your kids have to break into a song and dance routine reminiscent of "The Cosby Show" to help you feel better.

"The conclusion we came up with is that if there is perceived support—whether it's there or not—that's a major help," says Robert N. Jamison, Ph.D., a clinical psychologist and director of the Pain Treatment Service at Brigham and Women's Hospital, Boston, and an author of the Vanderbilt study.

For pain patients in the study, having supportive family members close by was a major insulator and helped them cope, says Dr. Jamison, who is an assistant professor at Harvard Medical School.

"Some people whose family is spread out or not helpful or at least not as available don't do as well," he says. "And that has implications for modern society. Most families are spread out a lot."

But what if your family is not only nearby but *too* close? Some family members will overdo it, raking the leaves, mowing the lawn, taking your temperature, and saying "poor you," says Dr. Jamison. "That's counterproductive, too."

"Family members can help, or they can completely discourage recovery. I think all family members should be involved in treatment. Family members and spouses are usually very interested in helping. But sometimes they don't know what to do."

How can you heal with a little help from your friends? Involve your spouse and other family members or the significant person in your life with your treatment and recovery, says Dr. Jamison. They should know about your medications and about what you need to do to get well. They can help you. Just don't let them do too much.

"If people surround themselves with upbeat people, they tend to do far better than if they surround themselves with people who bring them down," says Gerald M. Aronoff, M.D., director of the Boston Pain Center and assistant clinical professor at Tufts University School of Medicine. He advises therapy for people in troubled marriages and other unhealthy relationships and adds: "There's no shame in asking for help."

The payoff may be in tangible pain-relief terms. One

Canadian study showed that marriage therapy not only helps communication, it also may relieve chronic headaches. Ask your physician for a referral for counseling.

"Five or six couples told me that they learned to open up more and talk with each other, and it helped them cope with their pain," says Ann Gill Taylor, Ed.D., professor at the University of Virginia School of Nursing. Dr. Taylor is a researcher studying patients in pain and their spouses.

So keep talking—not fighting—and let your family work together to free you of pain.

Don't Pass On Pain

Researchers agree that people who are close to you can help you cope with pain. Just make sure you don't make them pay too dearly for the privilege.

People in chronic pain can be difficult to live with. They often are angry and afraid, depressed and demoralized, isolated not only from the world but from their families, says Dr. Taylor.

Both tensions and tempers can easily heat up in the immediate family of a person in chronic pain. Family squabbles can worsen your pain and make your spouse and children hurt, too, says Dr. Taylor. In her study of 40 spouses of chronic pain patients, 83 percent reported health problems they attributed to their partner's pain. She got similar responses when interviewing couples for an upcoming study.

"Anytime you have someone in pain, there is at least one other concerned person who is influenced by that pain, usually a spouse," says Dr. Taylor. "One spouse summed it up when she said, 'The pain has affected everything about us: him, me, the kids, our home, our money, everything.'"

A recent study by Dr. Jamison revealed that youngsters also suffer from their parents' pain. "Children of pain patients were reported to have more frequent abdominal pain and to use more medication than children of parents without pain," says Dr. Jamison. His study showed that 69 percent of the children of pain patients reported having stomachaches, 67 percent reported headaches, and 37 percent reported other pains in a three-month period. Twenty-four percent of the kids in the study missed more than one week of school because of physical illness.

"That says to me that other family members are involved," Dr. Jamison notes. "The illness actually affects the whole family."

So how can you help a family member deal with pain without shouldering that painful burden yourself? Dr. Taylor offers two pieces of advice: Be a good listener, and prevent the person in pain from being a patient.

"Have them participate in activities," Dr. Taylor says. Don't let yourself get caught in a trap of providing breakfast in bed every morning or slippers and a newspaper at day's end, she advises. Encourage them to be active and do things with other people. Strive to keep life normal.

Fido Fights Pain

Don't confine your pain-fighting partnerships to family and friends. One of your best helpers may be as close as your own heels.

He's your walking partner every day and your foot-warmer on winter nights. When it comes to listening to your woes, he has the best pair of ears on the planet. And when you come home from work, there's no sound you'd rather hear than his tail thumping on the floor.

From Lassie to Benji, from Trigger to Mister Ed, animals enthrall us, whether on television, in the movies, or curled up on the carpet at our feet. They make us feel good, or we wouldn't have them around.

But the fact is, pets really can affect our health in a positive manner.

A number of studies show that routine contact with pets can reduce blood pressure, heart rate, and pain-inducing stress. A study done at the University of Maryland showed that patients who suffer heart attacks fare better if they own dogs, cats, or birds.

Studies also show that bringing pets into the lives of the elderly and of patients with serious medical problems has beneficial effects, among them pain relief.

In a study involving 33 pain patients, the late psychiatrist Michael McCulloch, M.D., of Portland, Oregon, found there was one quality that all patients said their pets provided—comic relief.

"Every single patient said that at least on occasion, the animal was a source of humor or laughter or comic relief 'in my otherwise less-than-perfect life,' " recalls Alan Beck, Sc.D., of the Purdue University School of Veterinary Medicine. Dr. Beck, a professor of ecology, is a former colleague of Dr. McCulloch.

Fishy Findings

You don't have to put up with Fido's off-the-newspaper puppyhood mistakes to get the therapeutic benefits of pet ownership.

A case in point: Dr. Beck conducted a study showing that dental patients who watch fish in a tank before undergoing surgery on their teeth apparently have less pain and anxiety during the procedure.

"The observers in the study could not distinguish any anxiety in the patients as measured in terms of how often they asked for water, how often they gripped the arm of the dental chair, how often they pushed away the dentist—all of the things we do when we're uncomfortable at the dentist's office," says Dr. Beck. "Thinking about the fish, at least [as indicated] in overt behaviors, alleviated pain."

The therapeutic value of animals lies in the distraction they provide, plus the sense of familiarity and safety they offer, says Dr. Beck.

"When you come home to an empty house, there's a certain level of anxiety," he says. "If you come home to an animal behaving normally, you probably unconsciously feel more relaxed. We're not talking about protection. We're talking about a bird singing away. There is an assumption that the environment is as you left it."

Are there people in pain who shouldn't have pets? "If animals are not part of their experience, it's just another thing to have to deal with," Dr. Beck admits. A dog may

---

PAIN-FREE PET CARE

The joys of pet ownership are reputed to help distract you from pain. But taking care of your pet can become troublesome if your joints are stiff from arthritis. You need to walk your dog, but it hurts your hands when the exuberant animal pulls you down the street. Jodi Maron-Barth, a physical therapist in private practice in Maryland, offers these tips for pet care for people with arthritis.

Change your pet's schedule so that the animal is active when you are. Let him out before you go to bed at night so he can wait until later in the morning to go out again. This gives you time to get moving before he needs his morning walk.

To make brushing your pet easier, use a brush with a large handle and a loop that fits around your wrist.

Avoid thin leads and collars that can be hard on your hands. Install a pet door so you don't have to fuss with letting your pet outside.

Have a neighborhood child walk your pet, which will ease the strain on you.

---

be too much to handle while you're ill, so perhaps a low-maintenance pet is better.

Feeding fish can be a nurturing experience in a pain-filled day, says Dr. Beck. "We spend so much of our life trying to nurture, and losing that is really a painful experience for many people. To be a caregiver, even if it's only symbolic, is very important."

So drop a pinch of food in your fish tank. Move on over to the fireplace and give Fido a hug. Don't you feel better?

Forty Winks for Relief

Sleep that knits up the ravell'd sleeve of care,
The death of each day's life, sore labour's bath,
Balm of hurt minds, great nature's second course,
Chief nourisher in life's feast.

—*Macbeth*

Your relationship with others can have a profound effect on your pain—how you interact with your family, how you communicate with your doctor. But there's no getting around the notion that how you treat yourself is also important. Even the great minds of long ago knew that getting enough sleep is an important part of any pain-control strategy.

We've all felt the deep satisfaction of waking up after a good night's sleep. And we've also felt the thick-tongued, heavy-headed trauma of starting the day cursing the blasted alarm clock.

Doctors, who experience plenty of sleep deprivation first-hand during medical training, are quick to mention sleep's benefits. They say it can help you relieve headaches; relieve fibrositis or stiff, painful muscles; and, in time, improve cases of arthritis, peptic ulcer disease, and colitis and help you heal faster. It also helps you keep your overall immunity up to par.

It seems sleep truly can help a life unraveled by pain become whole again. "There's no doubt that a good night's sleep is the best preparation for the day," says Fred B. Rogers, M.D., professor emeritus, Temple University School of Medicine, Philadelphia. "We've all experienced that. Mother was right."

Adds Dr. Jamison, "There's a major relationship between sleep disturbances and chronic pain. It's fair to say that if chronic pain patients can get a good night's sleep, they can handle anything."

Does Sleep Help?
Does all this enthusiasm for the benefits of sleep mean the wall-banging, fist-in-your-skull, bashing headache will go away if you can simply shut your eyes and sleep?

People who suffer from migraine and other types of headaches can sometimes get relief from pain through sleep, according to James D. Dexter, M.D., of the University of Missouri's Columbia School of Medicine. But be forewarned: He and others agree that headaches can occur *during* various phases of sleep and immediately *after* sleep, as well.

Researchers are still sorting out the mystery of the headache/sleep connection. Headaches may occur when we relax following a period of excitement, notes Dr. Dexter. Ever get a headache after a big exam or job interview? Your body was reacting to your nervous system's fall from excitation to relaxation, according to Dr. Dexter.

What does all this mean for you? If sleep relieves your headaches, sleep. If it doesn't, try keeping track of how your sleep habits seem to affect your headache. Talk to your doctor if you think you see a connection.

Sleep to Soothe Muscles

Restorative sleep—the kind that leaves you feeling refreshed the next day—can help relieve fibrositis, or chronic muscle pain, according to Harvey Moldofsky, M.D., professor of psychiatry and medicine at the University of Toronto. Patients with fibrositis so commonly report poor, unrefreshing sleep that Dr. Moldofsky suggests that this kind of disturbed sleep is a feature of the sore muscle condition.

There's no secret to the pain-relieving powers of sleep. Injured tissues and tissues broken down during the day heal faster while you snooze.

"I see chronic pain as sapping a lot of your energy. It just drains you," Dr. Jamison says. "I see sleep as allowing you to recharge."

How Much Is Enough?

Although Washington Irving penned a lengthy slumber for Rip Van Winkle, doctors say there's no set amount of sleep every person needs. They recommend 6 to 8 hours for most people, says Dr. Aronoff.

But catching even 5 hours of rest can be difficult if you're in pain. "Pain often prevents normal sleep," says Edward J. Resnick, M.D., director of the Pain Control Center at Temple University Hospital in Philadelphia. Sometimes you may feel pain more at night, he notes.

"People who have sleep disturbances often are exhausted the next day. They're very short-fused, and it contributes to more anxiety and depression," explains Dr. Jamison. And anxiety and depression only make pain worse.

You easily can get caught in a cycle of not sleeping at night, taking naps the following day, and not being able to sleep again the next night. Dr. Jamison offers this advice for breaking the cycle: Try staying active all day long, even if you're tired. Once it's time to go to bed, you'll probably have no problem falling asleep. Forcing yourself to stay awake for one full day sets the stage for a schedule of more active days and peaceful nights.

Catching Some Z's

Here are some additional tips from the American Sleep Disorders Association for getting a good night's sleep.

- Get up at about the same time every day, regardless of when you go to bed.
- Go to bed only when you're sleepy.
- Establish relaxing presleep rituals like taking a warm bath, watching television, or reading.
- Take a walk or stretch 2 to 3 hours before going to bed.
- Organize your day, setting regular times for meals, naps, and exercise to keep your internal clock running smoothly.
- Avoid caffeine within 6 hours of bedtime, and don't drink alcohol or smoke at bedtime.
- Use alcohol sparingly, especially if you're sleepy, when it can have a more potent effect.
- Use sleeping pills with caution. (If you're on pain medication, ask your doctor before taking any over-the-counter medication.)

Don't forget, if you're having persistent problems sleeping, see your doctor.

The Perils of Caffeine

Getting a good night's sleep may or may not be a problem for you, but if you're like more than half of the U.S. population, you reach for a cup of coffee to help you wake up in the morning. Each morning, caffeine helps you pry your eyelids apart, removes the pasty taste of morning tongue from your mouth, and generally perks you up to meet a new day. If you go ahead and enjoy that aromatic brew, just be aware that caffeine may have an impact on pain perception.

When it comes to headaches, caffeine has both a dark side and a bright side. Caffeine can cause headaches—including migraines—because as a stimulant, it can "tire out" brain cells and make them reluctant to release pain-soothing brain chemicals. And as caffeine leaves the body, blood vessels may dilate, setting the stage for a migraine, headache researchers say.

On the bright side, a couple of cups of strong coffee or several glasses of caffeinated sodas, combined with over-the-counter pain medication, may stop migraine pain, headache researchers say. That's because caffeine enhances the absorption of pain medication from the intestine. That's why caffeine is included in many painkillers. Take note: This caffeine boost should be used no more than twice a month. And it won't work if you're a long-time caffeine user with a built-up tolerance to its effects.

Caffeine may also have a negative effect on breast pain. In a study of breast pain associated with fibrocystic breast disease, Linda C. Russell, a family nurse practitioner at Duke University Medical Center, found that 61 percent of the women who gave up or reduced caffeine consumption for one year experienced less breast pain or felt it vanish entirely. This study does not represent the last word on caffeine's effect on breast pain, if any, but cutting back on caffeine might be worth a try.

Caffeine also has been shown to cause anxiety and may reduce the effectiveness of antianxiety medication.

Not Even a Cup?

How much caffeine can you consume safely? Doctors say that 200 milligrams daily (about two cups of coffee) is probably safe. "You should stay on that moderate to low dose and adjust yourself or go off completely and don't play with it," says John W. Farquhar, M.D., director of the Stanford Center for Research in Disease Prevention at Stanford University.

If you do give up caffeine cold turkey, be prepared for headaches that may arrive 12 to 24 hours after your last dose. It's your choice to ease off gradually or stop completely. You'll notice a draggy feeling without your jolt of coffee, says Dr. Farquhar. In five or six days, your body will adjust and you won't need the caffeine kick.

Ale for What Ails You?

Coffee and caffeinated colas are not the only beverages that can have an impact on your pain. One of author William Faulkner's favorite things to do as a child was to listen to stories about the Civil War exploits of his great-grandfather, William Clark Faulkner, known as the Old Colonel. The young boy imagined men wearing blue and gray, fighting, getting wounded, then biting bullets and drinking whiskey to keep from passing out from the pain.

Today doctors know that alcohol's effectiveness for pain relief is almost entirely fiction. While heavy drinking can anesthetize you by putting you in a light coma, alcohol has no other role in relieving pain, says Henry Lahmeyer, M.D., director of the Sleep Disorders Center at the University of Illinois at Chicago. You might as well bite on a ball from a Civil War musket.

And as you may have experienced after a night of too many Harvey Wallbangers, alcohol can *cause* pain. The hangover you'll get if you overdo it can cause headaches and will worsen any other pains you may have, such as arthritis, rheumatic pain, or muscle pains, explains Dr. Lahmeyer. Alcohol, even one or two drinks a day, can irritate ulcer pain. It is also a direct toxin to the stomach and the liver and can irritate the pancreas, all of which can cause pain, says gastroenterologist Samuel Klein, M.D., of the University of Texas Medical School at Galveston.

Alcohol causes pain because of the neurotoxic or damaging effect it has on your cells, Dr. Lahmeyer explains. Because of its soluble properties, alcohol penetrates every organ in your body and interferes with every physiological system, he says. Several studies show that besides altering the activity of your brain, prolonged drinking affects levels of neurotransmitters, alters cellular membrane structures, and causes destruction of certain nerve pathways. Drinking can also impair your immune system, decreasing your ability to fight disease.

You won't know this is going on at the cellular level, of course, but you'll know something is different the day after the night before. During alcohol withdrawal (during the hangover), there is increased firing of nerve and muscle cells, Dr. Lahmeyer explains. "All cells are involved, so those involved in the pain are going to be intensified in their pain-sending capacity that day," he says. That means you're going to feel it.

Dr. Lahmeyer recommends the traditional, common-sense hangover medicines of aspirin, antacids, "hot baths, or whatever works for you."

Not a Pain Chaser

Don't make the mistake of reaching for a drink or two to dull your pain, advises Dr. Lahmeyer. "One or two drinks can intensify pain, and of course, as soon as the alcohol wears off, the effects intensify," he says.

"Using alcohol as a way to relax and relieve pain is really bad news for a lot of reasons, including the fact that you could become an alcoholic," says Dr. Farquhar. "If you have a pain problem, it's tragic to compound that problem with another one."

If a person in pain finds relief in the bottle, it's all too easy for alcohol consumption to become a problem. If you think alcohol is becoming a problem for you, ask your physician or call your local hospital for help in dealing with it.

Toss Cigarettes to Dump Pain

While we're on the subject of giving things up, there's one more indulgence that may have an impact on pain.

You've heard it so often, it might as well be our new national anthem. You probably remember its words clearly: *The Surgeon General has warned that cigarette smoking may be hazardous to your health*—and to your pain level, we might add.

You know you should stub out that last butt and never light up again. *Of course you know that.* But cutting back or quitting smoking is really tough when you're in pain. In fact, in a recent study at the Vanderbilt Pain Control Center, researchers found that 57 percent of chronic pain patients feel the *need* to smoke more when they're in pain. Yet 91 percent believed that smoking had no effect on their pain.

"That was the real surprise of the study, that people didn't think smoking made their pain worse or better," says Dr. Jamison, a leader of the study. "Still, if you ask people, they'll say they need to smoke more because they're hurting."

However, studies have shown that cigarette smoking may *worsen* pain because of nicotine's effects on your body. As a stimulant and vasoconstrictor, nicotine heightens pain sensations, Dr. Jamison says. Smoking one or two cigarettes increases resting heart rate and blood pressure, making your pain worse, he explains.

"You'd think there are lots of reasons why smoking should make things worse for people in pain," he says. "But nicotine is a powerful drug. It may make you feel good."

Smoking also seems to cause certain kinds of pain. One national health survey revealed that smokers have more low back pain and that smoking clearly preceded the onset of the pain in 63 percent of the cases. Not only that, but smoking has been linked to disk disease, because smoking restricts an already skimpy disk blood supply, says Augustus A. White III, M.D., professor of orthopedic surgery at Harvard Medical School.

Smoking may affect ulcers, making them more likely to occur, slower to heal, and more likely to come back, says Dr. Klein. It takes only a few cigarettes per day to aggravate already tender tummies caused by ulcers, he says.

Smoking also can cause angina, a dull, heavy chest pain

that can also be felt in the arms, back, and even the throat and jaw. If you have angina and you smoke, your doctor will tell you to cut back or stop smoking entirely.

Researchers are also finding evidence that smoking worsens migraine headaches. How? Carbon monoxide released by cigarettes can give people headaches. Also, once nicotine enters your system, it may interfere with some of the drugs used to control migraines. You may need more migraine medication (which would increase the likelihood of side effects) if you can't stop smoking.

Stubbing Out the Habit

If you decide to quit smoking, it may help you to realize that you are not alone. More than 1.5 million people quit smoking each year, with 40 million Americans identifying themselves as former smokers, the American Lung Association reports. And nearly half of adults who have ever smoked have quit, the association reports. It can be done!

Call your local chapter of the American Lung Association or ask your doctor about getting help to stop smoking. The minute you stop, your body starts repairing itself. Your cough won't be so annoying because it will disappear. Your circulation will improve, your energy level will rise, even your sense of taste and smell will improve. And you'll breathe easier knowing that quitting may help alleviate your pain.

Life Goes On

Just about everything you do in life has an impact on pain, including how you spend your leisure time.

Which of the following would be impossible for you? (a) riding a bike, (b) joining a continuing education art class, (c) learning to crochet, or (d) walking up the outside of the Statue of Liberty and kissing her on the nose.

If you're in enough pain, the answer may be (e) all of the above.

To a person in pain, bike riding, taking an art class,

or learning to crochet may seem as impossible as getting intimate with Miss Liberty.

On the other hand, recreation, hobbies, and taking vacations can be your allies in the fight against pain. "The more someone in pain can live a normal life, the better," says Dr. Jamison.

Exercise (see chapter 20), other recreational activities, and hobbies get you up and moving around, giving you something else to think about besides pain, says Ronald Lawrence, M.D., assistant clinical professor of neuropsychiatry at UCLA School of Medicine and author of numerous books, including *Goodbye Pain!*

Through his 38-year medical practice, Dr. Lawrence has found several recreational activities he advocates for pain relief.

For arthritis, the doctor recommends ballroom dancing and working with clay. Dancing combines mental and physical stimulation. Clay modeling is excellent for stimulating stiff fingers and hands.

For relieving headache pain, Dr. Lawrence recommends mild exercise such as walking, which he says is one of the best leisure activities for pain relief.

People with pain problems, especially those that limit mobility and range of motion, may benefit mentally and physically from painting or sculpting, says Dr. Lawrence. "Creating a painting, a drawing, or a piece of sculpture absorbs a person's mind probably more than anything," he says.

Turn on the television or go to a movie, he advises. Besides the distraction quality, television and movies may have an additional benefit, but only if you tune in to a tearjerker.

"For some reason, when people cry, it helps reduce pain," Dr. Lawrence says. It seems that tears release chemicals that help relieve pain. "Maybe that's why people with pain cry or agonize," he says. "Nature builds it in."

Noncompetitive activities such as stamp collecting are good, as is tossing basketballs or beach balls back and forth or moving about gently in a swimming pool, he notes.

A vacation or weekend trip may be just the thing to get your mind off pain, says Dr. Jamison. "Some folks need to get away, from both the house and their surroundings. It is important to change your environment and keep yourself mentally and physically occupied," he explains.

CHAPTER
24

MASSAGE:
HERE'S THE RUB

J oan lived with an aching back for so long, she almost lost faith that any kind of therapy could significantly relieve her pain. Then, on her doctor's recommendation, she found herself relaxing under the firm, sure touch of a massage therapist. At the end of her first professional massage, she was a true believer.

What is it about massage that helped relieve Joan's pain? Here's what the medical experts on this ancient form of therapy say.

Massage confuses the body's pain signals. Rubbing may interfere with pain signals' pathways to your brain, a process called the "gate control theory," according to Edward Resnick, M.D., professor of orthopedic surgery and director of the Pain Control Center at Temple University Hospital, Philadelphia. "Pain impulses run toward the spinal cord and then up the cord and into the brain," he says. "It's only when they reach the brain that these impulses are perceived as pain. Rubbing can send other impulses along the same nerves and interfere with the pain impulses. In this way, rubbing can 'close the gate' that pain impulses have to pass through."

Massage calls up the body's natural painkillers. It stimulates the release of endorphins, the morphinelike substances that the body manufactures, into the brain and nervous system.

Massage relieves muscle tension, spasm, and stiffness. All of these contribute to pain, and deep relaxation is the classic effect for which most people seek massage. "A tense muscle is usually one that's deprived of oxygen, because the tightness reduces blood circulation to the area," says Bill Mueller, a registered massage therapist and director of the Mueller College of Holistic Studies in San Diego. "Massage improves blood circulation, bringing with it what the muscle needs—oxygen and other forms of nourishment. The muscle then relaxes, and pain decreases."

Massage relieves mental stress and anxiety. The therapeutic value of touching for helping a person in pain is coming under increasing study, according to K. M. Doehring, R.N., a nursing instructor who writes about relieving pain through touch. Doehring cites research showing that even touch lasting for *less than 1 second* has the ability to make people feel better. Just think of what an hour could do!

Beyond Backs

What kinds of pain does massage relieve?

If it helped Joan's back pain, can it help yours, too? If the source of your pain is muscle tension—as is the case in many kinds of head, back, neck, and shoulder pain—then massage may be your ticket to freedom from pain. Releasing tightness and tension in muscles is the most obvious effect of a good massage.

Massage experts recommend it for relieving pain from other conditions as well, including arthritis, injuries, or even recent surgery. "Almost any kind of pain can cause your muscles to tighten in response," says Ronald Clark, registered massage therapist and director of the Austin School of Massage Therapy in Texas. Those tense muscles then cause more pain. And anxiety can increase pain intensity, too. A massage that reduces muscle tension and relieves anxiety can be a powerful weapon in the arsenal of pain-relieving techniques you can turn to for a wide variety of conditions, says Clark.

When Not to Rub

It's important to remember that there are certain kinds of painful conditions *not* to treat with massage, unless you get your doctor's approval first, according to American Massage Therapy Association (AMTA) guidelines. These conditions include phlebitis and other circulatory ailments, high fevers, infectious diseases, some kinds of cancer, certain cardiac problems, injuries that are inflamed or infected, and injuries to areas of the body that involved heavy bleeding or tissue damage. Fractures or sprains should not be massaged for 48 to 72 hours following the injury; after that, massage may be beneficial.

How to Give a Massage

Whether you're giving yourself a massage or learning how to help a loved one in pain, you'll have to learn a few basic techniques that can be used on any area of the body. These techniques are based on Swedish massage, the kind familiar to most people. Here are four basic techniques to use.

Effleurage, or Stroking

Effleurage is the "rub" in "rubdown."

"These are slow, smooth strokes in which you begin by pressing lightly, then increase to deeper pressure as the massage continues," says Jocelyn Granger, a registered massage therapist from Michigan who is a spokesperson for AMTA. Stroking forms the basis for a massage on any area of the body, and you can give a whole massage just using this one technique, says Clare Maxwell-Hudson, a British massage therapist and author of *The Complete Book of Massage*. You can begin any massage by stroking on a light vegetable oil. Oil helps keep your massage strokes fluid and protects the skin from irritation. To begin, place your palms on the skin surface; then press as you stroke upward, to the side, around in a circle, or down. On smaller areas, Maxwell-Hudson recommends stroking with your thumbs.

Petrissage, or Kneading

Petrissage penetrates deeper than stroking.

"This movement is just like kneading dough and is useful on the shoulders and fleshy areas such as the hips and thighs," says Maxwell-Hudson. Kneading can include lifting, squeezing, and rolling flesh, says Granger.

Begin this type of movement by pressing down with the palm of one hand. Then grasp the flesh between the fingers and thumb of the other hand and push it toward the flat hand. Release the flesh and grasp it with the other hand. Repeat these two steps back and forth rhythmically.

Tapotement, or Tapping

Light tapping on fleshy areas is the third basic massage technique. You can use your fingertips, the side of your hand (making karate chop-like motions), or the sides of your fists, says Granger. "This technique is fantastic for interrupting pain signals," she says.

Remember to check with your partner about how each movement feels. The taps may be brisk but should not hurt.

Vibration

Get ready to turn the flesh under your fingers into quivering Jell-O.

The next technique involves grasping the flesh lightly between your fingers and thumbs and shaking it, according to Granger. You can get the same beneficial effects by shaking and vibrating your own arms and legs, she says.

Putting It All Together

Whether to perform the strokes gently or vigorously depends on who's receiving the massage, therapists agree. Some people respond better to gentle movements, while others like more vigorous ones. "The body knows what it needs," says Mueller. "People are so complex . . . it's like opening a safe. You have to find the right combination of movements and locations before you can help someone."

You should always encourage the person you're massaging to tell you if a movement is painful, advises Mueller. Or if you're receiving the massage, let the therapist know. "A person has to be able to relax into a massage. If they're in too much pain, they can't do that," he says. Massage therapists agree that there is definitely what Mueller calls "good, or sweet, pain" in which the person being massaged can tell that the movement is "untying the knot," even if it causes a bit of discomfort. "But a good massage should never make you flinch," Clark points out. "If a massage is doing that, it should be stopped."

Where to Rub

If your pain is localized—in your head, shoulders, back, or legs, for example—should you concentrate on massaging only those areas? Probably not, massage therapists agree. Muscles in the area of an injury may be the first to feel pain, but other, more distant muscles quickly get involved, says Clark. Granger tells of a patient whose head was turned to the side for 6 hours during an ear operation. At first, only his neck hurt. But the pain soon spread to his shoulders, back, and leg. Granger had to give him a full body massage to relieve it.

Many kinds of pain are really a reaction to pain and muscle tension that begins elsewhere, says Granger. Headaches are a good example. "Neck and shoulder pain trigger headaches the most, but the pain can be triggered from as far away as the hips," she says. "The body is so interconnected—that's why a full body massage can really help a headache."

The lower back is another vulnerable spot for receiving referred pain, says Clark. So in many cases, a full body massage is the best way to hit all the potential hot spots that cause and receive tension and pain.

Finding a Professional Massage Therapist

If your pain is intense, ask your doctor if massage might offer some relief. Your doctor may be able to refer you to a professional massage therapist. You can also call the AMTA (312-761-AMTA) for a referral to one of its members in your area. Members of the AMTA have to meet strict membership requirements, which include either 500 hours of training in massage therapy or a demonstrated knowledge of massage therapy that's tested through practical and written exams.

Massage therapists are located in a variety of settings, says the AMTA, including:

• Private practice clinics and offices
• Health clubs, fitness centers, and YMCAs

- Chiropractors' offices
- Nursing homes and hospitals
- Spas, salons, and resorts
- On-site locations at the workplace

Many massage therapists will even visit you in your own home.

Whether the therapist is a member of the AMTA or not, you should ask her or him about schooling, certifications (the AMTA is just beginning a program), and the approaches she or he employs in massage therapy. In states that have licensing requirements, you can ask if the therapist is licensed. Those states are Arkansas, Delaware, Florida, Hawaii, Nebraska, New Hampshire, New York, North Dakota, Ohio, Oregon, Rhode Island, Texas, Utah, and Washington.

Depending on the area of the country, average fees for a massage range from $30 to $65 an hour, says Granger. You can request a longer or shorter massage time period, such as 30 minutes or 90 minutes.

If you're wondering why your doctor hasn't recommended massage therapy for your pain, it may be because he or she isn't yet aware of how effective it can be. Although massage therapists are commonly on the staffs of hospitals in the Soviet Union, West Germany, China, and Japan, they aren't as readily recognized here, says the AMTA. Increasing numbers of doctors are recommending massage as its value in pain relief continues to be studied. Some insurance companies now recognize massage as legitimate therapy for pain relief, says Granger, so you may want to see if your doctor can write a prescription for treatments for you so that you can try to receive insurance reimbursement.

SPORTS MASSAGE: SWEET RELIEF FOR THE WEEKEND ATHLETE

You've been totally sedentary all winter. Yesterday the spring sunshine invited you outdoors to exercise for an hour. Today you hurt. How do you spell relief? Try "m-a-s-s-a-g-e."

Sports massage can help everyone from top Olympic athletes to weekend sports enthusiasts. It's the best thing to happen in the locker room since the "no pain, no gain" theory went out the window. You'd be hard pressed to find a professional athlete who does without it, especially after vigorous exercise.

"Why do muscles hurt after vigorous exercise? There are several theories," says Bill Mueller, a national consultant to the American Massage Therapy Association (AMTA) and a sports massage therapist. "Some say it's due to the waste products that collect in muscles. Others say that the muscle is hungry for more nutrients and isn't getting them fast enough. Still others believe that it's due to muscle tearing. If the first two theories are correct, massage is a logical way to seek relief.

"When you exercise, the demands your muscles make are greater than your blood circulatory system can handle. But massage following exercise can increase the speed of your circulation, thus removing waste products and absorbing them faster, while at the same time delivering more nutrients to your hungry tissues."

Massage can help warm and ready your muscles for vigorous activity *before* a sporting event and loosen tight muscles *after* the event to reduce pain, say members of the AMTA's National Sports Massage Team, which provides finish line sports massages at major U.S. marathons as well as at the Olympics.

If you're nursing a sports-related injury such as a muscle tear, strain, or sprain, massage can make a tremendous difference in your recovery, says Mueller. "But you must wait 48 to 72 hours before getting the massage," he says. "When you have an injury, you can have broken blood vessels, damaged nerves, and torn tissue, and your body needs time to repair them. If you got in there and started massaging right away, you'd be likely to cause more damage."

Once you're ready to begin massage, Mueller recommends that you ice the area before starting. "Often tissue that's been injured goes into low-grade spasm," he says. "You're afraid it's going to hurt if you move it. Ice numbs the pain so that you can start moving the muscle without tension. Once the muscle begins to relax, circulation improves and you start to feel better."

The AMTA certifies sports massage therapists, so if you're looking for one in your area, call the association's national hotline (312-761-AMTA).

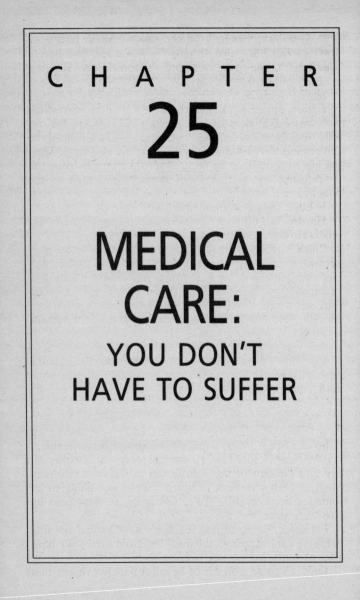

C H A P T E R
25

MEDICAL
CARE:
YOU DON'T
HAVE TO SUFFER

Edith lies in her hospital bed, staring at the ceiling or watching the people pass by her door. She barely moves. She tries not to breathe too deeply. Sleeping is nearly impossible for her.

She's in pain.

Edith's doctor left a prescription for pain-relief medication, but Edith must ring the nurse's desk to ask for her pills. She doesn't want to be a bother, so she waits until she can't stand the pain a minute more before she rings. Then she has to wait 10 or 15 minutes for the nurse to bring the medication. She must then wait another 20 minutes for the pills to begin working.

Is Edith the perfect patient?

Hardly, say doctors and nurses who specialize in pain relief. However, Edith is typical.

Edith is afraid to complain to her doctor about her pain because she doesn't want to bother "the busy physician." Her prescription is for a narcotic, and Edith is afraid of becoming an addict. And even if she got her medication on time, she would still be in pain. Her doctor hasn't prescribed *enough* medication. He, too, is afraid Edith might become an addict.

Are you an Edith?

You don't have to put up with pain, say the experts, especially in the hospital, where pain relief should be at your fingertips.

Don't Just Lie There—Ask

"The idea in the 1990s is that no one should be miserable," says Michael Gold, M.D., assistant professor of anesthesiology and director of the pain center at Tulane University Medical Center in New Orleans. "We're not going to let someone be miserable. We're not going to treat pain by passive neglect."

However, "most physicians don't have formal training in taking care of pain problems," Dr. Gold says. "We have a lot of tools, but no one is using them."

Only 25 to 65 percent of hospital patients report that

they are satisfied with the pain relief they get, says Dr. Gold. Additionally, studies show that even when doctors know how to use medications effectively, they tend to underprescribe. And sometimes nurses lack the training that helps them have a consistent approach to assessing and treating pain, says Dr. Gold.

So if you want the best pain relief possible while you are in the hospital, you have to approach it as a consumer, he advises.

You need to know when to complain about pain and how to describe your pain so that you get the right amount of medication at the right time. You also need to know that there are strong medications that eliminate pain, but there are also other things that can be done to give you the pain relief you need. And you need to know how to ask for help.

Tell It Like It Is

Medications are the first choice for pain relief, says Richard Gilbert, M.D., director of pain management services at the Carolinas Medical Center, Charlotte, North Carolina.

However, in addition to those medications, there is a wide array of other pain-relief tools and techniques that are available to make pain beat a retreat.

Doctors can recommend acupuncture, biofeedback, exercise, trigger-point therapy, physical therapy, relaxation therapy, whirlpool, massage, hypnosis, TENS, nerve blocks, and surgery (all of which are described in detail in other chapters) to boost or supplement your pain-relief medication.

In order to take advantage of your options, though, you must tell your doctor exactly how and where it hurts.

In the hospital, you get pain medication based on an estimate—a guess—of how much pain you may be having or how much pain your doctor thinks you probably have, based on the nature of your condition. However, it's only a guess, and what you get may not be what you need, says Dr. Gold. That's not too comforting a thought when something hurts.

"Doctors prescribe pain relief based on experience about what kind of medication is likely to be helpful and how much is usually needed. We're usually pretty close, but in some patients we can be way off," says Dr. Gold.

"If you prescribe just the right amount, the patient is all right," he says. "But that's just one little point on a long line of pain-relief possibilities. If you prescribe too much, the patient may get the side effects of the drug—and that can include difficulty breathing. If you prescribe too little, all you get is a patient who hurts."

Doctors, of course, prefer to have a patient who hurts over a patient who has to be revived because he's gotten too much "pain relief."

"That's why, given the option, a doctor would rather give too little than give too much," Dr. Gold says. Prescribing too little pain medication may make the job easier for doctors; however, you don't have to settle for a halfway measure.

Accurately describing your pain is the key, says Margo McCaffery, R.N., author of five books on pain relief and a frequent lecturer on pain control. She has some suggestions that take a lot of the guesswork out of measuring your pain.

Rate Your Pain

Think of your pain on a scale of 0 to 10, she says. Zero is no pain, 10 is the worst pain. Figure where your pain ranks on the scale. Then decide which number would be an acceptable level of pain for you. If your pain is a searing number 8, would you be happy if your doctor could give you enough medication to ease it back to a 2? Tell your doctor or nurse both of those numbers as a starting point.

Paint a Pain Picture

Next think of words to describe your pain. Sometimes the description can help your doctor pinpoint why you hurt —different things can cause different kinds of pain—and prescribe just the right measures to alleviate the pain.

Here are some words from the McGill Pain Questionnaire, a scale that pain-relief experts sometimes use to help them better understand pain: throbbing, shooting, stabbing, sharp, cramping, gnawing, hot/burning, aching, heavy, tender, splitting, tiring/exhausting, sickening, fearful, and punishing/cruel. Use as many or as few of these descriptions as necessary to draw a word picture of your pain.

Then tell your doctor how long you have had the pain. Has the intensity changed? Is it worse during the day or night? If you lie still, does your pain fade? If you sit up, do you feel better? Do small movements make the pain worse?

If you've had medication, how far down the scale did it make your pain number fall? How long after you took your medication did you feel pain again? If you still hurt after taking a pain reliever, you may need a different drug or a more frequent or larger dose of medication.

From this description, your doctor or nurse should be able to come closer to giving you the right dose of pain medication.

Getting More When You Need It

You've heard the joke about nurses waking you up to take a sleeping pill. Well, if you're awakened during the night to take a pill, it's more likely to be a pain pill. The ideal medication schedule in the hospital keeps a constant level of pain-killing medicine in your bloodstream, says Judith Garbush, R.N., patient care director for Lehigh Valley Hospice in Pennsylvania.

So if you are on a regular schedule for pain reliever (say, a pill or shot every 4 hours), you want to stick strictly to the schedule—even if it means waking up at night to do it (although there are some timed-release pain relievers that can work for as long as 12 hours).

Doctors say that if you prolong the period between doses of medication, you allow the pain to get worse. That means it takes longer to control your pain and you may need a higher dose of medication than if you put a stop to pain early.

Doctors also say that you should douse the pain even

before it gets started. If you take medication only when it hurts, ring for the nurse as soon as you begin to feel heaviness or warmth or any other symptom that you recognize as the approach of pain.

If you are still in pain after taking your medication or if you have pain before your next dose, don't hesitate to request an adjustment in your pain medication. Nurses give you what the doctor orders, but they have some flexibility of their own, too. Giving aspirin or acetaminophen in addition to a narcotic, for instance, can make pain relief more complete and longer lasting.

Try the Self-Service Pump

If you don't want to be at the mercy of someone else's time schedule, there may be other options. For instance, in many hospitals, doctors use patient-controlled analgesia (PCA), allowing postsurgical patients to control their own painkillers. PCA is also used in the hospital for chronic pain.

"There are a lot of new techniques available to us. We first looked at PCA in the 1960s, but the technology wasn't there. Now it's fairly popular," says Michael Levy, M.D., Ph.D., co-director of the Pain Management Center at Fox Chase Cancer Center in Philadelphia.

In PCA, typically, a pump is attached to an intravenous line and delivers a prescribed amount of painkiller each hour. If you feel your pain-relief medication wearing thin, all you have to do is push a button to release more medication. Using PCA means medication levels stay within a narrow range in your bloodstream, says Dr. Gold.

PCA reduces the risk of tolerance to certain drugs. Tolerance builds when your body becomes so used to the drug you're taking that your dose doesn't relieve your pain anymore. As a result, you need to take more of the medication. With PCA, you push the button only when you are in pain. As your body heals and has less pain, you need less and less medication.

PCA also eliminates middle-of-the-night calls to the doctor or nurse. That could be very good for you because, unfortunately, pain relief may be based on politics and politeness—even in the hospital, admits Dr. Gold.

"Doctors vary with empathy. If you're on the night shift and some guy keeps buzzing and buzzing and saying, 'I hurt,' and you don't personally believe him, then you're not going to move quite as fast. If it's a sweet little old lady who says you did a good job on her surgery and, by the way, she hurts just a little, you're going to do whatever you can for her. I'd like to think that it doesn't happen like that, but it does. If you show courtesy, you will get what you want."

Canceling Cancer Pain

Cancer pain can be the worst pain of all in the hospital, says Dr. Levy. Some of the cancer-fighting techniques, such as radiation or surgery, can make the pain temporarily feel worse. And yet between 90 and 95 percent of patients with advanced cancer can be pain-free, he says.

That's excellent news for people with this disease—and it's good news for you when you check into the hospital with any painful problem.

Doctors are learning how to better control all kinds of painful conditions through the artful use of narcotics and new techniques in giving painkillers. Hospitals are making pain management a priority now, according to Dr. Levy.

"We're starting to see a positive ripple effect," Dr. Levy says. "We've made pain therapy a subspecialty, and now it's reaching out to other chronic pain syndromes." For instance, in one new technique available to people with cancer pain, the doctor places a medication reservoir under the skin. The reservoir carries a month's worth of painkiller, so you are never without the medication you need.

Tuning In the Soothe Tube

You may not realize that one of the best high-tech pain relievers is right there in the hospital room with you. You probably thought the television was hung in front of your bed just to entertain you during those long hours between medical procedures and food trays. Yet the television—with the game show blaring—can be a good temporary pain reliever.

How?

It offers distraction from your pain. When you are concentrating on something besides your pain, your attention is focused away from your hurt and pain moves from center stage to the edge of your awareness.

No one says pain fizzles as easily as the game show starlet turns over the letters in the puzzle. However, pain can be more bearable and your pain tolerance may go up when you aren't concentrating on how much you hurt. For short-term pain relief, distraction helps you focus on something pleasant, say pain-relief experts. And it gives you a better sense of control over your pain, which makes pain easier to bear.

Soothing Strokes

It may take 20 minutes to a full hour for some medications to kick in, says Garbush. While you wait for your pain medication to work, you need some kind of relief. She suggests a combination of distraction and relaxation. Here's what she does to help a person in pain. You can try it on a loved one who needs relief.

"You hold the hand of the person in pain and stroke their arm upward, from the hand to the heart. You get them to focus on your voice," she says. "You talk in a monotone about something pleasant, about a happy vacation or a favorite walk. It's a fairy tale dialogue that takes them there and puts them in that picture. You're stroking and they are following the dialogue."

Distraction—anything from a television newscast to visualizing yourself at the beach—can help while you get through an uncomfortable medical procedure. Women have even used distraction—focusing their eyes and breathing rhythmically—successfully during labor and childbirth.

McCaffery advises distracting yourself or helping someone in your family with the following techniques:

- Look through a series of pictures or through a magazine and describe, out loud, each object you see.
- Sing silently, whispering or mouthing the words to a familiar song such as "Jingle Bells" or "Happy Birthday." Tap your fingers to keep time with the music.
- When you hurt more, talk or sing faster. Slow down when the pain is less. Be sure to begin your distraction before the pain starts, if possible.

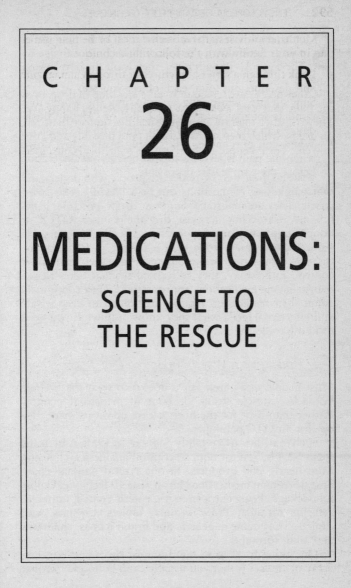

CHAPTER
26

MEDICATIONS:
SCIENCE TO
THE RESCUE

S ome people run to the medicine chest at the first hint of pain and toss down a couple of their favorite analgesic. The Type A's of pain relief, they want the hurt to stop now!

Other people are reluctant to take any kind of drug, even for pain that eats away at a normally active, happy life. They'd rather tolerate some physical discomfort than rely on drugs, which they see as a crutch (and possibly addictive as well). These people are the Puritans of medical consumerism.

Between these two extremes are people who understand that painkilling medications can be a blessing when used wisely. They are realistic about these drugs' potential benefits and risks. They may use over-the-counter (OTC), or nonprescription, drugs for occasional headaches or muscle pain. Or they may work with a doctor to find just the right prescription to bring long-term or severe pain under control. Either way, they've learned what it takes to use pain-relieving medications appropriately. They continually adapt their medication regimen as needed to keep it safe and effective. Here's what they know, and what you need to know to do the same.

Finding Your Way Through the OTC Maze

Most people don't seek out a doctor to treat the average headache, muscle strain, or bout of menstrual cramps. Rather than wait for the hurt to ease up on its own, they opt for an OTC painkiller.

Such remedies are certainly popular. In 1989, Americans spent $2.4 billion for nonprescription analgesics, choosing from nearly 200 products. In one typical national-chain drugstore, pain medications fill an aisle 10 feet long. Colorful packages boast extra strength, enteric coated, buffered, arthritis formula, PMS formula, tablets, capsules, and caplets. They come in generic and brand names, children's and adult formulas . . .

One thing to keep in mind amidst this mind-boggling array of choices is that you usually can't go too far wrong.

For relieving mild to moderate pain, most doctors (and the Food and Drug Administration, the FDA) agree that the recommended dose of one product usually works as well as another. (One exception is that ibuprofen appears to be tops for menstrual pain.) And for the vast majority, occasional use of OTC painkillers is safe, says William T. Beaver, M.D., professor of pharmacology at Georgetown University School of Medicine and Dentistry in Washington, D.C. But each can cause unpleasant or serious side effects. Let your doctor know if you experience any side effects from nonprescription medications.

Of course, that doesn't mean that the various types of pain-relieving compounds don't have differences that may make one your best choice for a particular kind of pain. They do. One may fight inflammation better, while another soothes fever better. And you may have a health problem or sensitivity that limits your choice of drugs. Stomach ulcers, heart disease, liver or kidney damage, even asthma and allergies can turn random pill-popping into a pharmaceutical Russian roulette, as you'll soon see.

What's on the Label?

Almost all nonprescription pain relievers contain one or more of these ingredients: aspirin, acetaminophen, or ibuprofen. A few, like Doan's, contain aspirin-related compounds such as magnesium salicylate, which are slightly less irritating to the stomach than regular aspirin but also have less pain-relieving power.

Reading the list of ingredients on the drug package will tell you the active ingredients in the product. It will also make you aware of all the *other* ingredients in the product—some of which you may not want or need. You may be surprised to find that a product contains caffeine, an antihistamine, or a diuretic, for example. Ask the pharmacist to explain the purpose and possible side effects of any unfamiliar ingredients.

Your pharmacist can supply you with a good deal of helpful information, but it's a good idea to talk with your doctor before you take any drug, even a nonprescription

WHAT'S IN A DRUG?

If you've ever found yourself trying to read the fine print while you're juggling several packages of drugs in some supermarket aisle, you'll be glad to know about the *Physician's Desk Reference for Nonprescription Drugs*. This book, which may be available in the reference section of your public library or local hospital library, lets you easily compare brands of over-the-counter drugs. It includes indications for use, recommended dosages, and possible side effects.

A similar volume, the *Physician's Desk Reference*, gives the same information for drugs prescribed by your doctor. It also ranks drugs by their potential for abuse or addiction and their safety during pregnancy. This information is also available on an information sheet you can get from your pharmacist for any prescription drug.

one, for the first time. This precaution is especially wise if you are older and taking other medications.

The OTC Lineup

It's always a good idea to discuss new pains with your doctor. If you aren't sure when it's okay to reach for an OTC medication, here are some guidelines that medical experts use.

OTC medications are usually more effective in relieving pain arising from the skin, teeth, muscles, and skeleton. Doctors call this kind of pain "somatic pain." Stronger, prescription drugs are often needed for controlling pain from the organs in the chest or abdomen.

Somatic pain is usually dull and aching, not sharp or breath-taking, experts explain. Somatic pain includes a wide range of all-too-common ailments: mild to moderate tension headaches, menstrual cramps, toothaches, and all sorts of nerve and muscle pain.

The Way They Work

All three of the most popular OTC pain relievers—aspirin, acetaminophen, and ibuprofen—work in a somewhat similar way, most experts agree. Understanding how they work will help you decide which one to reach for the next time you want to zap a particular pain. All three affect the body's manufacture or use of a group of chemicals, known as prostaglandins, that act as a type of emergency telegraph system for your body. When injured, your body uses pain to alert you to the danger, and it uses the prostaglandins to deliver the pain message.

Prostaglandins serve an important purpose, says Dr. Beaver. Because these chemicals sensitize an injured area to even the slightest touch, they encourage you to protect it, which aids in healing. Prostaglandins also call in your body's tissue repair crew. Once prostaglandins have done their beneficial work, their continuing action causes you a lot of grief, explains Dr. Beaver. They are a lot like a burglar alarm that won't turn off.

Aspirin and ibuprofen inhibit prostaglandin production both at the site of pain and generally throughout the body, says Dr. Beaver. The action of acetaminophen isn't quite so clear. It apparently also affects prostaglandins but in a less broad-ranging way. One theory is that acetaminophen blocks prostaglandin action only in the brain, not at the site of the pain, so it interferes with fewer of prostaglandin's beneficial actions. It is also less likely to irritate your stomach than aspirin and ibuprofen.

Easing the "-itis"

Aspirin and ibuprofen have a talent that acetaminophen lacks, however. When taken in higher-than-usual analgesic doses, these two drugs cool the inflammation that accompanies arthritis or injury. So besides relieving pain, they soothe swelling, redness, and burning.

That's why some athletes use either of these drugs in relatively high amounts for up to a week for muscle strains (along with ice, compression, and rest). As anyone who's ever sprained an ankle knows, injured muscles can balloon before your eyes.

People with joint-swelling rheumatoid arthritis also find aspirin and ibuprofen very helpful. But treating arthritis yourself with OTC medications can be risky business, warns Charles F. Seifert, Pharm.D., associate professor at the University of Oklahoma College of Pharmacy. Relief may come only with long-term high doses that have serious side effects, such as life-threatening stomach bleeding, he says.

"Anyone who thinks they have arthritis should be diagnosed by a doctor and should use drugs only with medical supervision," Dr. Seifert says.

An OTC Checklist

Before you take any nonprescription drug, you may want to ask yourself the same questions a pharmacist or doctor should ask you. Better yet, discuss these questions with your pharmacist or doctor, suggests Dr. Seifert.

- Do you have any idea what may be causing the pain? Is it related to an injury, migraine headache, arthritis?
- What kind of painkiller usually works for you? If it worked before, chances are good it will work again.
- What have you already taken? How much and for how long? If it's not working, you should see your doctor.
- Does aspirin or ibuprofen upset your stomach? If so, you may want to try acetaminophen, or take the drug with a meal.
- Are you allergic to anything? Respiratory allergies could mean you're aspirin-sensitive.
- Do you have asthma or an ulcer or have you had either in the past? Either would make acetaminophen your wisest choice.
- Are you currently taking medication for high blood pressure, gout, arthritis, or diabetes, or one that makes your blood thinner? If so, you should have your doctor's okay before taking any nonprescription drug.

Sidestepping Side Effects

OTC medications are considered safe; otherwise they wouldn't be on the market. But they're not perfect. They do cause side effects that you should be aware of.

While you may enjoy the relief that aspirin and ibuprofen offer, for example, your stomach doesn't necessarily share your enthusiasm.

There's no doubt that acetaminophen is easier on the stomach than either aspirin or ibuprofen. Research shows that even with long-time daily use, acetaminophen causes practically none of the stomach irritation, ulcers, or even life-threatening bleeding that ibuprofen and especially aspirin can cause. Acetaminophen's kindness to the stomach is a big reason for its popularity. And it's why doctors often tell their patients to try acetaminophen first for their pain, especially chronic pain. Make sure you check with your doctor before changing your medications.

Taken daily, aspirin—and to a lesser extent, ibuprofen—can make your stomach feel like base camp for an army of fire ants. The antiprostaglandin effect of these drugs is to blame, says Dr. Seifert. Prostaglandins help to maintain a healthy stomach lining; so when prostaglandin production is inhibited, the stomach lining begins to break down, leaving it exposed to the corrosive effect of its own acids. This excruciating effect occurs because of the drug's contact not only directly with the stomach but also through the bloodstream. The effect occurs even when the drug is taken with food, buffered, or enteric coated—covered with a film that lets it dissolve only after it has reached the small intestine.

"With long-term use [of aspirin or ibuprofen], you are going to have stomach problems. And the higher the dosage, the worse the problem," Dr. Seifert says. That's why he suggests taking a prescription anti-inflammatory drug with fewer stomach-searing properties instead.

Soothing the Stomach

Besides playing havoc with your stomach through the bloodstream, aspirin can eat right into your stomach lining if it stays in direct contact for too long. If you take aspirin with only a small amount of fluid, you're asking for trouble. After all, it is an acid. (People who resort to a risky toothache remedy—placing an aspirin on their gum by the bad tooth—can attest to its ability to "burn" mucous membranes.)

To limit this stomach-burning effect, doctors recommend that you take aspirin with food. Eat a bit, take the aspirin, and then finish eating. Or you can take the aspirin with a glass of milk.

The problem with taking any drug with food, however, is that food delays the drug's absorption into the bloodstream, says Dr. Seifert. A drug that might provide relief in 45 minutes or less when taken with only water may take hours to kick in if you down it with a few slices of pepperoni pizza. That delayed reaction doesn't matter if you are taking a drug regularly to maintain a constant blood level, as you might for rheumatoid arthritis, he says. But if you're taking it for hopefully quick relief from, say, a night of overindulgence, washing it down with a big glass of water or choosing the fizzle version of a drug (like Alka-Seltzer) will give you maximum relief in minimum time, moving it through your stomach and into your bloodstream without delay, says Dr. Seifert.

Enteric-coated aspirin avoids direct contact with the stomach and may cause less stomach irritation, says Dr. Seifert. Buffered aspirin, on the other hand, is "all hype," he maintains. "We used to think it reduced stomach irritation. Now we know there is no convincing data to support that it buffers."

Avoiding Aspirin

Medical researchers give their vote to acetaminophen when it comes to avoiding "allergic" reactions, or sensitivities. It seldom causes a problem. Fewer than 5 percent of the people who react to aspirin or related compounds also have allergies to acetaminophen.

Who's aspirin-sensitive? People with asthma, hay fever, or nasal polyps are at highest risk, says Dr. Beaver. Signs of a sensitivity, which can occur within minutes of taking aspirin, include a stuffy, runny nose, swollen throat, itching and hives, and asthma attacks. In rare cases, life-threatening shock can occur. Aspirin-sensitive people should also avoid

LOVE THAT ASPIRIN, HATE THAT ULCER
There's no doubt that nonsteroidal anti-inflammatory drugs
(NSAIDs) such as aspirin help many people lead more active,
pain-free lives. But even just a few weeks of use can lead to
serious problems of stomach irritation, ulcers, and bleeding,
especially in people ages 60 and over. Because these drugs
mask the aching pain of stomach irritation, many older people realize they have a bleeding ulcer only when they develop
anemia, notice black, tarry bowel movements, or vomit
blood. By then, they have a serious problem.

That's why rheumatologists are now prescribing a drug
called misoprostol (Cytotec). This unique drug stimulates the
growth of mucus-producing cells that form the stomach
lining. It helps to prevent the stomach ulcers that are always
a threat with long-term anti-inflammatory use.

"Many rheumatologists are now routinely prescribing
Cytotec to their arthritis patients age 60 or older, whether
they've had stomach problems in the past or not," says
Charles F. Seifert, Pharm.D., associate professor at the University of Oklahoma College of Pharmacy.

He says many doctors, usually general practitioners, incorrectly prescribe ulcer medications (histamine blockers like
Tagamet or Zantac) to their patients who are taking NSAIDs.
These drugs can help heal an ulcer that's already formed if
NSAIDs are stopped during the two- to three-month healing
process, but there is no proof that they help to stop stomach
ulcers from forming, says Dr. Seifert. "Currently, Cytotec is
the only drug clearly shown to prevent ulcers caused by anti-
inflammatories," he says.

ibuprofen and check every OTC product for "hidden" aspirin, usually listed on the label as some form of salicylate or
salicylic acid, says Dr. Beaver.

If aspirin or ibuprofen makes your ears ring, hiss, or
roar, it's time to back off, says Dr. Seifert. It means you're
nearing what for you is a toxic level of this drug. Some
supersensitive people experience ringing with just a few
pills. Usually the bells stop as soon as the blood level of the
drug drops to a safe level.

Protecting the Liver and Kidneys

Your liver and kidneys are responsible for breaking down and clearing toxins out of your body. These cleanup chores expose them to the toxic side effects of drugs.

Medical research shows that problems can develop when people take more than the recommended dosage for long periods of time or take even one extremely high dose, especially of acetaminophen. Some studies report that 7 to 10 percent of end-stage kidney disease (which requires use of a kidney machine) is linked to the misuse of analgesics.

Even a few days of taking the recommended dosage can cause total kidney failure in people with congestive heart failure, severe high blood pressure, or kidney or liver disease. People with these problems should take *nothing* without their doctor's okay. And people taking diuretics for any reason should also consult with their doctor before taking an OTC pain reliever, as diuretics combined with analgesics can damage kidneys. (The diuretics found in some menstrual-pain formulas, though, are so weak they present no hazards, says Dr. Seifert.)

Alcoholics, too, are at high risk. "Studies clearly show that acetaminophen is extremely toxic to the liver in alcoholics, even in normal doses," Dr. Seifert says. Because heavy drinkers also tend to have stomach ulcers and other problems, he suggests they use ibuprofen rather than aspirin.

Presurgery Precautions

Scheduled for surgery? You'll want to stop taking any aspirin at least two weeks before the big day, and ibuprofen a day or two before, says Dr. Seifert. Both drugs make blood much slower to clot, which means you could lose more blood during your operation. Discuss this problem with your doctor. If you need pain relief, he or she may have you switch to acetaminophen. After surgery, many doctors continue to prefer acetaminophen because it has no effect on blood clotting.

Dousing a Fever Safely

Aspirin, ibuprofen, and acetaminophen are considered equally good at cooling the aches and pains of fever, most experts agree.

In adults, any of these medications will do. But in children, acetaminophen is your safest bet, says Ralph Kauffman, M.D., professor of pediatrics and pharmacology at Wayne State University in Detroit. That's because several studies have linked the use of aspirin in children or teenagers with a potentially fatal disease—Reye's syndrome.

If a child shows signs of dehydration—fewer wet diapers, no tears—due to vomiting, diarrhea, or fever, stop giving acetaminophen or other drugs and call your doctor. Dehydration makes a child's kidneys particularly vulnerable to a drug's toxic side effects, says Dr. Kauffman.

Champion for Cramps

For menstrual discomfort, some women swear by ibuprofen, and apparently with good reason. In several studies, ibuprofen beat out aspirin and acetaminophen in relieving menstrual cramps, backache, and headache. Some women also report that it helps reduce the diarrhea and nausea that they have during the first day or two of their period.

"Ibuprofen is the only nonprescription drug that makes any sense for menstrual cramps," Dr. Beaver says. The theory is that women get cramps because they produce excess amounts of prostaglandins in the uterus during their periods. Prostaglandins are thought to stimulate uterine contractions, which in turn can cause pain.

"Most women know their own pattern of pain and can figure out when they need to start taking the drug, and for how long, to control their pain," Dr. Beaver says. He believes that taking 400 milligrams of ibuprofen every 4 hours, up to 1,600 milligrams a day for 24 to 48 hours, relieves most women's pain. This amount exceeds the recommended nonprescription dosage, but, he says, "for this occasional short-term use that's not a problem." Ask your doctor if higher doses of ibuprofen may help relieve your menstrual discomfort.

As Easy as One, Two, Three

When you want fast relief, you reach for your OTC drug of choice. When you want faster relief or stronger relief, you may be tempted to grab a couple more tablets. That may not be such a good idea. Here's why.

The recommended single dose for acetaminophen and aspirin, whether you're taking regular or extra strength, is two tablets.

Most "regular" formulas of acetaminophen and aspirin contain 325 milligrams. A few (Anacin, for instance) contain 400 milligrams. "Extra" or "maximum strength" and arthritis formulas usually contain 500 milligrams.

Every over-the-counter ibuprofen brand comes in 200-milligram strength. The recommended dose is one tablet, but the directions for most formulas say to take one, and if that doesn't do the trick, take another. "In other words, take the lowest effective dose, but no more than two tablets, or six in a 24-hour period," Dr. Beaver explains. Because of possible side effects such as stomach irritation, the FDA limits its nonprescription dosage. "Extra strength" ibuprofen is available by prescription only, with good reason.

If they are going to relieve your pain, all three drugs will generally have an effect in 45 to 60 minutes, provided they are not timed-release, enteric coated, or taken with food, in which case they can take much longer to work, says Dr. Beaver. Experts say that aspirin and acetaminophen will usually provide relief for 3 to 4 hours, and ibuprofen for 6 hours.

If you're tempted to double-dose, take note: More is not necessarily better. Your body can metabolize only a certain amount of a drug in a given period of time. The recommended dosage exists for a reason: It balances pain relief against side effects. Taking more than that amount could cause toxicity without providing additional benefits. It's especially important to read the label on the medication that you're using and to not exceed the recommended daily dosage, notes Dr. Beaver.

Calling in the Big Guns

When nonprescription pain relievers no longer work, or if they simply don't help right from the start, it's time to see your doctor. He or she may recommend a stronger version of the same drug you could purchase over the counter. Or he or she may want to try a drug that relieves your pain in a way entirely different than nonprescription drugs do.

It's important that you and your doctor know exactly which physical ailment is causing your pain and what can be done about it. You don't want to be taking painkilling drugs, at least not for long, for a condition that hasn't been properly diagnosed or that could be corrected by surgery or some other medical treatment, warns Nelson Hendler, M.D., director of the Mensana Pain Clinic in Stevenson, Maryland. Don't accept a "diagnosis" of "psychosomatic pain" or "chronic pain syndrome," he says. "These are not medical diagnoses. They are simply a sign of lazy, sloppy medicine." In the hands of experts, it's rare that a cause of pain cannot be found, he stresses.

Protecting Yourself

In a "just say no" society, people are often wary of addiction. Sometimes their wariness is based on misconceptions; other times, it's for darn good reasons.

If you've been afraid to even discuss the possibility of a prescription pain-relieving drug with your doctor, keep in mind that some kinds of drugs ease pain very effectively with no hazard of physical addiction. Also, prescription drugs can be used in combination, or along with non-drug treatments, in order to keep doses low. Stronger prescription medications can also be reserved for acute flare-ups.

Studies show that when used properly, pain-relieving drugs, including narcotics, seldom cause addiction, even though they do have that potential. The key phrase here is "used properly." Any drug, including aspirin, can be abused, Dr. Hendler warns. And people can develop a psychological dependency (without physical dependency) to just about anything, including teddy bears.

With these things in mind, let's look at the prescription drugs that relieve pain—including narcotics.

Beyond Aspirin: Anti-Inflammatory Drugs

Aspirin and ibuprofen are just 2 of 20 or more nonsteroidal anti-inflammatory drugs (NSAIDs) now on the market. Most are available only through a doctor and have names only a chemist could love—or pronounce. (Some of the more popular ones: prescription-strength ibuprofen, diclofenac sodium, sulindac, indomethacin, and piroxicam.)

All NSAIDs relieve pain by reducing the swelling, redness, and burning associated with inflammation, Dr. Seifert explains. That's why they're the main arsenal against many kinds of arthritis as well as gout, Lyme disease (a rare disease transmitted by ticks), and ankylosing spondylitis (inflammation of the spinal vertebrae).

NSAIDs are also used to treat other painful inflammatory diseases, including ulcerative colitis (inflammation of the colon), arteritis (inflammation of the arteries), and such rare connective tissue diseases as systemic lupus erythematosus, says Dr. Seifert.

All of these drugs, at varying doses, also relieve pain independently of their anti-inflammatory effects and so are used for more general kinds of pain: severe headaches, cancer pain, postoperative pain, and pain caused by torn muscles or broken bones.

"These drugs are extremely versatile and useful, but they do have side effects," says Dr. Seifert. When they're taken for more than a few weeks at a time, each can cause stomach irritation, ulcers, and, occasionally, hard-to-control stomach bleeding. Some can even cause serious blood and bone marrow disorders that lead to anemia or lowered immunity. That's why it's crucial not only to take these drugs under the supervision of a doctor you trust but also to stay in close contact with your doctor while you're taking them, advises Dr. Seifert.

"Some anti-inflammatory drugs are more likely to have side effects than others, so you are depending on your doctor to choose the right one for you," Dr. Beaver says. Rheumatologists—doctors specializing in arthritis and other inflammatory diseases—are more likely to know these drugs inside out, since they prescribe them every day.

"Most rheumatologists have their own sequence of selection of drugs for a particular disease," Dr. Beaver says. "They may start with the one least likely to produce side effects. If that drug doesn't work, or if certain side effects begin to appear, they move on to another drug." Sometimes, though, experts say, the best strategy is to start with a heavy-duty drug (such as a steroid) to get inflammation under control quickly and then switch to a weaker but safer drug for long-term use.

Many people taking anti-inflammatories are age 60 or older and have sluggish kidneys and liver, notes Dr. Seifert. For these people, taking smaller amounts of a drug several times a day is often safer than taking a longer-acting drug once a day, he says. Longer-acting drugs are more likely to build up in the body to levels that hurt the liver or kidneys, he explains.

Raising Spirits . . . and Relieving Pain

People who've been hurting a long time are often depressed. Who can blame them? Continual pain can truly darken one's sense of pleasure. That's why treating depression is an important part of any pain-relief program.

But even when they're not depressed, some people with chronic pain can apparently benefit from taking certain kinds of mood-elevating drugs, called tricyclic antidepressants, according to Nagagopal Venna, M.D., associate professor of neurology at Boston University School of Medicine.

Unlike many other mood-altering drugs, antidepressants such as doxepin, amitriptyline, and imipramine are not narcotics, says Dr. Venna. They are not addictive. You do not have to take them in ever-larger doses to get the same amount of pain relief. Possible side effects, which are relatively mild compared to those of many other pain-relieving drugs, include dry mouth, drowsiness, poor concentration, urinary retention, and sometimes dizziness and low blood pressure. In some people, these drugs provide complete relief after years of troubling pain, says Dr. Venna.

Antidepressants seem to work by blocking pain messages traveling through the spinal cord. It's possible that some antidepressants may also change the way a nerve acts at the site of an injury, explains Mitchell Max, M.D., a pioneer in pain research at the National Institute of Dental Research in Bethesda, Maryland. The drugs may act directly on injured nerves, stopping painful spasms or decreasing their sensitivity, he says.

So far, antidepressant drugs have been found to work best on pain caused by nerves that have been damaged. The damage may have been caused by diabetes, injuries, amputation, or viral infections that strike nerves—such as shingles. "Such pain has traditionally been considered hard to treat," Dr. Max says. "In the past, people often were told they'd just have to learn to live with it."

Antidepressants are also used, along with analgesics, to treat severe, recurrent headaches and for low back pain, especially pain related to a back injury, says Dr. Hendler.

Doctors vary in how they prescribe antidepressants, but most start at very low doses (10 to 25 milligrams) and over a period of weeks work up to a level that relieves pain, says Dr. Venna. The amount that relieves pain is usually below the dosage needed to treat depression and is likely to cause only mild side effects, if any, he notes.

"I ask my patients to try to stay on them for four to six weeks," Dr. Venna says. "If these are going to work, generally they will within that period of time."

Relaxing Muscle Spasms

A massage, hot bath, or gentle stroll can help relieve pain by relaxing tense muscles. A class of medications known as muscle relaxants can do the same. They are often used along with such treatments as rest, physical therapy, and biofeedback to stop muscle spasms causing low back pain, headaches, or neck pain. Some muscle relaxants work by inhibiting certain reflexes in the brain and spinal cord that cause painful contractions in the muscles, experts explain.

Muscle relaxants are relatively safe, but usually they're prescribed for only a week or two at a time, says Dr. Hendler. That's because they cause drowsiness and light-headedness and aren't necessary after the worst pain has loosened its grip, he says. Doctors often prescribe two particular muscle relaxants—carisoprodol (Soma) and cyclobenzaprine HCl (Flexeril)—because they have fewer mood-altering effects than other drugs that are sometimes prescribed to relax muscles—such as Valium and other tranquilizers and sleeping pills, according to Dr. Hendler.

Stop the Motion

Some of the most painful conditions known to humanity fall under the category of nerve disorders. Nerves carry pain messages, and when that message system itself goes awry, what comes through can be pretty excruciating.

Fortunately, experts agree, the same drugs that can block an epileptic seizure can also calm the sporadic nervous system misfirings of some of these disorders. These medications, known as anticonvulsants, are also used for pain caused by inflamed nerves where there is no mechanical problem.

Anyone taking one of these drugs needs careful monitoring and frequent blood tests, Dr. Hendler cautions. These drugs can conceivably cloud your mind and slow your movements. They can also cause liver and kidney damage and affect blood cells. Your doctor should have you stop taking the drug for a week or so every three months to see if your symptoms have disappeared, says Dr. Venna.

When All Else Fails

Doctors have used opium—the juice of the poppy plant—for more than 2,000 years to stop pain. It was a "wonder drug" back then, and the medicines derived from it today, called "opiates" or narcotics, still offer the strongest, fastest relief possible to people in teeth-gritting, breath-taking pain, says Dr. Hendler.

Injected narcotics aren't, and shouldn't be, used when other drugs or nondrug treatments will relieve pain, experts agree. Generally, they're used only when pain is intense but short-lived—for kidney stones, herniated spinal disks, severe burns, or compound fractures, or after surgery. Studies show that after an operation, people whose pain is relieved by regular, adequate doses of pain medication generally need fewer repeat doses and get off medication sooner than those whose pain is not adequately relieved or those who are required to ask for pain medications.

Narcotics are also used to relieve pain from cancer. For this, they may be used off and on over a period of years, along with other drugs, or continually if a cancer patient needs them, Dr. Beaver explains.

Unlike NSAIDs, narcotics do not work at the site of an injury; they work in your brain and spinal cord. Narcotics signal your brain to send pain-suppressing messages down to the part of the spinal cord that is relaying pain messages up to the brain. They also block the pain messages from reaching your brain, where they would be perceived as pain. This means they relieve pain everywhere in your body and can block pain deep in your organs and spinal cord.

Narcotics are unexcelled as pain-relieving agents. Unfortunately, they have a lot of other actions on the body. Compared to other nonsteroidal analgesics, narcotics have many more potential mood-altering side effects, such as euphoria and sedation. They affect the parts of the brain that control respiration and digestion. People taking narcotics often have problems with constipation and slowed breathing.

These drugs also have the potential for producing psychological and physical dependence as well as the development of tolerance. In other words, you can become addicted to them.

Tolerance means that the dosage must be repeatedly

increased in order to maintain the initial pain-relieving effect. A few terminal cancer patients, for instance, may reach a point where they need to double their dosage every week or two in order to stay ahead of their pain. These larger doses potentially carry a slew of side effects.

Dependence can be physical, psychological, or both. Physical dependence means that the user shows signs of withdrawal when the drug is stopped. Narcotics can produce a strong tendency for physical dependence. In people taking these drugs for pain relief, withdrawal may mean a temporary surge in pain and anxiety, along with sweating, agitation, and trouble sleeping.

For people with terminal cancer, tolerance and physical dependence shouldn't be considered a problem, Dr. Beaver stresses. Relieving pain is what matters most, he says.

For people with chronic pain not caused by cancer, though, narcotics often make things worse in the long run, doctors warn. Narcotics sedate you and make you dizzy and nauseated if you stand up and move around. They also make the pain seem worse, at least temporarily, when they wear off. If your goal is to function normally—perhaps with some pain—you need to ask your doctor to ration or stop your dose of narcotics, experts agree.

"Most chronic pain patients will tell you that the continued use of narcotics really doesn't help their pain," Dr. Hendler says. "They'll tell you it helps them cope with the pain or makes them feel good, but it really doesn't do much to modify the pain itself." Many admit they are using narcotics because they are depressed, anxious, and unable to sleep because of their pain, he says, "so it would be more appropriate to use other drugs to treat depression, sleep problems, and anxiety than to use narcotics."

Dr. Hendler says he will prescribe no more than ten narcotic pills a month for a patient to take during acute flare-ups of pain. He limits the prescription, he says, because he's seen too many patients who couldn't do without their pills and had to go through a drug withdrawal program.

Avoiding Addiction

How can you keep from getting stuck in the addiction trap? "Ask your doctor to avoid escalating the dose of a drug," Dr. Hendler answers. Most people can take a constant dose of a narcotic for seven to ten days for acute pain and then, in two to three days, decrease their dosage and then stop the drugs, he says. (Their doctors sometimes substitute non-narcotic analgesics or antidepressants.)

Here are the four warning signs of addiction.

- You find yourself looking forward to a dose for its mood-elevating high.
- You need to up the dosage to continue to relieve pain.
- You are taking it for more than ten days in a row.
- You have a hard time stopping the drugs within the period of a few days.

Always tell your doctor if you currently have or in the past have had a problem with alcohol or drugs. It may affect the prescription he or she writes, or whether he or she prescribes a drug at all.

Doctors tend to "rank" narcotics according to their pain-relieving ability and their potential for addiction, says Dr. Hendler. This ranking, though, is somewhat arbitrary. The dosage and whether the drug is given as a pill or an injection affect its strength. And all narcotics can be addictive. Perhaps the safest and most often prescribed narcotics are codeine and its derivatives.

Codeine is rarely sold alone; it's usually combined with a nonnarcotic pain reliever such as acetaminophen or aspirin. The number following the drug name, from one to four, indicates the amount of codeine in a formula. These drugs are frequently prescribed after dental surgery or other outpatient surgery or for other mild to moderately severe pain, experts say. Codeine combinations are considered to have some potential for abuse, but it is low.

Narcotics for severe pain include morphine and its derivatives, such as hydromorphone and oxymorphone, and totally synthetic drugs, such as meperidine and methadone. The strongest pain relievers available, they are used mostly after surgery or severe injuries and for cancer pain. They are considered to have high potential for abuse.

Be a Wise Consumer

If you find that pain-relieving drugs are necessary, you want to take precautions to use them wisely and protect yourself. Make sure you understand your doctor's prescription, read the label, and do not exceed the recommended dosage. It's up to you, with your doctor's help, to weigh the risks of taking a particular drug against the potential benefits, and then decide what's best for you.

Taking an anti-inflammatory drug for rheumatoid arthritis, for instance, will increase your chances of getting a stomach ulcer. But if the drug is the only thing that lets you go about your business without pain and stiffness, you may consider it well worth the risk, Dr. Seifert notes.

If you're taking narcotics for chronic back pain, on the other hand, and you find yourself not only needing more and more but becoming irritable or depressed, you may decide you're not really benefiting from the drug, says Dr. Hendler. You may look for something that offers more benefit: physical therapy, losing weight, or perhaps nonnarcotic analgesics or antidepressants, he says.

Don't assume that just because your doctor is writing a prescription for you, it's the right drug in the right dosage. Ask questions: Why are you prescribing this particular drug? (In other words, exactly what condition is it meant to treat?) What are its side effects? Is there a safer drug you could prescribe that would work as well? Is there something I can do to relieve my pain without drugs?

If you decide to take the drug, get a drug information sheet from the pharmacist. Read it, and keep it on hand to refer to later if necessary. Report any disturbing new symptoms to your doctor. They could be side effects. It may be necessary for you to stop, switch, or back off on the dosage of the drug.

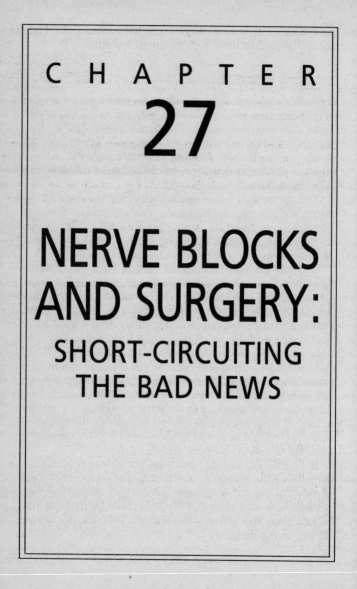

CHAPTER
27

NERVE BLOCKS AND SURGERY:
SHORT-CIRCUITING
THE BAD NEWS

The thinking behind surgery for pain relief is simple enough: Since nerves transmit pain signals from an injured body part to the brain, why not just cut the nerve? It seems that should stop the pain message from reaching the brain. In theory, it would be just like cutting the telephone wire to your house. You wouldn't be able to receive calls. You wouldn't even know someone was trying to get in touch with you, unless they decided to bypass the phone and come knocking at your door. Your calls would end up in electric limbo; so, it would seem, should your pain. Without the nerves, the pain message simply wouldn't get through.

Unfortunately, the body mechanics of such a scheme aren't so simple. It's true that temporary nerve blocks—injections of local anesthesia—are useful in diagnosing some types of pain, especially neck and back pain. And permanent nerve blocks—cutting, freezing, or chemically destroying part of the nerve—may stop severe pain, including some kinds of cancer pain.

But nerves are living tissue, not copper wire. They can grow back and reestablish connections. Cutting or burning them sometimes causes a new kind of pain that's difficult to relieve. These and other side effects make doctors cautious about using permanent nerve blocks. They are definitely not for everyone.

Temporary Tactics

If you've ever had a novocaine injection to kill the pain of dental work, you've had a temporary nerve block.

Temporary nerve blocks have none of the risky side effects of permanent nerve blocks. Because the anesthesia is injected into the tissue around the nerve, not directly into the nerve, a temporary nerve block can be done with comparative ease. A permanent nerve block, on the other hand, usually requires the use of a fluoroscope, an x-ray screen that allows the doctor to direct the needle toward the proper area.

In some cases, temporary nerve blocks are all it takes to

relieve pain: Doctors use them for rib fractures, pain around surgical incisions, compression fractures of the spine, and the searing pain of shingles. Temporary nerve blocks are particularly good at easing muscle spasms caused by whiplash or low back injuries, and they sometimes help resolve the strange prickly, sweating symptoms of sympathetic nerve pain.

"They break the cycle of pain and suffering, so that a person can get a good night's sleep and can start moving around again," says Raymond Maciewicz, M.D., Ph.D., director of Massachusetts General Hospital's Cancer Pain Center and its Pain Physiology Laboratory and associate professor of neurology at Harvard Medical School. "They often provide enough relief to get someone proceeding toward recovery."

If it's permanent pain relief you're after, it's important that your doctor do at least one temporary nerve block first, says Nelson Hendler, M.D., director of Mensana Clinic in Stevenson, Maryland. If the temporary nerve block provides good pain relief, a permanent nerve block in that same spot is likely to do the same, he says.

Permanent Solutions

A permanent nerve block, correctly performed, produces a sensation of numbness in an area of the body that previously felt pain, says Dr. Hendler.

Permanent nerve blocks can be done anywhere in the body, according to Peter Wilson, M.D., anesthesiologist at the Mayo Clinic's Pain Center. Usually, though, they're done near the spot where the nerve joins the spinal cord. That's because it's easier to find the nerve there: It's right by a particular vertebra and it's right under the skin, not buried in inches of muscle or fat.

These days, an anesthesiologist or neurosurgeon usually blocks nerves in one of two ways, says Dr. Wilson. Using an insulated probe that looks like a needle, he or she either cooks the nerve with microwaves (radiocoagulation) or freezes it with liquid nitrogen (cryosurgery).

The tricky part is controlling the amount of heat or cold applied, so that only the nerve fibers carrying pain messages are destroyed, leaving the nerve fibers that carry other sensory messages like touch or muscle control mostly unharmed. Some loss may result if there is too much nerve fiber destruction. But if too few of the fibers are destroyed, some pain may remain, says Dr. Hendler.

A surgeon determines if the nerve block has worked by asking the patient if they still feel pain. A person can usually tell immediately if the pain is gone. (The procedure reproduces the pain for the few seconds it takes to destroy the nerve.)

To Block or Not to Block

There's no doubt that permanent nerve blocks are a proper treatment for cancer pain originating from a localized spot in the body, such as an arm, a leg, or the abdomen, says Dr. Wilson. Generally, a nerve block is done when a patient is terminally ill and is not expected to live more than six months. In such cases, the procedure provides quick, sweet relief. "I do them all the time here, but only for cancer patients," says Dr. Wilson. Cancer patients are also good candidates for certain spinal cord blocks, he says.

Aside from people with these specific conditions, each person has to be evaluated individually to determine whether the procedure would be truly beneficial.

"It's very hard to generalize about who would benefit from a permanent nerve block," says Carol Warfield, M.D., director of the Pain Management Center at Beth Israel Hospital in Boston. "You can't just say doctors always do a permanent nerve block for a certain condition and that they never do one for some other condition. You need to weigh the risks against the benefits for each particular patient. How much pain do they have? How disabled are they? What's already been tried? How close are they to the end of their rope?"

Here are some chronic pain conditions that some doctors say may improve with a permanent nerve block.

Injury to a single nerve or nerve root. This type of injury could occur when a nerve has been squeezed for so long by a slipped spinal disk or by swollen tendons that it is permanently injured. Surgery may ease the pressure, but it doesn't stop the nerve from continuing to send pain messages.

Carpal tunnel syndrome is one such condition in which tendons and bones pinch the median nerve in the wrist. Trigeminal neuralgia, in which the main sensory nerve to the face is irritated or squeezed, is another, says Dr. Maciewicz.

Posttraumatic reflex sympathetic dystrophy. This is a strange and rare (or at least, rarely diagnosed) condition that can start with even a slight injury to the hand or foot— a sprain or cut, for instance. It can also start as a result of a fracture or even surgery. It causes diffuse burning pain; cool, tight, shiny skin; and, often, sweating in the affected area. Treatment with drugs and physical therapy doesn't always work. Since temporary nerve blocks do provide some relief, a permanent nerve block may be tried if this pain is severe, says Dr. Hendler.

Facet joint pain. Facets are the bony outcroppings from each side of your vertebrae. Facets have smooth, spongy "disks" of cartilage separating them, as do vertebrae. Facet pain occurs when the facet disks are ruptured, due to a blow or fall. This type of pain is aggravated by arching backward.

A word of caution here, though. Many doctors believe back pain is seldom due to facet injury alone and that a permanent nerve block to a facet is no better than an injection of an anti-inflammatory drug such as cortisone. Some, though, say a carefully done facet nerve block can relieve pain after years of suffering, reports Dr. Hendler. There's no good proof that either side is right, he says.

Weigh the Risks

Why do most doctors keep permanent nerve blocks stashed away in their bag of tricks? Because they know that the possible complications are considerable.

Cutting or permanently blocking a nerve (technical term: *rhizotomy*) can create its own type of pain, one that is very difficult to treat. Called dysesthesia, this disorder causes unpleasant tingling, prickling, and burning sensations at the lightest touch, even though the skin feels numb. Published reports indicate that this type of pain occurs in about 5 percent of patients with permanent nerve blocks. This pain doesn't occur at the time of the nerve block; it starts three to six months later, the result of abnormal nerve regrowth, says Dr. Wilson.

Even when a nerve is permanently blocked and the procedure initially relieves pain, the pain usually returns. The pain signal finds an alternate route, just like the persistent caller who knocks at the door or sends a letter when they can't get through by phone. The nerve may even grow new fibers, reconnecting the original route. Even "permanent" nerve blocks that are considered successful usually last only about six months, and seldom beyond two years. Of course, if the treatment worked well during that time, the nerve can always be blocked again, says Dr. Wilson. But the decision to try again depends on many factors. If the nerve was blocked to relieve cancer pain, for instance, the return of pain could mean that the cancer has spread beyond the range of that nerve.

Ask the Right Questions

If your doctor—in this case, an anesthesiologist or neurosurgeon—does recommend a permanent nerve block, you need to ask some important questions: What exactly is my diagnosis? Exactly which nerve or nerves do you intend to block? Is this the usual treatment for this kind of pain? What other treatments are available? How often do you do this kind of surgery? What is your success rate? What kinds of complications do your patients have? How often do they have complications?

If your doctor can't or won't answer these questions, find one who will. And even if your doctor's answers seem reasonable, you may want to get a second, independent opinion from another, equally qualified doctor.

Cutting the Spinal Cord

Sometimes, instead of blocking a nerve, a surgeon will destroy a bundle of pain-transmitting nerve fibers in the spinal cord itself to relieve pain. The particular nerve bundle involved in this procedure is called the spinothalamic tract. It ends in the thalamus and relays information to the part of the brain that perceives pain. Two nerve tracts in this bundle—one on each side of the spine—send pain messages up to the brain. Usually only one tract is cut, says Dr. Maciewicz.

This procedure, called a cordotomy, provides total pain relief on the side of the body opposite the block. It wipes out pain from the site of the block all the way down to the feet. Dr. Maciewicz explains that cordotomy used to be performed for a variety of painful conditions, but that now it's reserved for a few special instances, such as cancer pain. Since it may cause muscle weakness and loss of sensation in the affected side, it's seldom used for chronic pain not caused by cancer.

Like permanent nerve blocks, cordotomy may only be effective for six months to two years, says Dr. Maciewicz. Sometimes when the pain returns, doctors will try cutting additional spinal cord pathways. However, this may result in extreme side effects, including loss of bladder and bowel function, inability to walk, and, if the cut is high on the spinal cord, trouble breathing. It truly is a last resort.

Push-Button Relief

Imagine being able to press the button on a small radio transmitter in your breast pocket and have pain anywhere in your body melt away into a warm, pleasurable sensation. That's not science fiction; it's modern medicine. Those little radio transmitters really exist. Once installed, they allow a return to life for people with pain so bad that suicide seems like a reasonable alternative. The installation, by the way, involves brain surgery.

Several thousand people in the United States alone have

a wire-thin, 4-inch-long electrode implanted in their brain near the area where pain is perceived. A wire from the electrode, placed under the skin, runs from the scalp down behind the ear and down the neck to just below the collarbone. There, a radio receiver about the size of a pacemaker (3 inches in diameter) is implanted. When it is activated, the receiver sends a tiny electrical current through the electrode to the brain.

Depending on the type of model, the electrode may work automatically for, say, 5 minutes each hour. It may also be set up so that you operate it yourself as necessary. The only hint that you're using a deep-brain stimulator is a lump on your chest that's visible only when you are wearing your skivvies (or less).

How does deep-brain stimulation work to relieve pain? Experts say the mild electrical current may stimulate brain cells to release feel-good, pain-relieving endorphins. Or it may send an electrical current from the brain down the "pain tract" of the spine to block pain messages coming up to the brain.

As you might suspect, doctors say that deep-brain stimulation isn't for everyone with pain, or even for everyone who wants the treatment.

Good candidates for this surgery, they maintain, are people who've had pain for years, who've tried every medicine and every medical treatment under the sun, who've had surgical procedures, including nerve blocks, and who are still disabled by severe pain. These people often have also been in a multidisciplinary pain clinic and have been examined by a psychiatrist, a neurologist, and an anesthesiologist before seeking this form of treatment. It tends to be offered after all other options are exhausted.

Deep-brain stimulation is an accepted therapy for the most stubborn types of chronic pain. It's used for what's called "failed back syndrome," to treat pain caused by a stroke in the thalamus, and for some other rare kinds of pain associated with brain damage.

Oddly enough, deep-brain stimulation is not often used for cancer pain. Only patients who are medically fit and who are expected to live longer than three months are considered candidates for this kind of treatment.

Getting Wired

The operation to insert the electrode takes 1 or 2 hours. It's inserted through a small hole drilled through the skull about 6 inches back from the bridge of the nose (hidden in your hair, unless you're bald). The patient receives local anesthesia but is awake for the procedure. This is necessary because the patient needs to be able to tell the doctor what sorts of sensations they are feeling as the electrode goes in. The spot that provides the best pain relief with fewest side effects is where the surgeon permanently secures the electrode.

The greatest risk is the remote possibility (2 percent) of having a stroke during the operation. Infection and problems with blurred vision are other possible complications. Unlike cordotomy, this operation does not produce muscle weakness or paralysis, and with proper placement, it does not make the pain worse. Incorrectly placed electrodes can produce pain relief but also generate a feeling of anxiety.

Possibly the biggest limitation to this high-tech solution is the development of tolerance. Just as people who take narcotics to ease their pain have to take bigger and bigger doses to get the same pain relief, so people with deep-brain stimulation usually have to use higher currents more frequently to get the same pain relief as time goes on. They do not become addicted to the stimulation, however. Addiction takes place in a different part of your brain.

Studies show that some people are still able to get good pain relief ten years after their implant and that some get relief for no more than two years.

A large number of people apparently get significant long-term benefits. They can lead relatively normal lives. They can't have magnetic resonance imaging (MRI) scans or be exposed to very strong magnetic fields, but that's about their only limitation.

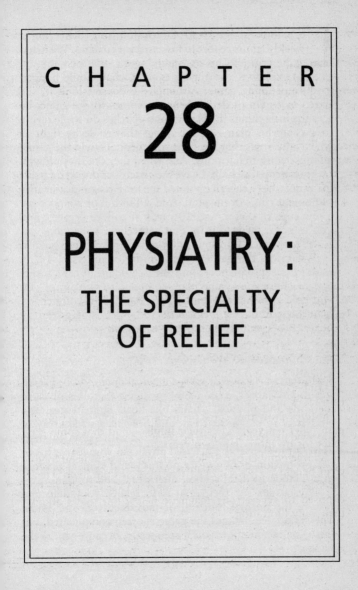

C H A P T E R

28

PHYSIATRY:
THE SPECIALTY
OF RELIEF

Let's look in on Head Coach Johnson, delivering a weekly status report to his assistant coaches. We listen as he critiques his assistants' work. It's their job, he says, to explain to the players exactly what should happen in the upcoming game. Although he doesn't look it, the coach is a man of detail. When it comes to the game, he sees the little things the players and coaches do while trying to execute his plan—all the things they're doing right as well as the areas that need improvement. To win the game, all must work in harmony. And when they do, they *all* win.

Now drop the chalk. Leave the coach's cramped quarters for a dust-free, cheerily painted meeting room at a nearby outpatient clinic or hospital. Add a handful of white coats, a few cups of coffee, and 10 yards of college degrees, and you've got a medical team that can relieve your pain.

As for Coach Johnson, call him Doc. He's a physiatrist. What does this gathering mean for you in terms of pain relief? It means you have someone to guide your care, someone to chart your game plan, someone to encourage you and hold your hand or nudge your backside if you need it. It means you have a *medical doctor* supervising a team of health professionals working to ease your pain.

Someone to Watch Over You

A physiatrist (fizzy-A-trist) is a medical doctor who specializes in physiatrics, a branch of medicine that uses physical methods and physical agents like heat, light, water, and electricity to diagnose, treat, and prevent a wide array of physical problems. Not to be confused with a physical therapist, a physiatrist is a licensed physician who learns his or her profession during years of study and clinical practice that include medical school, internship, and residency.

Physiatrists say their goal is to relieve your pain and restore the normal function or movement of your body. The stakes are big and the game is often complicated, but this is one team effort you'll appreciate, because *you're* the winner.

A physiatrist accomplishes those goals by working with you and with physical, speech, or occupational therapists, psychologists, nurses, and any other health-care professionals needed to execute a game plan he or she's drawn up to relieve your pain. He or she knows how each of these health professionals can help you. Like Coach Johnson and his assistants working with the players, the physiatrist and the other health professionals will work with you to help you beat your pain.

What Physiatry Fixes

Physiatrists work in two broad areas that often overlap: physical medicine and rehabilitation. You may benefit from the physiatrist's expertise in physical medicine if you have low back pain; neck pain; sore shoulders, elbows, knees, or feet; or any number of other kinds of *musculoskeletal* pain or pain from damaged nerves.

In the area of rehabilitation, physiatrists help restore normal movement and function in people with severe impairments like spinal cord injury, amputation, cancer, or severe arthritis.

Keep in mind the physiatrist's team approach. He'll stay in contact with the health professionals he's enlisted to help you, and he'll work with you as well. If this sounds like more attention than your average family doctor can offer, it is. And this is part of the advantage of turning to physiatry. You still have to play the game against pain, but you're not alone.

A physiatrist guides the patient along. "It's not just a high-tech office visit," says Willibald Nagler, M.D., physiatrist-in-chief at New York Hospital—Cornell Medical Center. "A physiatrist has to tell the patient why they got this way, what they have to do to get better, and how long it will take. It's a field that goes far beyond giving medication for something. It's a field that is constructive and leads people back to independence."

How the Job Gets Done

Physiatrists use physical exams, x-rays, and lab studies when they work with patients. They also rely on special diagnostic techniques, such as electromyography (EMG). EMG makes use of a device that measures muscle activity and can, for example, pinpoint the pinched nerves of carpal tunnel syndrome—a painful nerve condition in the wrists, fingers, and hands. Physiatrists plan treatment programs using "modalities" such as heat, cold, and electrical stimulation; exercises; and biofeedback. They can do the physical treatment themselves, but they usually refer you to a physical therapist for the more lengthy procedures that may be necessary.

Hold it. Why not just go to a physical therapist in the first place? "Physical therapists are professionals and experts in evaluating the musculoskeletal system, but they're not medical diagnosticians," says Randall Braddom, M.D., a physiatrist and vice president of medical affairs at Philadelphia's Moss Rehabilitation Hospital. They can't diagnose medical problems or provide medication. If you're in pain, Dr. Braddom says, "you need to make sure you don't have a neurologic problem or cancer or some other problem. The main disadvantage of going directly to a physical therapist is that you miss the diagnostic step that's so important."

Physiatrists will do whatever is necessary, short of surgery, to relieve your pain. "We have a full armament available," says Dr. Braddom. "It's not just a matter of prescribing some therapy and if that doesn't work, goodbye. It's a matter of using any kind of treatment modality that's out there, except for surgery. And if surgery is what you need, we'll send you to a surgeon. We use everyone necessary because the most important thing is getting a person better. We're trying to get a person back to work or back on the playing field or whatever it is they do at the earliest possible moment."

Getting Back to Normal

One of the most common reasons people find their fingers walking through the phone directory in search of a physiatrist is for relief of low back pain, Dr. Braddom says.

When you gingerly open the door of the physiatrist's office, trying not to stir the back monster that's clutching you in its vertebral fingers, what can you expect from the doctor inside?

The physiatrist's approach to low back pain is conservative. After taking a complete medical history, the doctor will have you hop (make that ease yourself carefully) onto the exam table.

During the physical, he or she may use EMG to help figure out what's wrong. During EMG, he or she inserts tiny needle electrodes into your muscles to record electrical impulses. You'll feel the pricks of the EMG "pins" in your muscles, but Dr. Braddom says that's all; the pricks cause only minor discomfort, if any. Here's the theory behind the EMG: When a normal muscle is at rest, it is electrically silent; but when the muscle is active, it generates an electrical current. By reading the electrical impulses picked up by the EMG, a physiatrist can tell what's going on in your muscles. "We can tell if a person has pinched nerves or nerve or muscle disease," Dr. Braddom says.

After making the diagnosis, the physiatrist usually prescribes a treatment program of physical therapy, including various modalities and exercises. He'll probably refer you to a physical therapist or other therapist who specializes in the kind of pain you have. Your physiatrist will also follow up on your physical therapy and any other treatments to make sure you're getting better and to make sure the problem doesn't recur.

Back to Exercise Basics

Physiatrist Leonard B. Kamen, D.O., physical medicine and rehabilitation medical director at Moss Rehabilitation Outpatient Services in Philadelphia, describes the experience of one typical back pain patient. The man was a middle-aged college professor who'd been treating himself for back pain with stretches and exercise. With no relief for two years, the professor finally was referred for an appointment with Dr. Kamen.

"I spent time with him, going over the specifics of his exercises and working on simplifying his approach to his daily stretching routine, which was appropriate but not well balanced. We straightened that out, and I gave him a list of things to do at home," Dr. Kamen explains.

"I had him perform the home exercises for me before he left. I corrected his technique, and I gave him some additional suggestions." The doctor then performed a spray and stretch technique on the professor's sore back—a modality that involves applying a vapocoolant spray to a muscle while it is passively stretched.

Soon the professor was ready to go with an open-ended prescription. "I left it completely up to him. If he wants to give me a call and intensify his exercise in a couple of months, that's fine," Dr. Kamen explains. "If he's not having any discomfort, I don't need to see him."

Sitting Down on the Job

Low back problems may also be corrected by examining a person's posture and discussing how they sit or stand on the job, says Dr. Kamen. It's not uncommon for a physiatrist to ask you to demonstrate how you sit or position yourself at work.

"I often recommend better seating to support the lumbar area," Dr. Kamen says. "I'm often able to make suggestions to change posture or position to reduce the stress on a person's back.

"I do a lot of hands-on. With each patient I see for pain, I do my darndest to do a very dynamic, provoking type of examination. I don't just sit there and talk to them and take their blood pressure. I want them to perform maneuvers that demonstrate for me where their pain is. I want them to show me what makes their pain worse and what relieves their pain. And by doing so, I can help devise appropriate postural and exercise techniques to correct that."

Playing a Rehab Role

Aside from working in physical medicine, the physiatrist works in rehabilitating more severely disabled people, patients that other medical disciplines can't always help.

"The goal is to have the person become independent, or as independent as possible," Dr. Braddom says. "Our goal is not necessarily to cure the individual or the impairment, because usually that's impossible. We want to lower their level of disability and handicap."

A physiatrist involved in rehabilitation works in a clinic, a hospital rehabilitation unit, or a special rehabilitation hospital. His or her patients have disabilities or significant physical problems that they must learn to live with. A physiatrist, with the allied health team he or she supervises, helps these people cope.

"With my team, I can take a person who is paralyzed from the waist down with spinal cord injury, who doesn't have control of their bowels and bladder, who doesn't feel anything below their injury, and can teach them how to manage their bowels and bladder, how to protect their skin, how to get around and drive a car, how to live completely independently if they wish," Dr. Braddom explains.

Why Physiatry?

Why might you take something like a sore shoulder to a physiatrist rather than to your regular family doctor?

"If someone comes in with a sore neck or a bad back," explains Dr. Braddom, "we feel we're the best people to treat these conditions because we're diagnosticians and treatment specialists."

If you have a painful muscle condition, a bad back, or a sore knee or shoulder, physiatrists are specially trained to use their hands, x-rays, lab tests, or EMG to pinpoint the exact nature of the muscle or nerve problem and write your prescription for care and followup, he says.

"While I highly respect family physicians," Dr. Braddom says, "they can't know about every physical problem. The main advantage of seeing a physiatrist is our increased level of expertise in these areas. Part of our increased experience and expertise is designing a plan to get rid of your pain and prevent its recurrence." While a family physician *may* do this, a competent physiatrist *must* do this, says Dr. Braddom. It's part of their job.

Perhaps you've already decided to go beyond your family doctor, to an orthopedic surgeon. Keep in mind that this kind of doctor is trained for *surgery*, says Dr. Nagler.

"In most instances it is worthwhile to see a physiatrist before an orthopedic surgeon because many situations can be handled more successfully without surgery than with surgery," he says.

Dr. Braddom agrees. "We do a careful diagnosis," he says. "What happens with low back pain is that it's so common, the average physician you might see for it, especially if they're not interested in low back pain, tends to lump it all together as 'back pain.' They don't attempt to sort it out as to the exact cause. We do a careful diagnostic study of each person to try to determine the *exact* cause of low back pain."

Indeed, doctors often refer their patients to physiatrists, Dr. Braddom says. Your doctor may refer you if you ask. You also may be referred to a physiatrist by a rehabilitation nurse or social worker, although a referral is not necessary.

Selecting Your Physiatrist

Physiatry is a rather new specialty, created in the United States during World War II because of the need to care for injured servicemen, says Ernest W. Johnson, M.D., physiatrist and professor of physical medicine and rehabilitation at Ohio State University, in Columbus.

There are currently 4,000 physiatrists in this country, according to the Association of Academic Physiatrists.

While the field is growing, the number of physiatrists is still limited, which means you may experience a bit of difficulty in finding one, says Dr. Braddom.

To find a physiatrist in your area, Dr. Braddom suggests you look in the Yellow Pages under physical medicine and rehabilitation. Physiatrists' fees vary by geographic regions but are similar to what your internist charges, he says.

If there is a rehabilitation center in your area, call and ask if there are physiatrists on staff. You might also try calling your local hospital.

You may also contact one of these organizations: The American Academy of Physical Medicine and Rehabilitation, 122 South Michigan Avenue, Suite 1300, Chicago, IL 60603, (312) 922-9366; or the Association of Academic Physiatrists, 7100 Lakewood Building, Suite 112, 5987 East 71st Street, Indianapolis, IN 46220, (317) 845-4200.

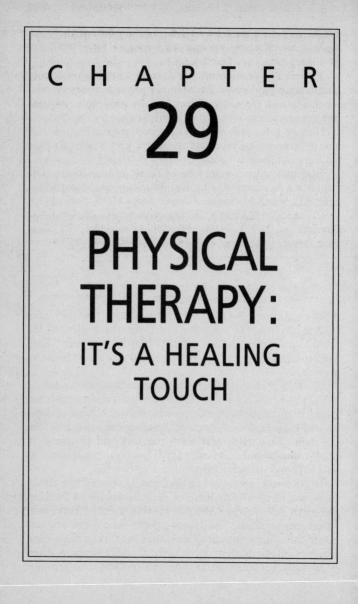

CHAPTER
29

PHYSICAL THERAPY:
IT'S A HEALING TOUCH

P icture Soldier Field in Chicago before a football game, the stadium filled to the very last row. Now file those people out and run a new group in, once again filling the 65,793-seat stadium to capacity. Watch as this happens *three* more times.

That's just about the number of people that physical therapists treat *every day*: 350,000, according to the American Physical Therapy Association (APTA).

APTA estimates there are a whopping 70,000 physical therapists out there actually doing the hands-on work—manipulating sore mastoids, repositioning wayward patellas, and in general soothing millions of aches and pains each year.

Yet physical therapists work under a shadow of anonymity. The words "Bart" and "Simpson" probably get more name recognition than "physical" and "therapy."

Rodney Dangerfields of Medicine

"The chief complaint of physical therapists is that they have such a low profile," says Stanley L. Grosshandler, M.D., chronic pain specialist in Raleigh, North Carolina. "They need to alert the public to the tremendous benefits they can give."

Physical therapists use technology, intuition, and their own two hands to treat a wide variety of pain problems: strained and sprained muscles, whiplash or other accident-related injuries, low back pain, postsurgical pain, and cancer pain. They also treat burn patients and people with temporomandibular disorder (TMD, sometimes referred to as TMJ) and diabetes pain.

Physical therapist Jim Griffin sees problems like these. In his job in the Department of Anesthesiology at the University of Texas at San Antonio Health Science Center Pain Management Clinic, he treats people who have trigger-point pain—tiny muscle spasms that hurt like crazy—and reflex sympathetic dystrophy, or RSD. RSD happens when your body produces an exaggerated response to a minor injury like a bruise. Your arms might swell because of a bruise on your hand, for example.

"A lot of the people we see have a diagnosis of exclusion," Griffin says. "That means everything else has been ruled out. They've had the million-dollar workups. What do they have left? Maybe a little joint problem that I can deal with or subclinical RSDs."

The work with cancer patients has grown and changed from its beginnings in the 1960s with breast cancer patients, says physical therapist Wayne F. Gray, consultant to Holly Hill Hospital in Raleigh, North Carolina.

The physical therapist can be of particular assistance following cancer treatment, says Gray. The therapy can help in rehabilitating people from the damage done by both the disease and the treatments.

Tools of the Trade

The treatments physical therapists use to relieve pain include customized exercise programs, traction, ultrasound, and applications of heat and cold.

"Nobody else in medicine does what we do," says Tim Meyer, a Brockton, Massachusetts, physical therapist. "We have our own area of treatment. One of the skills we have is a personal, hands-on approach where we apply something warm and we massage and we palpate and we touch. People just love that. It's very relaxing and settling."

"I think one simple definition of physical therapy and what physical therapists are for is helping the disabled— whatever type of disability—to facilitate and bring about restoration of the body's ability to function following a physical injury, illness, or surgery," says Gray.

Meet the Physical Therapist

By now you've probably got a picture in your mind of a typical physical therapist: *Bruno's muscles rise like ridges underneath his black T-shirt. His blond hair is closely cropped on top and looks soft as a sheepskin rug, but who'd dare touch it? As he stands before you, popping his knuckles and chewing gum, your mind wanders back to the Old Country, where Bruno learned the trade from his uncles, Sven and Thor . . .*

Whoa. Stop that mental tape.

In fact, you'd be more accurate if you changed Bruno a bit. According to the APTA, the average physical therapist is a woman under 34 years old with a bachelor's degree. She spends most of her time in direct patient care and usually sees patients after a doctor's referral, although she may work in private practice. She also takes continuing education classes to update her training. Think Betty instead of Bruno.

"Physical therapists have good evaluative skills, especially involving the musculoskeletal area," says Lynn Palmer, Ph.D., professor of physical therapy at Simmons College in Boston. "While a physician is responsible for medical and surgical management of patients, physical therapists are highly skilled at evaluating the muscles, bones, and joints. Unlike physical therapists, a physician uses additional tools, such as x-rays and blood tests, to evaluate patients, and may depend on surgery and drugs to deal with the patient's problems."

Many people these days opt for physical therapy as an alternative to surgery, says Dr. Palmer. "We are conservative and try to correct problems without the need for surgery," she says. "People would rather have conservative treatment than surgery, where they'll be laid up for six weeks or more."

You Don't Just Hang a Shingle

Betty begins to sound a lot less threatening, but that's hardly sufficient reason to trust your sore shoulder to her hands. Just where do physical therapists learn their skills?

A physical therapist, according to the APTA, is a graduate of an accredited college or university and has passed a licensing test. Physical therapists work in hospitals, nursing homes, home health agencies, public and private schools, and hospices, as well as in private practice.

It's not an easy profession to enter. Betty was selected from hundreds of applicants to go through rigorous academic training, including 18 to 32 weeks in a clinical setting.

"The minimum academic requirement is a bachelor of science degree in physical therapy," Dr. Palmer explains. Some physical therapists earn a post-baccalaureate degree in physical therapy if they already have a bachelor's degree in a related field. Many physical therapists also specialize and take additional courses at the master's and doctoral levels, says Dr. Palmer.

What's an Office Visit Like?

What can you expect from Betty before you hop up onto her examining table at the clinic for the first time? The typical physical therapist, according to the APTA, will talk with you about your problem and take your medical history. She may consult with your doctor or a specialist. Then she'll create a game plan for your therapy, establishing objectives and goals for treatment.

"We try to establish a reasonable program for each patient. We try to set it up for two to three times per week for about four weeks. Then we reassess what we're seeing," says Meyer. "Hopefully, at the end of that time, we'll see some improvement. And then we'll go on to the next step. If the patient shows no improvement in a four- to eight-week period and physical therapy isn't helping, then we refer to a specialist and direct the patient a different way, medically. If the patient is showing improvement, therapy continues."

Hands-On Help

Manual manipulation plays a large role in a typical session with a physical therapist. Here's where Betty's strong-looking forearms and fingers can seem foreboding. "She's not going to let her fingers walk up and down on *my* sore back," you may feel like shouting as you back toward the door. But wait a minute. This "hands-on" treatment can give you relief—sometimes the very same day. Manipulation loosens restrictions that lead to pain and stiffness, according to the APTA. You'll experience fuller movement with less pain if you let the therapist work on your aching body.

"A physical therapist's training can include high-velocity thrusting maneuvers," says Scott Hasson, Ed.D., associate professor and director of research at the School of Physical Therapy, Texas Women's University Medical Center, Houston. "But traditionally, the therapist performs gentle glides and oscillation with the joint."

Therapists also use massage to ease muscle spasms and provide relief of soft tissue, skeletal, and muscular pain, Dr. Hasson says.

"As a practicing therapist, I like to get the hands-on approach of feeling a tissue," says Dr. Hasson. "I have a good feel for how normal tissue should feel. If I touch the area where a person has pain, then the surrounding areas, often I can get a feel of whether there is an increase in muscle tone, since it's much harder compared to normal tissue. So therapists are very much into seeing with their hands."

What therapists want to see is your muscles—and you— moving freely and painlessly.

"My goal is to restore normal motion in the system. Then the joint works better, all the soft tissues attached to the joint move better, and all the muscles move better," Griffin says. "Generally, the more normally they move, the better they are. The bottom line is, you want to get the patients moving comfortably and freely, and let them go on about their business."

Mini-Manipulation

Mobilization is a fingertip technique similar to manipulation, but it's much gentler, Meyer says. For example, raise your arm: As your arm goes up, your shoulder joint moves down into the socket. When your muscles are stiff and tight, that motion doesn't take place, Meyer says. The physical therapist uses gentle movements to train the joint to move the way it should.

"Mobilization feels good because it's a movement pattern the body wants to feel," Meyer explains. "The skill of the therapist is to retrain that movement pattern that's been lost."

Thus, mobilization may be used to increase your range of motion, which can be impaired after illness, injury, or surgery, the APTA says. Therapists may assess your range of motion during your initial visit.

"We do a physical exam using our fingers, doing palpations, nerve and reflex testing, range of motion, and muscle strength," Meyer explains. "Then we go through movement testing. How is the patient able to move? Where are the restrictions in their movement? We observe the quality of movement. With a back patient, we'll ask them to bend forward, then side to side, then backward, and we see what happens. We're always assessing a person's response to the activity that we're putting them through. The specific exercise is dependent upon the patient's restrictions."

Although you may desire a high-tech treatment, the elbow-grease approach is special to a therapist. She or he's earned the ability to sense what is right and wrong with a body through hours and hours of hard work.

"The technology is helping us to develop a whole new way of looking at our patients objectively," Meyer says. "Yet we always go back to our skills of touch and feel and examination and range of motion and strength evaluation."

Exercise to Feel Good

You've heard of exercise to lose weight or stay in shape. Your physical therapist may give you a set of exercises that will give you an entirely new reason to get your body moving—pain relief.

"Exercise is the most effective way of getting blood flow to an area," Dr. Hasson says. "It's even better than hot packs or paraffin or other types of heat. Exercise can alleviate pain."

Even pains that are *caused* by exercising the wrong way can be treated with exercise, physical therapists say. For example, physical therapists often see people with tennis elbow, a form of tendinitis.

"We can approach pain relief for tendinitis from one of several ways. We can immobilize the person, give them anti-inflammatories, and eventually they'll get healthy again," explains Dr. Hasson. But the problem is that once they feel better, "they'll get out there and overdo again, and because they've been immobilized and the muscle tendon has gotten weaker, they end up causing this chronic problem again rather rapidly."

The better solution, according to Dr. Hasson, is using what he calls gentle movements. "If the tennis player, for example, is exercising their arm or doing active motion—without holding a racquet—and that's not causing pain, that's good. With gentle movements the tissues are still allowed to keep their flexibility. And you're going to increase the amount of blood flow to the area and that's going to promote healing," Dr. Hasson explains. "Then, when you get them back to the actual activity, you need a commonsense approach to building it up. So they go out after a couple of weeks and play some tennis, but only 20 percent of the time they used to play. Then after a six-week period, they can be back to 100 percent."

Exercise is often the physical therapist's chief weapon against pain. "My goal as a therapist is not to have the individual dependent upon me to do something passively to them," says Dr. Hasson. "My goal is that they are independent. So a lot of my therapy is teaching them techniques to exercise, as well as educating them about why I'm doing things. I spend a lot of time as I'm working with them, teaching them about what is going on so they become a much greater part of the therapeutic intervention. Because when it comes down to it, with physical therapy, it's the patient's compliance that is the critical thing."

A physical therapist will give you stretching and

strengthening exercises designed to treat your specific problem. She or he may also have you work with weight machines or other exercise equipment to increase muscle strength and improve coordination, endurance, and circulation.

You don't have to be afraid that you'll be asked to start right in with exercise, however. Physical therapists usually begin treatment with something soothing like heat, says Meyer. This helps to prepare the muscle tissues for exercise. They also change the exercises throughout the healing process.

"As the injury resolves itself, physical therapists begin stretching you to improve muscle and joint flexibility," says Meyer. "When appropriate, you will begin what is known as progressive resistance exercise—using resistance or weights in a specific movement pattern for strengthening.

"You start testing the muscle to see if it can take a little extra loading," says Meyer. "And if it can, then you can progress to the next level."

"This level may involve isokinetics," says Meyer. This is a high-tech means of exercising the muscles. It relies upon the speed of muscle contraction rather than resistance to the weights. "I think isokinetics is a safer way to exercise because there is less tendency to overload and reinjure. All the patient has to do is slow the exercise unit down, and the patient receives less resistance from the unit," says Meyer.

A good physical therapist will give you something else to take home besides a bill (usually about $50 per hour) tucked under your sweaty arm.

"A physical therapist will generally provide you with a home exercise program," Meyer says. "That's really important. We want to give patients a program that's going to help them take care of themselves at home."

Modalities to Maul Pain

If you're a chronic pain patient, you may also experience any number of pain-relief treatments known as "modalities" at the hands of your physical therapist.

Therapists use traction, ultrasound (sound waves), diathermy (electrical heat), electrotherapy, cryotherapy (cold), and hydrotherapy (water). (See chapter 21 for more information on hot and cold therapy and hydrotherapy and chapter 32 for more on electrical stimulation.)

"We use traction, either cervical traction for neck injuries or pelvic traction for low back problems," Griffin says.

Traction involves pulling to lift the natural weight of one part of your body (your head, for example) from another part (your shoulders). Traction, which can be done either mechanically or by hand, is gentle and should not hurt, says Meyer. Traction equipment is programmed to pull at varying weights and times. The machine may pull for 15 seconds, then rest for 5 seconds. Or it may pull to a certain level and hold for 15 to 20 minutes. When traction is done by hand, your therapist relies on touch to move joints to get the same pulling effect.

Making Waves

Ultrasound uses high-frequency sound waves to heat the deep tissues in your muscles. The only sensation you're likely to feel during a 5- to 10-minute session will be the comforting touch of the therapist as she or he smoothes a gel on the area to be treated with a metal sound head applicator. The sound head applicator is a round disk attached to what looks like a telephone receiver. The therapist directs the ultrasound waves through your skin, causing the muscles beneath to heat up by about 5 degrees. This increases blood flow, relaxing your muscles and getting rid of inflammation, Meyer explains.

Ultrasound can be continuous—a constant bombardment of ultrasound waves to the muscle. A pulsating mode can also be used, involving extremely small interruptions in the waves.

Your therapist might choose pulsating ultrasound if you have problems with a bony area—such as your jaw, knee, or shoulder—where there's not much soft tissue to absorb the ultrasound waves, Meyer says. Pulsed ultrasound also can be more gentle to sensitive tissues.

Mixing and Matching

Therapists may use different modalities or a combination of modalities to treat various problems. Although treatment programs vary, the result is the same—getting you back to normal.

"Everybody is different," Griffin says, adding that he doesn't have a "cookbook approach" to modalities. "Some people may have been to physical therapy before. If they tell me somebody put a TENS (transcutaneous electrical nerve stimulation) unit on them for three months and tried every combination of settings in the world and it didn't work, I'm not going to make them put a TENS unit on for three more months. If three months of hot packs, ultrasound, and massage didn't work, six months isn't going to work either. I will try to do something they haven't had before."

Time Is in Your Hands

Physical therapists have so many things they can do for and with you, it's natural to wonder how long it's going to take before you experience some relief. How long should it take?

You can count on spending anywhere from 30 minutes to many hours working on your treatment program. The initial visit and exam will take an hour or so, Meyer says. You can work out two or three times per week under your therapist's supervision, or more if she or he believes it is appropriate. You may also work on appropriate exercises at home.

"People come to our clinic with standing appointments. Most are treated for at least 1 hour each time they're in," Meyer says. "Once a treatment program is established, they come in on a regular basis for hot packs, ultrasound, stimulation, and other modalities. Then, every patient receives some type of physical activity program or physical prescription of exercise."

Meyer says he treats acute pain problems for up to two months. Then he refers a patient to another physical therapist or to a specialist if the problem is not resolved. Chronic pain patients may be in for a longer haul.

"We see lots and lots of people who've been to three, four, five, six, ten other doctors," says Griffin of his work at the Pain Management Clinic. "Our goal is to treat them as efficaciously as possible. Sadly, we see many people who've had problems for years. And if we can't help them 100 percent, we can at least make them feel better and make them less dependent on doctors and the health-care system—teach them how to manage their pain, be active and independent."

Some Tales of Relief

When physical therapy works, results can be swift and dramatic. While Griffin sees people who've gone around the medical track and back with their pain problems, he sometimes sees spectacular results.

A Kansas City woman came to the clinic one day, walking on a sore knee. She had injured her back lifting a box out of the trunk of her car three years before. A visit to the chiropractor fixed her back, but soon after, she developed knee pain. She then went to an orthopedic surgeon. "They took lots of pictures of her, but nobody put their hands on her," says Griffin. Using sensitive touch techniques developed through years of training, the physical therapist discovered a tiny strain in the hamstring muscle behind her knee. He stretched out her hamstring, and in three days, the three-year knee pain was gone.

In another case, Griffin tells of a woman who was injured in a fall and had pain in the groin area and down the inside of her leg for nine years. "She'd been everywhere, and nobody knew what to do with her. In fact, OB/GYN sent her to us. She had a pretty simple musculoskeletal problem that I worked on. We had her stretch the muscle on the inside of her leg. We didn't get rid of all of her pain, but she was 90 percent better. She had been seeking relief for nine years."

The point? Physical therapists are trained to observe the way you move and to feel the way your muscles and bones move. According to Griffin, part of their job is not overlooking the obvious things others miss.

Let Your Fingers Walk

Finding a physical therapist can be tricky. In 24 states, you may walk into a physical therapist's office for treatment without a physician's referral. These "direct access" states are: Alaska, Arizona, California, Colorado, Idaho, Illinois, Iowa, Kentucky, Maryland, Massachusetts, Minnesota, Montana, Nebraska, Nevada, New Hampshire, New Mexico, North Carolina, North Dakota, South Dakota, Utah, Vermont, Washington, West Virginia, and Wisconsin.

In these states, you can locate a physical therapist on your own by looking in the telephone book, asking your doctor, or calling your local hospital.

In the remaining 26 states, a physician must refer you to a physical therapist for treatment.

Physical therapy costs are covered by most insurance companies as part of a major medical plan, says the APTA. The amount covered depends on your plan, so call your insurance company if you have any questions.

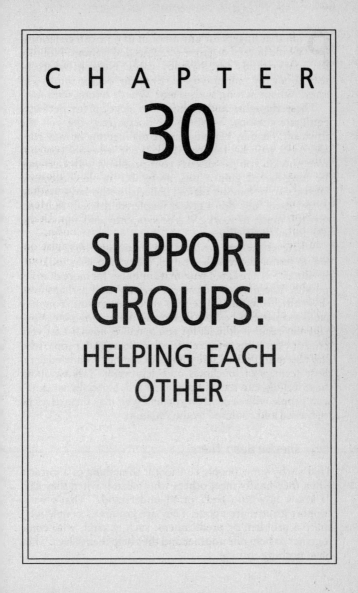

CHAPTER
30

SUPPORT GROUPS:
HELPING EACH OTHER

P ain that lingers for any amount of time can generate a whole host of negative thoughts and feelings: Nobody understands me. Nobody cares. Nobody wants to hear about my pain anymore. Even my doctor thinks I'm crazy. What's wrong with them? What's wrong with *me*?

These thoughts and feelings can develop for perfectly legitimate reasons. Maybe your doctor *is* giving you the brush-off. He may believe you are malingering or may consider your pain his failure. Maybe your wife told you that from now on you can discuss your problems with Gertrude the long-haired guinea pig, preferably in the basement. Maybe you're fending off bill collectors who have made it crystal clear they don't give a (expletive deleted) that you hurt too much to work. Maybe sympathy and support really *are* in short supply.

Whatever the case, experts say it's possible that you can end up feeling depressed—fearful, angry, hopeless, and terribly alone—as a result of pain that continues for more than six months. You may withdraw emotionally, and perhaps even physically, from the people who are closest to you. You may avoid social events because they're just not fun anymore. Your pain may make it difficult for you to dance, bowl, sit for very long, or even focus on a conversation. Being with people who don't seem to understand your pain can put a knife-edge on those feelings of loneliness and depression. Talking about those feelings can seem impossibly hard, especially when it's with people who depend on you and who may themselves be frightened and confused by the situation.

They've Been There

That's why some people consider it something of a miracle when they finally meet others who mean it when they say, "I know how you feel" or "I understand." That's what support groups are about. They are groups of people who share a problem or predicament, such as pain, who come together to help one another and thus help themselves. They have nothing to hide.

Two different kinds of gatherings may be called support groups.

Professional Leadership

Some support groups are actually therapy or counseling sessions, although they offer support as well. Led by a psychologist, a social worker, or a nurse, such groups are offered mostly through pain clinics or rehabilitation hospitals to patients going through a pain treatment program. These groups may be run like a four- to eight-week course, with group discussions on a new subject at each meeting. Discussions may revolve around such topics as recognizing and expressing your feelings, your pain's impact on your family, or receiving and giving help. The therapist's role is to guide the conversation in a way that hopefully provides everyone in the group with some insight into their own situation and behavior.

Occasionally, the therapist himself or herself has chronic pain and may run the group as more of a self-help group, as you'll see below. Laura Hitchcock, Ph.D., executive director of the National Chronic Pain Outreach Association in Bethesda, Maryland, is one such therapist. "There are not very many of us," she says. "And fewer will state it publicly, because chronic pain is so stigmatized."

Self-Help Gathering

Other support groups are led by the same people who are its members. Known as self-help or mutual-help groups, they depend on the relationships that develop and the exchange of information that occurs among members as their main means of providing help. Some meet weekly or monthly in a church or home; some are correspondence or phone networks of people confined to their home. Some even offer computer hookups.

What are these groups like? How do they help people deal with their pain?

"Our goal is to help people determine what they need to do in order to regain control of their lives," explains

Penney Cowan, founder and executive director of the American Chronic Pain Association. With some 13,000 members and almost 450 chapters nationwide (in every state but Nevada), her organization is the largest network for chronic pain support groups.

How Groups Help

"We don't promise to take anyone's pain away," Cowan adds. "We don't offer any medical advice or treatments. We do offer coping skills, which can help people become more involved in their recovery and, hopefully, reduce their pain. What's most important is that we are trying to help people get out of their patient role and become people again, by example and by helping them improve the quality of their lives."

Karen Moss, who along with her husband founded the Chronic Pain Support Group (with more than 2,000 participants and support groups in Ohio and California), voices similar goals.

"We encourage you to find ways to do all the things you want to do, perhaps on a limited basis," Moss says. "Many people who suffer from chronic pain have the tendency to lose their self-identity and become very passive. Their pain limits them. They can recall that at one point in their lives they stood up for themselves, but now the pain has become so bad they have given in to it.

"I recently talked with a man who said when he and his wife traveled they used to like walking around. He had stopped walking because of back problems. I asked him how long he could walk now. He said about 15 minutes at a time. I encouraged him to walk for that amount of time. It's true that he won't see as much as he would if he could walk longer, but he will have seen something. He will have gotten out. He won't have given in to the pain."

Lending a Shoulder

Even though local groups sometimes struggle to stay in existence, the support often goes beyond the emotional to whatever it takes to keep a person afloat.

"One friend has offered to come over and hold me, in my pain, even if it's three o'clock in the morning," says Gloria Bellanca, a member of a chronic pain group that meets every week in Harrisburg, Pennsylvania. Living alone and on crutches, faced with daily pain from an incurable bone disease, it makes all the difference in the world to her to know she can call for such all-out support. Her friend, Dennis Town, the group's oldest member, has faced many painful, sleepless nights himself and admits he's as likely as not to be up at that hour. "I offer that kind of support to anyone who asks for it," he says. As someone who once contemplated suicide because of unrelenting pain, he takes every request for help seriously.

Lending a Hand

"I've organized food drives for people in my group who could pay for either rent or the groceries, but not both," says Gloria Bryan, a leader of groups sponsored by the Southern Maryland Chronic Pain Outreach Association. "We have people in our groups who have lost everything as a result of their pain."

She, like Dennis Town, has more than once offered the ultimate support: helping someone in pain make the choice to continue living. "Oh, yes, I've met people who have said they would rather be dead than to live the life they were living. We try to give them a little bit of hope."

She knows all too well what it's like to stay home all day long, with the curtains closed. The 36-year-old former auto mechanic did just that herself for a full year after a bad back injury. "That's the kind of person I try to reach my hand out to now and grab," she says.

Information Exchange

Mutual-help groups also provide a way for people to share with others what they have learned about their pain or illness, to pass along information about medical treatments, lifestyle changes, or other things that have worked for them. The thinking is: The more you know, the less likely you are to overlook important options in your medical treatment.

And ultimately, it may be easier to accept the pain you continue to have if you believe you truly have explored all possible options and are doing everything you can to relieve your pain.

"If you find someone with the same sort of problem you have, as you often do, you can compare notes on what you've tried and haven't tried, and that can be really useful," Dr. Hitchcock says. People often exchange the names of helpful doctors and clinics and discuss the pros and cons of medications and treatments.

Consumer savvy is sometimes promoted in reaction to what is perceived as haphazard medical care for chronic pain patients.

"One of our goals is helping people to obtain better medical treatment," Moss says. "A lot of people with chronic pain have been going to the same doctor year after year with no help. That doctor may not know about new treatments. He may not want to try anything different. He may not even believe your pain is real. We tell people they have the right to go shopping for a doctor to find the treatment that is going to suit them."

Many newcomers to a group learn for the first time that there are national pain-management clinics that deal with specific types of pain or offer a certain kind of treatment. "Many people, once they are directed into the hands of the proper pain-management unit, do get some relief from their pain," Moss contends.

No Pity Parties, Please

One thing support groups work to avoid is swapping horror stories.

"It's not that misery loves company, but when you find out you are not the only one suffering from pain, you can say, 'Okay, my pain is real—now how do I get on with my life from here?' " says Moss. "You can present a problem and discuss with others how to solve it, but we won't allow you to complain about it."

Talking about their pain per se may be what the people

in a group feel they need, but in the long run it is not at all helpful, Dr. Hitchcock agrees. Her association's suggested guidelines state that except for a brief statement of the cause of your pain, it is not a good idea to talk about your particular kind of pain. But you *are* encouraged to convey information that could be helpful to the whole group. "You might talk about how being in pain makes it difficult for you to get along with your family and what you could do about that," Dr. Hitchcock explains.

Giving to Get

Is a support group for you? Both professional and volunteer group leaders agree on this: You get something out of a support group only if you're willing, and able, to put something into it. That something doesn't necessarily have to be spilling your guts, editing a newsletter, or organizing a fund-raiser, Dr. Hitchcock explains. It may simply mean that you invest your emotional energy into being there with the intention of learning how to cope better.

"We've had people come to support groups who sit back and the attitude is, 'Okay, save me now. Do something for me,'" Dr. Hitchcock says. "Those people will never get any help from the support group, because they want someone else to take care of them. On the other hand, we've had people who hardly say anything but who still get an awful lot out of it."

If, for whatever reason, you can't or won't put anything into the group, you may need professional help, Dr. Hitchcock says. "Support groups are not a good place for people who are seriously depressed or seriously angry. It's one thing to have trouble coping and to be depressed, but if you are so depressed that you can barely get out of bed to get to the support group, you ought to go see a mental health professional."

If, on the other hand, you know you just need support, a group could be ideal. Why pay a psychologist $70 an hour to hold your hand? You can get it held for free at a support group. (Actually, it's in exchange for one of your own body parts—an attentive ear, perhaps, or a steady shoulder.)

"These groups aren't a substitute for competent medical care, or psychological counseling, if that's what is needed, but they can substitute for private psychological care if the person just needs support," Dr. Hitchcock says.

SELF-HELP RESOURCES GUIDE

At least three national groups deal with chronic pain. Such groups may sponsor support groups and provide startup materials and information. They are listed below.

Other support groups deal with specific painful conditions such as carpal tunnel syndrome and temporomandibular disorder (TMD, sometimes referred to as TMJ). For information about these groups, you may want to contact The American Self-Help Clearinghouse, St. Clares—Riverside Medical Center, Denville, NJ 07834, (201) 625-7101. Or look at your local library for a copy of their book, *The Self-Help Sourcebook*, 3d edition, which includes contacts for over 600 national and model self-help groups, contacts for local self-help clearinghouses, national toll-free numbers, and ideas and resources for starting a group.

The national groups are:

The American Chronic Pain Association
P.O. Box 850
Rocklin, CA 95677
(916) 632-0922

Penney Cowan is the executive director. With at least 13,000 members and almost 450 chapters (in every state except Nevada), this is currently the largest sponsor of chronic pain support groups in the United States. It offers referrals to support groups near you, a workbook for self-help recovery, a quarterly newsletter, group development guidelines, a phone network, and an outreach program to clinics. There are no dues, but you are asked to pay for the workbook.

The Chronic Pain Support Group
P.O. Box 148
Peninsula, OH 44264
(216) 657-2948

Karen Moss is the director. The group has 2,000 participants and six affiliated groups in Ohio and California. It holds monthly meetings and seminars and publishes a newsletter. Assistance is available for starting groups. There are no dues, but a donation is requested to receive the newsletter.

National Chronic Pain Outreach Association
7979 Old Georgetown Road
Suite 100
Bethesda, MD 20814
(301) 652-4948

Laura Hitchcock, Ph.D., is the executive director. An information clearinghouse for chronic pain, the association may refer you to other organizations that can help more specifically. It provides startup information to support groups and can put you in touch with the nearest existing group.

Finding the Right Group

Do shop around, Dr. Hitchcock suggests. Every support group is different. Some may be mostly made up of professional people; others may be blue-collar workers. Some follow an established program; others are informal. Some are well run, others are not. "A lot depends on the group's leader," Dr. Hitchcock says.

A mutual-help group may have sponsorship and professional guidance from a national office, which provides it with a startup manual, workbooks, and leader training. Some have strict rules about professional involvement. The American Chronic Pain Association, for instance, discourages groups from meeting in a medical building or doctor's or psychologist's office, and it does not allow doctors or psychologists to attend meetings, except as guest speakers.

There is a high dropout rate among newcomers, Dr.

Hitchcock notes. They may realize they are functioning too poorly themselves to benefit from a group. Or they may become depressed because many of the people they meet are worse off than they are.

"I'd suggest going to a few meetings before writing a group off," Dr. Hitchcock suggests. "You should find one that you feel comfortable in, and where you feel you are getting support."

Ultimately, you may have to make a decision based on gut instincts, she says. "If you go three times and each time you feel worse after it's over, I wouldn't recommend going back. You may need professional help, or you may want to try a different kind of group." Within six to ten meetings, you should feel as if you're really benefiting from being part of the group.

CHAPTER
31

SURGERY:
BEFORE, DURING,
AND AFTER

I n 1841, Swiss surgeon Emil Theodor Kocher took a knife and carefully slit a patient's throat. Then he removed the man's thyroid gland. Afterward, the skillful surgeon sewed his patient's throat back up and bandaged it. Dr. Kocher's surgery represented an innovative cure for goiter that would be noted in medical history books.

But was the patient grateful?

Probably not—at least not that day.

The good doctor didn't use anesthesia—which blocks pain messages from reaching the brain—because 150 years ago there was no such thing as anesthesia.

Fortunately, we've come a long way since those hold-'em-down days. Today, if you're faced with surgery, there are a number of things that you can do—before, during, and after—to assure a minimum of pain and discomfort.

Ask the Right Questions

Ideally, pain relief should begin long before you're wheeled into the operating room—and it should begin in your mind. Studies show the better prepared you are *psychologically* before surgery, the less pain you will have afterward.

What we're talking about is *stress*—worry, anxiety, fear, the very thought of being invaded by a knife. Feeling emotionally comfortable before your surgery may actually help you feel physically comfortable during your recovery. One study at Notre Dame University showed that surgical patients recover an average of three and a half days faster when they are taught to deal with the mental stress their operations generate. De-stressed people have less pain and require less pain medication. Antistress techniques include deep breathing, muscle relaxation, and thinking soothing thoughts. (See chapter 22 for more on these techniques.)

So ask your surgeon and, if possible, your anesthesiologist to tell you exactly what is going to happen during your operation. Get details about the kind of pain relief you'll receive during surgery. Find out exactly what will be done to ease your discomfort afterward. Ask questions that will give you the whole picture: When will pain relief begin?

Will you be on a medication schedule or will you have to ring for a nurse when you feel pain? What happens if you feel pain and it isn't time for more medication? How many days will the pain last?

Knowing how you will be treated gives you a feeling of control. That feeling is a powerful tool, doctors say. Not knowing what is going to happen can cause tension that stays with you through surgery and increases your pain afterward.

"The more anxiety, the more anticipation, the more exaggerated the pain," says anesthesiologist Jeffrey Ngeow, M.D., director of the pain management program at The Hospital of Special Surgery in New York City. "The more relaxed you are, the easier it is for you to deal with it."

"The doctor needs to say, 'This is a painful procedure and this is what we will be doing for the pain,' " says David Rosen, M.D., assistant professor of anesthesiology at the University of Michigan Medical Center in Ann Arbor.

The Power of Anesthesia

Today, thank goodness, you can take for granted that when you have surgery, you'll get some type of anesthesia. The three types usually given are local, regional, or general. The drug will be administered by a specialist, a medical doctor called an anesthesiologist. Or you may be treated by a specially trained nurse, an anesthetist.

X Marks the Spot

You get local anesthesia when you go to the dentist to have a cavity filled. It also can be used for minor operations—repairing an ingrown toenail, for instance.

Local anesthesia is injected directly into the area around the surgical site, where it numbs the nerves and blocks the pain right where it occurs. It may be given by the doctor performing the operation instead of by an anesthesiologist. Local anesthesia can last as little as 30 minutes or as long as 6 hours.

Wider Coverage

Regional anesthesia has been used for many years to relieve the pain of childbirth.

For regional anesthesia, a medication is injected into a *group* of nerves, which numbs larger portions of the body. For instance, a "saddle-block," given in the spine, numbs only the area that would touch a saddle while horseback riding.

For spinal anesthesia, medication is injected into the spinal fluid to block nerve impulses. You won't be able to feel any pain being relayed into the spinal area that receives the injection.

An epidural, another kind of regional pain-relieving injection, places medication outside the spinal canal, where it numbs nerves that fan out after they leave the spine.

When you have regional anesthesia, you are awake throughout the operation. If the procedure makes you tense or apprehensive, you can ask your doctor to give you a type of sedation that will help you relax, says Michael Gold, M.D., assistant professor of anesthesiology at Tulane University Medical Center in New Orleans.

It takes from 3 to 20 minutes before regional anesthesia begins working. First you'll feel warmth in the area affected. Then you'll feel numbness and, finally, a loss of sensation and movement in the area.

Regional anesthesia gradually wears off in 20 minutes to 2 hours, although your doctor can use an epidural or other technique to prolong pain relief for as long as necessary.

Total Blackout

You aren't "just asleep" when you get general anesthesia. If you were really asleep, then doctors could simply walk into your hospital room at night to operate.

Instead, an anesthesiologist gives you intravenous medication (or helps you breathe a gas) that puts you into a "controlled coma," which stops your brain from receiving pain signals, says Dr. Gold.

General anesthesia does *not* stop the pain of surgery, says Dr. Gold. The anesthetic does contain chemicals that prevent you from remembering the pain. The anesthesiologist, who carefully monitors the body's vital signs throughout the operation, may see changes in your breathing, heart rate, and blood pressure during surgery that signal your body is feeling discomfort. When you awaken, however, you usually won't be able to recall what happened, says Dr. Gold.

"Most of the general anesthetics given in the United States today involve a potent inhalational agent," he says. "Those drugs seem to have the ability to scramble your brain's signals to the point where it isn't aware of the pain." That's why you never open your eyes and say that it hurts. After the surgery, you don't remember it hurting.

"When the anesthesia is over, that brain scrambling is undone. It's a funny concept. The bottom line is you don't remember it later," says Dr. Gold.

You may become conscious again almost immediately after surgery or, instead, perhaps doze 18 hours more. Individual reaction to anesthesia can vary greatly.

Make the Choice

Your surgeon will probably choose your anesthesiologist, but you may have the choice between general anesthesia and regional anesthesia, says Dr. Gold. Your choice, of course, depends on the type of operation you have. You'll *want* general anesthesia for open-heart surgery. Your doctor usually will insist on general anesthesia for any surgery of the head, neck, spine, or chest. However, you may have the choice of anesthesia used for most surgery in the lower half of the body.

So which should you choose?

Studies show that no type of anesthesia is really safer than others, says Dr. Ngeow. "There is no great difference between general and regional now, because general has become so safe," he says.

However, when doctors are asked what *their* choice would be if they were having surgery, they usually say, "Make mine a regional anesthetic," notes Dr. Gold.

There's good reason, it seems. With regional, you automatically get pain relief. With general, you don't—pain relief may not begin until sometime after you're in the recovery room. Regional anesthesia offers continuous pain relief that begins before surgery and extends through the recovery room period, says Dr. Ngeow.

"If you talk about patient comfort and acceptance, regional is preferable," he says. "Patients really like it. They have no pain until the anesthetic wears off, and that's a gradual thing. They are wide awake and alert and can ask for medication before the pain becomes overwhelming."

Having general anesthesia is no guarantee that you will feel no pain after surgery. One of the things anesthesiologists like about general anesthesia is that the pain helps wake you up, says Dr. Rosen. "When your brain is no longer scrambled by the general anesthetic, you'll hurt, and that will wake you up," he says. "If you don't hurt, the doctor has to wait for you to wake up on your own. General anesthesia, where the patient wakes up quickly, offers a very fast turnover. It's a matter of ease."

"We hear moaning and crying in the recovery room because there's a period of feeling pain and not being able to vocalize it," Dr. Ngeow says. "When you're just waking up, you don't know where the pain is coming from or why. And when the nurse gives you a shot of morphine or Demerol, these medications can cause nausea. So you go through the sensation of not knowing where you are, then pain, and then nausea."

However, if you must have general anesthesia, you don't have to awaken in pain, says Dr. Rosen. He often gives his patients pain-relief medication while they are still under general anesthesia.

"This is not universally done. Most people don't get pain medication until the recovery room. But you're already behind in pain relief if you wait that long," he says. "I do what I can to make sure there is some pain relief. It's part of the anesthetic plan."

You can ask your doctor to give you pain-relief medication *before* you wake up, he says.

How Far Out?

Before you enter the operating room, you'll want to know the answer to a couple of the more frequently asked questions: How 'out' are you *really* under anesthesia? What are the chances of feeling pain?

You're out. Way, way out, says Dr. Gold. The anesthesiologist can tell if you are starting to "wake up" from general anesthesia and will give you additional medication to lull you back into unconsciousness.

If you are under regional anesthesia and start to feel something during the operation—a very rare occurrence, Dr. Gold says—the word "ouch" is appropriate. Your surgery will stop immediately and one of the doctors will add more anesthesia or give you local anesthesia directly in the area being operated on. If nothing else works, the anesthesiologist can give you general anesthesia for the remainder of the surgery.

"This happens, but not very often," Dr. Gold stresses.

Some Precautions

Your doctor will have some questions for you, too, to assure your safety during anesthesia. If your doctor doesn't ask these questions, be sure to volunteer the information.

The anesthesiologist needs to know about any previous experience you've had with anesthesia—whether you had a reaction or problem. If someone in your family—parents, siblings, children—has had problems with anesthesia, be sure to mention it. Sometimes reactions to anesthesia are inherited.

Also, your doctor needs to know whether you smoke and whether you take any drugs—over-the-counter, prescription, or illegal. But don't quit taking regular medications unless you are told to do so. Chronic illnesses such as high blood pressure and diabetes must be kept under control.

Beyond Anesthesia

Anesthesia is not the only thing that can help with pain relief during surgery.

Some doctors talk to their patients during surgery. Fred Schwartz, M.D., for example, sits at the head of the operating table at Piedmont Hospital in Atlanta and whispers sweet words of pain-relieving encouragement into the ears of some of his patients.

"Surgery is going well," he might say. "You'll recover from this very quickly. You'll feel well rested, energetic. You'll be very comfortable when you wake up."

Dr. Schwartz is an anesthesiologist, and his patients are asleep under general anesthesia when they hear this message. While they won't remember his exact words after the operation, Dr. Schwartz maintains that their body remembers the message and they feel better than those people who hear only the usual sounds in an operating room.

He has been using this positive suggestion method as an adjunct to traditional anesthesia since about 1988. He read in the British medical journal *Lancet* about an experiment using positive suggestions during surgery. Women, unconscious under anesthesia, wore headphones during surgery. They heard positive messages, like Dr. Schwartz's, or they heard only a blank tape. Those who heard the positive messages recovered faster and requested less pain medication than those who heard nothing, says Dr. Schwartz.

If we're "out, way out" under anesthesia, how do these messages get through?

Evidence shows that "the central nervous system is active even under anesthetic and that it responds to the stress of surgery," says psychologist Henry Bennett, Ph.D., of the University of California, Davis, Medical Center. And while part of you is aware of what is happening during surgery—

an idea that might be unnerving to you—that same awareness also can serve you, says Dr. Bennett. Even though you are unconscious, you can still hear and respond to positive instructions your doctor might whisper, he says.

Dr. Bennett, too, has tested the suggestibility of people under general anesthesia during surgery and discovered that learning *can* go on while people are anesthetized.

His study looked at people undergoing abdominal surgery, who ordinarily would have been uncomfortable for days afterward, until their digestive tract began working again. Before and during surgery he told them, "Your stomach and intestines will start moving and churning and gurgling soon after your operation." The people studied began experiencing intestinal movement 40 percent sooner than those who had no preoperative instruction, he says.

If you are interested in hearing positive messages, though, you'll have to ask for them.

"Most doctors have their own routine that they don't vary that much," Dr. Schwartz says. "If people ask for it enough, we may begin to see it used more routinely."

The Pillow Trick and Other Painkillers

Once back in your room after surgery, there are tricks you can use to feel more comfortable.

For instance, there seem to be hundreds of ways to use pillows to support your body and relieve pain. Holding a pillow against your chest and abdomen when you cough helps reduce pain wherever you have stitches, says Dr. Ngeow.

If your surgery was in your abdomen and those sore muscles are sagging, tuck one pillow in front and another behind you to support yourself while lying on your side. If you want to keep your legs straight, put a pillow between your knees. Experiment a little, tucking your pillows in and around your body until you find something that feels good.

Another tip: You may be especially thirsty after surgery and look forward to that first glass of water. Sip the water straight from the glass; don't be tempted to use a straw.

Using a straw pulls in air with the water, and that extra air can cause gas pains.

Also, when you stand after surgery, be sure to support yourself with both hands as you climb out of bed, says Dr. Ngeow. To make the job easier, sit up first. Swing your legs to the side and over the edge of the bed, as if you were sitting in a chair. Lean forward and slide to your feet. Push the rest of the way up with your hands.

For other easy pain-relief tricks after surgery, ask your nurse, who has undoubtedly seen lots of people come and go and has discovered the best pain-relief tricks for your particular kind of surgery.

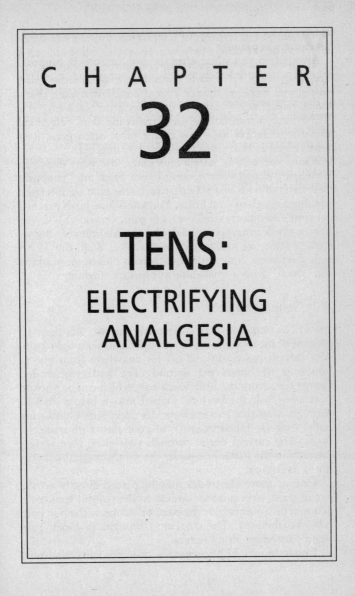

C H A P T E R
32

TENS:
ELECTRIFYING
ANALGESIA

Your physical therapist has just told you she has something she thinks may help your pain. She holds up a little black box with dials and buttons, about the size and shape of a TV remote control unit. What's she going to do, you wonder, change your channel? In a way, that's exactly what she's going to do. That little black box is a TENS unit, a transcutaneous ("across the skin") electrical nerve stimulation unit, one of the most often prescribed pain remedies that's not swallowed or injected.

Once the unit is wired into place, the pain messages traveling through your nerves to your brain are "jammed" —interfered with in a way that keeps the pain signals from getting through to your brain. You know how birds perched on your antenna create showers of static on your TV screen that make Vanna White look like the Abominable Snowman? (Yeah, we know, you have cable.) Well, the TENS unit does something similar with pain messages, masking the "ouch" with a mild, almost pleasant tingling.

Stimulating Relief

All TENS units use a tiny electrical current, less than 10 percent of the amount it takes to light a 60-watt light bulb. The current pulses on and off for anywhere from one to hundreds of bursts per second. The battery-generated charge runs from the little black box, which can be hooked over your belt (or bra) or slipped into a breast pocket, through wires that end in electrodes (electricity-conducting pads) that are taped or stuck to your skin with a special paste. The current enters through your skin, then travels laterally in the tissue just under the skin, stimulating nerve fibers as it goes.

One or more electrodes may be placed directly on the site of pain, over a nerve leading to the painful spot, over acupuncture points near the pain, or wherever the best pain relief is obtained. The current is thought to block pain signals traveling along nerves.

Conventional TENS generally provides pain relief only

while it's being used and for a short time afterward. (One physical therapist uses what he calls the two-for-one rule. "If I use TENS on a patient for half an hour, I want to see at least an additional hour's worth of relief," he says.) For some patients, though, it provides much longer relief. Conventional TENS produces a "pins and needles" sensation, but it's set low enough to avoid the muscle contractions that result from a stronger electric current.

Longer-Lasting Relief

Another form of stimulation, called "acupuncture-like" TENS, is thought to stimulate the release of pain-killing endorphins in the brain. Its pulsing current is strong and slow compared to conventional TENS, and in addition to tingling, it produces visible muscle twitching. It reportedly provides pain relief for many hours after the stimulation is stopped.

Most TENS units these days can be set to provide either conventional or acupuncture-like stimulation, although they can't do both at the same time.

Despite hundreds of studies on the use of TENS, few studies compare one type (or modality) of TENS stimulation with another. "There's no agreement on whether a particular kind of stimulation works best, or whether particular types of electrical stimulation should be selected to treat certain kinds of pain," says Michael Nolan, Ph.D., a physical therapist and associate professor of anatomy and neurology at the University of South Florida in Tampa. Some physical therapists use conventional TENS for acute pain and acupuncture-like TENS for chronic pain, he notes. Others try conventional TENS first, then switch to other modalities if conventional TENS fails to relieve the pain.

"It really comes down to trial and error," says Joseph Kahn, Ph.D., a physical therapist and professor of physical therapy at the State University of New York at Stony Brook. "A physical therapist selects a starting point based on the characteristics of the patient's pain, the therapist's own experience, even the kind of equipment that's available."

Black Box Appeal

TENS units have proved popular because they are relatively easy to use—people are more likely to use one than they are to follow an exercise program, for instance. Doctors say they involve little risk to the user—certainly less risk than most pain-killing medications. There is a variety of TENS units available in a wide range of price and quality. Consult your doctor or therapist about the kind of unit that may be appropriate for your condition. Although some are not cheap, they are cheaper than, say, back surgery or a month-long stay at a chronic pain clinic. And studies say they do work . . . at least sometimes . . . for some people . . . for some types of pain. Their ability to ease pain after surgery or during dental procedures is fairly well accepted.

Catalogs full of TENS units attest to this treatment's popularity. Manufacturers apparently try to find a "market niche" for their line of units. One is advertised as being designed just for menstrual cramps; another's big dials make adjusting the controls easier for people with arthritis; yet another is supposedly perfect for people who haven't gotten pain relief from previous TENS treatment.

Despite the plethora of products and manufacturers' claims, all TENS units are pretty much the same and work about equally well, Dr. Kahn contends. "One's a Cadillac, another's a Chevrolet. They'll both get you to Chicago," he says.

Off to a Great Start

TENS has been tried for just about every imaginable type of pain: nerve injuries in the hands, feet, arms, or legs; shingles (a painful viral infection of nerves); wound pain; face, mouth, and tooth pain; diabetic nerve damage; itching; cancer pain; phantom limb pain; labor pain; post-operative pain; phlebitis; rheumatoid arthritis; pancreatitis; chest pain; headaches; multiple sclerosis; low back pain; neck pain; and bursitis, among others.

Just how well does TENS work for any of these conditions? One study done at the University of Colorado Medical Center found that at least half of people in pain had an initial good response to TENS. They experienced a reduction of 50 percent or more in their pain, although they may have tried several different types of TENS before they hit on one that worked for them.

But studies also show that the initial good response drops off dramatically during the first year of use, so that by the end of that time, only about 30 percent are still having good results. In a process called accommodation, the nervous system begins to ignore the therapeutic electrical stimulation and allows the pain message to break through. It takes stronger and stronger stimulation, or a change in the electrical stimulation pattern, to achieve continued pain relief.

Few studies follow TENS patients beyond their first year of use, so no one really knows what percentage continue to have good results. Individual therapists, however, report that at least a small number of people with chronic pain remain comfortable for years by periodically changing the settings on the TENS machine. Switching to a new brand that creates a different pattern of stimulation may help when all options on one machine have been used.

"Change is the name of the game," says Dr. Kahn. "It allows my patients to use TENS to control their pain for longer periods of time."

When to Try TENS

In the case of acute pain, TENS may be particularly suited to the treatment of fractured ribs, postoperative pain, childbirth pain, and acute dental pain.

Breathe Easy

Fractured ribs can make it painful to breathe deeply and to cough. Doctors say being able to cough comfortably is important, especially when you are confined to bed. It helps you clear fluid from your lungs and thus reduces your risk of developing pneumonia. While narcotics can relieve the pain of fractured ribs, these drugs also suppress breathing and can cause as many problems as they relieve, says Dr. Nolan. Strapping or taping the ribs also interferes with deep breathing. In many cases, TENS applied to the muscles between broken ribs relieves pain well enough so that you can breathe deeply and cough, notes Dr. Nolan. It does not slow or impair breathing.

Postoperative Comfort

TENS has been used in several kinds of postoperative pain, including hip replacement, spinal disk removal, chest and abdominal surgery, knee surgery, and cesarean section. Many studies show that people who use TENS after surgery require fewer painkillers than people undergoing similar surgery who don't use TENS. Some studies also report that TENS users breathe easier and are less likely to develop a collapsed lung or pneumonia. Other studies indicate that TENS users are less likely to develop paralyzed bowels—a common and painful consequence of abdominal surgery that can be aggravated by narcotics use.

A study of people who had knee surgery showed a dramatic drop in narcotics use in those using TENS compared to those not using TENS. Some people were able to stop taking the medications entirely. TENS users also had better motion in the knee and were able to walk sooner after surgery. They were able to leave the hospital in an average of 2.5 days, compared to 3.9 for those not using TENS.

Despite their apparent benefits, TENS units are not routinely used for postoperative pain. If you're planning to have surgery and would like to use a TENS unit afterward, you'll have to make prior arrangements with your surgeon. Generally, TENS is used continually for 24 to 48 hours after surgery, and then as needed for an additional seven to ten days.

The Baby Electric

Dozens of studies worldwide suggest TENS is effective in relieving the pain of childbirth. TENS is not approved by the Food and Drug Administration (FDA) for this use, and there has been little U.S. research to verify the positive findings of researchers in Scandinavia, where TENS is often used during childbirth.

These studies show no adverse effects to mother or fetus. Researchers who conducted these studies say TENS has obvious benefits compared to pain-killing drugs or spinal anesthesia, which can slow and even temporarily stop labor, making a forceps delivery or cesarean section more likely.

Using TENS allows perhaps one woman in ten to have her baby without requiring pain-killing drugs, says Laurie Arne, one of four physical therapists who attend births at Lake Forest Hospital in Lake Forest, Illinois.

"It's not that they don't have any pain, or that they don't take any painkillers at all," she explains. "It's more that they feel in control of their pain and often require less pain medication than women not using TENS."

If you are interested in using TENS as a pain-relief technique during your delivery, ask your physician if it's appropriate for you.

Gentle Dental Work

Dentists have tried TENS for all kinds of painful dental procedures—drilling, extractions, minor surgery. One dentist even designed a drill that delivered a tiny electrical impulse to the tooth during drilling.

TENS has been used to control pain after wisdom tooth extractions and to temporarily ease the pain of temporomandibular disorder (TMD, sometimes referred to as TMJ).

You won't find most dentists routinely using TENS, though. Most are more comfortable and familiar with other means of pain control. (And so, probably, are their patients.) Some dentists offer TENS to patients who are allergic to local anesthesia or are afraid of needles. That's the kind of dentist you'll have to seek out if you think you might prefer TENS to novocaine.

Using TENS for Chronic Pain

In the United States, TENS is most often prescribed for pain that has persisted six months or more despite medical care, says Dr. Kahn. It may be added to a treatment program in an attempt to avoid or limit the use of painkilling drugs, or to enable someone to exercise with less pain. While it's most often prescribed for back problems, TENS is also recommended for rheumatoid arthritis, osteoarthritis, diabetic neuropathy, knee and hip pain, and some kinds of cancer pain.

Does TENS help chronic pain? A skilled physical therapist may be able to help you continue to use TENS successfully for years, says Dr. Kahn. Most, though, adopt a different strategy. They try to limit TENS treatment to six months to a year and use additional treatments such as strengthening and limbering exercises, limb mobilizing therapy, correct movement and posture, and weight loss as ways to permanently decrease pain.

"TENS is not a curative procedure," Dr. Nolan emphasizes. "If you have a patient in pain, and you know what the cause is, then you treat the cause and cure the pain."

Most of the chronic pain patients he sees have been trying other forms of therapy for months, perhaps for years, Dr. Nolan says. "They may have been taking medications and doing physical therapy. You can't help asking yourself, 'Why haven't any of those other things worked?' That's one question I ask myself. And if those other things haven't worked, what makes you think TENS is going to work?"

Those who see the little black box as a magic cure and a substitute for lifestyle changes, weight loss, or exercise may find relief, at least temporarily, Dr. Nolan says. But six months or a year down the road, they may once again face the same painful symptoms.

People who are realistic about what TENS can and can't do for them, and who acknowledge what they need to do for themselves and begin doing it, are most likely to benefit from TENS, Dr. Nolan says. They will use TENS to help them cut back on pain medications or to help them seriously tackle an exercise/weight loss program.

CURRENT HEALING

Electricity has been used practically since the beginning of medicine for all sorts of amazing, alarming, and—in more than a few cases—phony cures.

Can you imagine standing calf-high in salt water, atop a squirming electric eel, to cure your painful gout? Or sitting in a kind of "electric potty chair" to cure your constipation—instantly? How about donning a battery-powered jockstrap to recharge your sexual potency?

While the medical use of electricity has fallen in and out of favor over the centuries, there always seem to be at least a few "mad scientists" out there, fiddling with some sort of device or another. And there have been enough fascinating discoveries to keep fueling an interest in electricity's healing potential. For instance:

- Certain electrical devices have been approved by the Food and Drug Administration (FDA) since 1979 to help heal recalcitrant fractures. The devices coax the body to create new bone tissue.
- An electrical device was given the U.S. federal government's stamp of approval for use following spinal surgery and for treating spondylolisthesis (a spine disease).
- Researchers are exploring electrical stimulation as a way to halt osteoporosis, a bone-weakening condition that most often strikes post-menopausal women, and to reverse osteonecrosis, a crippling hip condition.
- Certain kinds of electrical currents are used to maintain strength in muscles confined in casts. Applied via leads threaded through a hole cut in the cast, the electricity stimulates the muscle to contract and relax. Similar devices are sometimes used after surgery on the chest and belly to stimulate the muscles around the lungs and intestines, and thus improve breathing and bowel function.
- Certain kinds of electrical currents may one day help heal injuries and surgical incisions, prevent swelling, perhaps even coax the regrowth of damaged nerve fibers and boost immune function.

While some of these medical uses of electricity are backed by legitimate research, other uses are considered dubious at best. For instance, units that stimulate the scalp or earlobes are being plugged as a way to curb drug addictions and smoking, as well as to enhance learning. There is no proof that they work.

If you're considering trying or buying an electrical medical device, check it out first. Ask for published studies that show it works. (Write to the manufacturer for such information if necessary.) Ask for your doctor's opinion. Call a physical therapist for an opinion. Write to the FDA at its Freedom of Information office, 5600 Fisher's Lane, HFI-35, Rockville, MD 20857, or phone (301) 443-4190. The people there can tell you if a device has FDA approval for a particular use.

Does It Hurt the Pocketbook?

Expect to pay $500 or more for a basic TENS unit and up to $900 for the latest in high-tech, take-home TENS. (Office models cost even more.) Or you can pay about $100 a month to rent a unit.

Most private and group insurance plans, as well as Medicare, will reimburse patients for up to 80 percent of the costs of TENS treatment, provided the unit has been prescribed by a doctor. A doctor may suggest you try one or may send you to a physical therapist, who will evaluate your condition and decide whether or not it's worthwhile to try TENS.

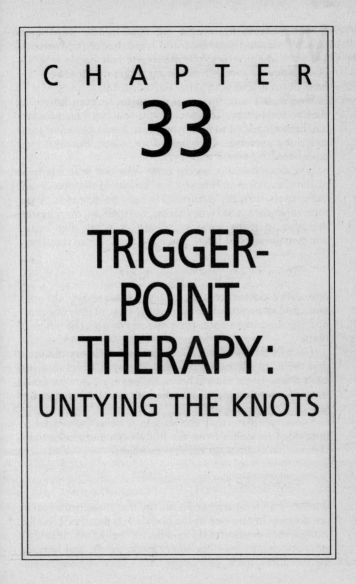

CHAPTER
33

TRIGGER-POINT THERAPY:
UNTYING THE KNOTS

What in the world are those tender hard spots around your hips and lower back? A couple feel like marbles; the others are stiff bands with the consistency of partly frozen meat. Press on those sensitive little buttons and your pain alarms go off.

You're not sure how you got them, or even how long they've been there. The doctor you saw last year said you had tight muscles and prescribed muscle relaxants and some stretching exercises. That helped for a time, but then your pain flared up worse than ever.

The doctor you're seeing now—the one who has been probing and questioning you for the last 45 minutes—calls these spots "trigger points." He says he wants to inject them and then send you across the hall to the physical therapist to learn some stretching exercises. But before you're willing to go for it, you have a number of questions.

What Exactly Is a Trigger Point?

Not every doctor believes trigger points exist, although more and more do. Some think those painful little knots are nothing more than sore, tight muscles or areas of inflamed tissue.

Doctors who endorse the trigger-point theory maintain that the hard places are bundles of muscle fibers that just can't relax. These muscle fibers, they say, are in a continual state of contraction, all bunched up, just like a clenched jaw or a cramped calf.

Some speculate that the muscle is being influenced by misguided messages from the body's sympathetic nervous system that tighten up skeletal muscles.

Finding the Trigger

Doctors who treat trigger points say that these tender areas can develop in any one of the body's 400 muscles. Usually, though, they develop in the middle, or "belly," of the body's most active muscles—the lower back, pelvis, and hips, or the shoulders, neck, and upper back. They've been associated with many different kinds of musculoskeletal pain but especially with chronic pain of the upper and lower back, jaw, and face, and with headaches. If you're a tennis player, they say, you may develop trigger points in your forearm; if you're a runner, in your calves, groin, or hips.

Unless they're buried under fat or muscle, most trigger points can be felt by palpating a muscle with the tips of your fingers, says Willibald Nagler, M.D., physiatrist-in-chief at New York Hospital–Cornell Medical Center and author of *Dr. Nagler's Body Maintenance and Repair Book*. Trigger points can feel like little bumps, stiff bands, or lumps the shape and size of a small plum, he says.

A doctor may rely on the "jump" reflex to confirm his diagnosis. He knows he's found a trigger point when his patient hits the ceiling. You can find them, too, by the same method, says Dr. Nagler. You may be able to feel them in your own gluteus maximus—your buttock muscles. If pressing a tender spot there makes you snap to attention involuntarily, you know you've found one. You also might find some around the edges of your shoulder blades. Pressing or "strumming" the muscle may make it tighten up completely. It takes a great deal of expertise, though, for a doctor to pinpoint a trigger point accurately enough with his fingers to do an injection.

Aside from strumming, doctors may back up their diagnosis with more sophisticated tests. Thermography, which uses an infrared scanning device to show temperature variations on the skin, may detect trigger points as "hot spots," says David Zohn, M.D., a physiatrist in private practice in McLean, Virginia, and author of *Musculoskeletal Pain: Diagnosis and Physical Treatment*. A device called a "pressure threshold meter" can also reveal tender spots or trigger points as areas that produce pain under less pressure than normal tissue.

Not a Sore Muscle

What makes trigger-point pain different from a regular sore muscle? For one thing, the pain doesn't get better with traditional treatment. "A regular sore or tight muscle should respond to heat, rest, a little aspirin, things like that," says Dr. Zohn. "Trigger-point pain lingers on and on, and often will not be deactivated unless you actually treat it."

A more important distinction is that pressing on a trigger point causes what's known as referred pain, says Dr. Zohn. It produces a predictable pattern of pain, usually around the trigger point but sometimes in areas of the body nowhere near the trigger point, he says. Pressing on a trigger point on the back of your neck, for instance, can cause pain in your temples or on the top of your head. Pressing on one in your buttocks sometimes causes pain in your calf muscle. Pressing on one in your calf can cause heel pain.

East Meets West

The ability to cause referred pain is a quality that trigger points share with acupuncture points, says Dr. Nagler. Indeed, some 70 percent of trigger points are located at acupuncture sites, he notes. The connection between the two is a mystery. Indeed, acupuncture points are still pretty much of a puzzle, at least to Western science. Traditional Oriental healers maintain that acupuncture points are located along "energy pathways" within the body. These pathways do not correspond to nerve fiber pathways, though, or to anything else remotely anatomical in the body. One form of acupuncture, called "dry needling," is successfully used to treat trigger-point pain, as you'll see on page 680. To the probable consternation of disciples of this ancient medical technique, Dr. Zohn calls acupuncture "Eastern trigger-point therapy." (For more on acupuncture, see chapter 16.)

Mimics Other Pain

Sometimes trigger-point pain is mistaken for pain caused by nerve root pressure or damage, says Dr. Nagler. "In the hip and shoulder region, especially, trigger points can mimic the symptoms of nerve root pressure," he says. "They cause shooting or radiating pain in a specific region. For instance, trigger points in the lower back and the sacral area can send pain shooting down the leg, very similar to sciatica. In some cases, the knotted muscle can actually press on a peripheral nerve."

Trigger points can and often do occur along with other injuries that cause their own pain, says Dr. Nagler. If you are treated for a herniated disk, for instance, but still have muscle spasms and pain, it's possible that trigger-point therapy may help, he maintains.

Priming the Triggers

Just about any kind of muscle injury can create trigger points, says Dr. Zohn. They can result from a severe muscle strain or tear, even one that is years old. Whiplash from an automobile crash, which tears neck muscles, is a common cause. So are falls that snap your back. Slipping on ice and landing hard on your bottom is a particularly good way to create trigger points.

Doctors who treat trigger-point pain say the points can be created by all kinds of everyday activities: repetitive motions such as heavy lifting or hammering; unusual pressure, such as sitting on a fat wallet or carrying a heavy purse; extreme heat or cold; surgery, which often creates scar tissue; nerve entrapment; certain fever-producing infections; even scrunching up your shoulder and neck muscles or clenching your jaw. One noteworthy culprit is "bird-watcher's pose," a posture that has you sitting on the ground for hours with binoculars to your eyes, your elbows on your bent knees, and your head craned forward.

If they're caused by an injury, trigger points can develop within weeks, says Dr. Zohn. Your doctor may suspect you have one or more if your muscle pain lingers on instead of slowly improving. Usually, though, trigger points develop over a period of two to three months or longer, as a chronic ache that slowly gets worse and worse. If they're caused by a postural problem, they can take years to develop, says Dr. Zohn.

They seem to occur less frequently in people who exercise regularly or have heavy manual labor jobs and more frequently in weekend warriors who indulge in occasional orgies of activity but who may not be particularly fit. Stretching or warming up before beginning exercise might help prevent trigger-point pain, says Dr. Zohn.

Older, inactive people also develop trigger points, but they complain less of pain and more of stiffness and reduced range of motion in joints.

Finding Release

Okay, you've strummed your gluteus maximus and it not only twitches, it begs you for relief. How do you get that annoying knot of pain untied?

Trigger points can be treated by deep tissue massage, anti-inflammatory medication, and injection therapy, by "dry needling"—a Western form of acupuncture—or by certain types of pressure-point massage such as deep muscle therapy or acupressure, says Dr. Nagler.

Injection, needling, and pressure-point massage do basically the same thing: They temporarily block the pain in the muscle so it relaxes somewhat on its own and can be stretched with less pain, explains Dr. Nagler. Some doctors also say that these three forms of therapy help separate clumped muscle fibers and so restore the muscle to normal.

Numbing by Injection

With injection therapy, the doctor shoots a local anesthetic, such as lidocaine or novocaine, or a saline (salt) solution directly into the trigger point. Some doctors also inject inflammation-fighting corticosteroids; others save them as a last resort; and some, like Dr. Nagler, won't use them at all. (He believes they can damage muscle tissue.) Although the doctor inserts the needle only once into each trigger point, he or she does move the needle around within the area. With practice, a doctor can feel the needle hitting individual muscle bundles within the trigger-point areas, says Dr. Nagler. The doctor wants to try to inject as many muscle bundles as possible.

The injections can hurt, although as soon as the anesthesia goes to work, the pain stops, says Dr. Nagler. Some doctors do only one injection; they'll do a second if the pain returns in a few weeks. "Generally, two injections should resolve the problem," he says. Some physicians routinely (and admittedly, somewhat arbitrarily) do a series of injections. Dr. Zohn, for instance, does one a week for three weeks in each trigger point. If the therapy seems to be helping, he continues the treatment.

Numbing with Needles

To do dry needling, a doctor inserts a needle into the trigger point and moves it around. Like acupuncture, the needle is thought to cause local irritation that stimulates the release of the body's own pain-relieving endorphins.

Press Here for Relief

With pressure-point therapy, a therapist uses his or her knuckles, fingertips, or elbows or a small wooden dowel to apply pressure right on the trigger point. This can hurt, although some people say it "hurts good," says Kitty Spivak, M.D., a certified trigger-point myotherapist practicing in Greensboro, North Carolina. With time, the trigger point starts to relax and becomes less sensitive. "Some patients require 3 sessions; some require 30," says Dr. Spivak. "It depends on a person's age, the extent of their injury, and how long they've had the injury."

Stretching It Out

Whatever form of treatment you choose, doctors and physical therapists agree: You must follow it with limbering and stretching exercises targeted for the muscle groups involved. Those exercises help restore the muscle to its normal length and strength, says Dr. Nagler. They keep it from springing back into a tight knot.

"Injections alone don't solve the problem," he says.

"They are only part of a total rehabilitation program, although they are an important and effective part." Not only that, he says, the stretching exercises must be a lifelong commitment. If you stop doing them, your trigger points are likely to return—if not right away, sooner or later.

Will Therapy Work?

There are no studies comparing the success rates of the different forms of trigger-point therapy. (One small study does suggest that dry needling works as well as injection therapy.)

"They all work," Dr. Nagler says, "but injection therapy works the fastest." That's something New Yorkers appreciate. "They don't want to have to be coming back again and again for treatments. And some of the pressure-point therapies hurt, at least initially. Some people stop going just for that reason."

Unfortunately, no studies compare trigger-point therapy with other forms of therapy, such as exercise alone, massage, or even no medical treatment at all, says Dr. Zohn.

So is trigger-point therapy for you? Doctors who use this therapy say you may want to try it if

- Your pain does not seem to have a direct "structural" problem (arthritis or an out-of-whack spinal disk, for instance).
- Other simple forms of therapy, such as heat, massage, or aspirin, have not resolved the pain.
- Your structural problems have been controlled (with medications or surgery, say), but you continue to have pain.

The risks of trigger-point therapy are few, says Dr. Zohn. You are unlikely to develop more pain as a result of this therapy; at worst, you may try it, find it doesn't work, and look for a different diagnosis, he says.

The benefit of at least discussing trigger-point therapy

with a physiatrist or an experienced rheumatologist or orthopedist, notes Dr. Nagler, is that you may save yourself an expensive and possibly painful workup for spinal pathology, and a possible misdiagnosis.

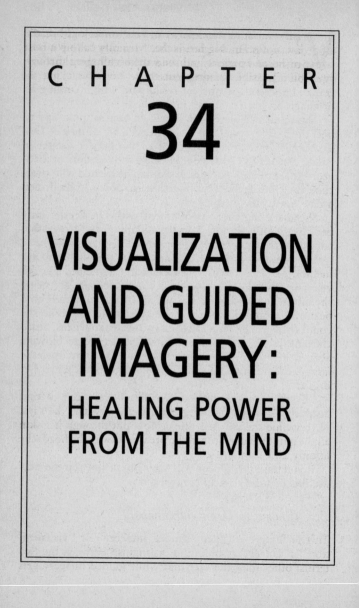

C H A P T E R
34

VISUALIZATION AND GUIDED IMAGERY:
HEALING POWER FROM THE MIND

Visit a mountain hideaway in your mind and breathe away a pounding headache. Mentally call up a host of fierce warriors and send them galloping through your bloodstream, routing out those body-wracking flu germs. Put out the flames of facial pain with a cooling jet of imaginary water. Sound far-fetched?

The mind has incredible power to control pain and to heal the body, says David E. Bresler, Ph.D., author of *Free Yourself from Pain* and director of the Bresler Center in Pacific Palisades, California. He cites the example of a 32-year-old, extremely successful woman he treated who overcame daily headaches that forced her to down 15 ibuprofen a day "as if they were candy."

She made her first appointment with Dr. Bresler only because the potentially dangerous daily dose of over-the-counter medication no longer stopped her headaches.

His solution was to teach her an increasingly popular method of pain control: visualization. He helped her develop her own imagery to combat the headaches. Whenever she felt the onset of a headache, she imagined herself on a beautiful mountain retreat—the most peaceful scene she could visualize. In her mind she saw the distant vistas, heard chirping birds, and actually felt a gentle breeze blowing against her face. It took her only three sessions to learn how to use this technique to banish her headaches, says Dr. Bresler.

"Every time she inhaled, she filled every cell of that headachy area with healing, nourishing oxygen," he says. "Every time she exhaled, she'd blow out through her skin all the painful feelings until she breathed away the headache in only 2 or 3 minutes."

If you have the approval of your physician, you too may use this method to help control pain.

Coming to Terms with Imagery

This technique is called "guided imagery" or "visualization." It is mere quibbling to distinguish between the two terms, other than the fact that while guided imagery gets all five of your senses involved, visualization involves just one—your ability to see things in your mind's eye, says John Lyons, Ph.D., coauthor of *You Can Relieve Pain: How Guided Imagery Can Help You Reduce Pain or Eliminate It Altogether*.

Definitions aside, let's take a look at this remarkable technique that allows mental images to chase away physical pain. First, each person creates their very own vision. This is an important point. Just as no two individuals think exactly alike, there are vast differences in the ways we all react to pain, says Dr. Lyons. A professional football player tolerates pain on a daily basis; the same pain might cause you to scream like a banshee.

Moreover, says Dr. Lyons, the pain that has you doubling over today might seem much less severe at another time. "Pain is whatever the mind decides it is," he notes in *You Can Relieve Pain*.

He points out that wounded soldiers in World War II often refused offers of morphine for the same types of pain for which civilians routinely requested painkillers. One researcher theorized that the soldiers' pain was eased naturally by the euphoria they felt over sustaining a wound that would send them home from the war.

You can take advantage of your mind's marvelous power to control pain by consciously creating your own healing images. Imagery may help your brain zap pain again and again.

Launching a Mental Guided Missile

Guided imagery accomplishes two things with regard to pain, says Kenneth L. Lichstein, Ph.D., professor of psychology at Memphis State University in Tennessee and author of *Clinical Relaxation Strategies*. Number one: It's a legitimate form of relaxation. "Any time you're relaxed, you're going to experience less pain than when you're tense," he says. Number two: It "diverts your attention from the pain."

The rationale behind guided imagery is that if our mind—beset with stress and worry—can make us hurt, it also can ease the pain. "If you can worry yourself sick—and we know you can with ulcers, cardiovascular diseases, and so on—you can think yourself well," says Dr. Bresler.

"We have a great deal of untapped power in our ability to control our body with our mind," says Dr. Lyons. He explains that all the sounds, tastes, touches, smells, and sights that we experience with our five senses are perceived in our unconscious mind as *images*. If you can control your imagery, you also can control pain, he says.

Imagery in Action

One respected practitioner of guided imagery, Carl Simonton, M.D., medical director of the Simonton Cancer Center in Pacific Palisades, California, uses it to help people fight cancer. He asks patients to conjure up mental images of their pain problem. (What does your pain look like?) If they picture their disease as invincible—a dragon, for example—and their white cells as weak and nonaggressive—say, cotton puffs—Dr. Simonton counsels them to alter the image. If people can give their body's defensive white cells a fiercer persona, such as warriors running roughshod over the malignant cells, they have a better shot at reducing their pain and even curing their illness, notes Dr. Simonton.

Dr. Bresler once asked a woman to come up with an image for her facial pain. She imagined that her mouth was on fire. Once she created a counterimage of clouds of water putting out the flickering flames, her pain began to lessen.

Regaining a Lost Art

Guided imagery is a simple process for some creative people but harder for those who have let the cares and concerns of adulthood bury that talent for imagining things, which most of us had as children.

"Some people are very developed in this area," says Dr. Lyons. "I spent a lot of time in grade school visualizing being somewhere else."

Even highly creative people can have trouble with guided

imagery, however, if chronic pain so overwhelms them that they have difficulty concentrating on their inner pictures, says Dr. Bresler.

Creating a healing image isn't the same thing as conjuring up a black-and-white freeze-frame photograph in your mind, says Dr. Lyons. Guided imagery can be enhanced by developing your awareness of how things smell, taste, feel, and sound—as well as how they look. Don't assume that you need the observational powers of a best-selling novelist, however. Dr. Bresler says that all you have to do is strive to experience your images vicariously and improve on the image-creating abilities you already possess. Other doctors say that imagery can be more of a "feeling" than an actual image.

As an exercise to show how quickly your mind can experience a taste, Dr. Bresler suggests that you imagine cutting a juicy lemon into quarters and sucking one piece dry.

Close your eyes and visualize that lemon passing between your lips . . . roll that sour, tart piece of lemon around in your mouth . . . chew it, suck it. Let your palate fully experience that sour lemon. Let your taste buds curdle.

Did you salivate? If so, says Dr. Bresler, you've tasted that lemon in your mind. You've just proved to yourself that you can create a physical response with a mental image. And you should have no problem using guided imagery as a tool for pain relief.

Picturing Relief

One of Dr. Bresler's patients was a woman who survived a bout with cancer but was plagued by postmastectomy pain. The image that she chose to represent her pain was that of an elephant sitting on her chest.

She cut a deal with the pesky pachyderm. They agreed that if she practiced her stress-management and relaxation techniques daily, the elephant would go on a diet.

"Over a period of several sessions she reported the elephant getting smaller and the pain being much less," Dr. Bresler says.

One day, the elephant's ears turned into wings like Dumbo's. Flap, flap. He literally flew off her chest.

"She was 100 percent free of pain," says Dr. Bresler. The pain vanished from her life as long as she remembered to do her mental exercises. When she lapsed for a time, she again had an unwelcome guest lounging on her chest: He returns to remind her.

A man with terrible back pain following cancer surgery told Dr. Bresler that his image was that of a dog chewing on his spine. He was pain-maddened to the point of feeling suicidal. Instead of battling the dog, the man reasoned with it. And once the man made some adjustments in his personal and professional life, the dog began to relax its grip, mercifully alleviating the pain in only a few weeks.

Another variation on this pain-relief technique, according to Dr. Lyons, is to develop an automatic healing image that you can call to mind every time you feel pain. If your back pain feels as if a sharp spike is being driven into your spinal cord, for example, your healing image might be a pair of steel-like hands jerking the spike out.

What does your pain feel like to you? Can you come up with an automatic image? If you have some difficulty visualizing either the pain or a healing image, a specialist in guided imagery might be able to help you.

Color Me Painless

Many specialists in guided imagery use slightly different techniques, but they all have the same end result in mind— to rid you of pain. Dr. Bresler has people draw three caricatures of themselves—one of themselves while feeling the worst possible pain, another of themselves when the pain is present but tolerable, and a third of themselves pain-free. He then supplies them with a cassette tape that contains an exercise that helps them transform their image of themselves in the worst possible pain into an image of themselves as pain-free. Often, these changing images are accompanied by actual pain relief, he says. (Tapes may be obtained from the Bresler Center, P.O. Box 967, Pacific Palisades, CA 90272.)

Another way to help people improve their ability to come up with effective imagery is by creating diagrams, says Neal Olshan, Ph.D., author of *The Scottsdale Pain Relief Program* and director of the Scottsdale Behavioral Health Center, Scottsdale, Arizona. He uses line drawings of people and asks his patients to color the areas where their pain lies. Most commonly, people color their pain red, black, deep blue, or purple. He then asks them to choose a color—such as yellow, green, or orange—that represents pain relief for them personally. The object of such imagery is to get the pain-relief colors to dominate and overpower the pain colors.

Pain-Specific Visualization

One of the most common reasons people turn to imagery is to relieve migraine headaches. One commonly used visualization technique takes care of the blood flow problem that leads to such headaches, according to Dr. Lyons.

"Picture your hands inside a warm sock, or picture your hands in a warm bath or holding something warm, such as a mug of coffee," he says. "To meet the expectations of your hands actually warming, your body sends more blood to your hands and therefore less blood to your head."

Adios, migraine. The decreased blood flow to the head often helps alleviate pain, Dr. Lyons explains.

Rub Yourself the Right Way

Yet another visualization technique is particularly valuable for people who are in so much pain that they can't seem to perform other guided imagery techniques, according to Dr. Bresler. In this exercise, patients imagine that they are wearing a glove that gives one of their hands the power to numb or anesthetize anything it touches. They then place this hand on any part of their body that hurts and keep it there until the physical symptoms of pain subside.

One of Dr. Bresler's patients was a woman in her early fifties named Judith. She had deep-rooted, ultrapainful joint disease in her neck, as well as numbness and tingling in her arms and hands. Her job required that she sit in front of a word processor all day. "She was just terribly uncomfortable," says Dr. Bresler.

Her salvation was the imaginary anesthetizing glove. She first imagined the glove on her left hand and rubbed it over her neck and shoulders to numb that area until she rid it of pain, says Dr. Bresler. She then shook her left hand to get rid of all the anesthesia in it, repeated the process with the other hand, and returned to work.

The technique worked slowly but surely. "She started off having pain relief that lasted maybe 3 or 4 minutes," recalls Dr. Bresler. "She was able to work up to where she could go 4 hours at a time. When the pain started, she would use it, and she'd be clear for the morning. The pain would come again after lunch, and she would use it so she'd be clear for the afternoon. She ended up managing her pain very well."

Relaxation Helps It Work

Relaxation is "essential" before guided imagery can be attempted, says Dr. Bresler. "If there's one thing that people in pain seem to have in common, it's the stress that's associated with having intractable pain," he says.

There is a Catch-22, unfortunately. Although you realize it is important for you to relax, you may be in too much pain to do the concentrating necessary to learn relaxation skills. If you are in terrible pain, choose times to learn these skills when your pain is at its lowest ebb, recommends Dr. Bresler. "Anybody can learn them," he says. (You can find additional information on relaxation techniques in chapter 22.)

Knowing What to Expect

Guided imagery is a relative newcomer to the field of medicine. Hence, some physicians still are skeptical about its value. Although many physicians swear by it, others are not yet familiar with guided imagery or are reluctant to accept personal success stories, which they call "anecdotal evidence." "At this stage it's a technique that's just beginning to be widely accepted by practitioners," says Dr. Lyons. Dr. Bresler says that in almost all cases, visualization is a safe, effective tool to relieve a wide variety of pain.

Visualization and guided imagery have a wider application than simple pain relief, however.

Imagery has already had a major impact in sports medicine—both to reduce pain and to help athletes enhance their performance by visualizing future success, says Dr. Lyons. Imagery can also help people in pain remain on the job, he notes.

One journalist told Dr. Lyons that she followed his suggestions about using imagery to help overcome the pain of arthritis in her hands so that she could bang away at a computer terminal hour after hour. "She developed her imagery to imagine lubrication coming through her joints," he says. "She got to the point where she could type without pain."

Picking a Pro

If you think you'd like to try visualization, ask your doctor if it's appropriate for you. Your doctor may be able to refer you to a health-care professional who can help you get started.

Finding just the right professional in your area can be tricky. One reputable source of information is the Academy for Guided Imagery in Mill Valley, California. It's toll-free phone number is (800) 726-2070.

You might also ask your religious leader if he or she knows of someone who gives training in visualization, says Dr. Lichstein. Your local college's psychology department may also be able to refer you to someone legitimate.

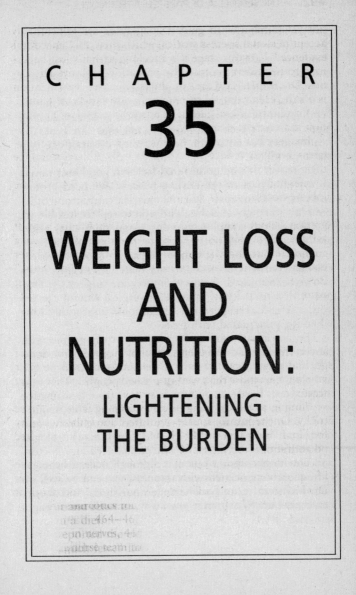

C H A P T E R
35

WEIGHT LOSS AND NUTRITION:
LIGHTENING THE BURDEN

It's true that special diets that eliminate or add certain foods can dramatically alleviate some types of pain. Migraine headaches, irritable bowel syndrome, and gout are just some of dozens of distressing conditions that may clear up with changes in eating habits.

It's also true that many nutrients are involved in preventing painful conditions such as cancer and heart disease. Since we can't pick our parents (and thus our genes), a healthy diet is one of the best ways to thwart these two common killers.

Moreover, it's an undisputed fact that good nutrition is an essential part of the healing process. We need protein and vitamin C to repair skin and muscles, calcium and other minerals to patch up bones, and iron to replace lost blood. We also need B-complex vitamins, magnesium, fatty acids, and a host of other nutrients to perform just about every function in our body. It's important to get enough of every essential nutrient in order to get better, especially when you've been injured or you've undergone surgery. As anyone with a recalcitrant fracture or surgical wound can tell you, a lengthy recuperation can become unbearably long when it's punctuated with pain.

The consensus among doctors who treat people with cancer, chronic back problems, alcohol-induced nerve damage, and other types of pain is that malnourished people just plain hurt more than well-nourished people. "They find medical tests harder to endure, may have trouble sitting for very long in a chair or lying on an examining table, require more pain medications, and are often apprehensive and depressed," says James F. Balch, M.D., an Indiana urologist and author of *Prescription for Nutritional Healing*. Doctors and nutritionists point out that although malnourishment is frequently associated with thinness, you can be well on your way to zaftig and still be undernourished. (And obesity can contribute to pain in its own way, as you'll see on pages 698 and 701.)

Can Deficiencies Cause Pain?

Can a nutritional deficiency actually lead to a painful condition? Some deficiencies can, if they are severe enough, although all are likely to cause other symptoms first, says Mona Sutnick, Ed.D., a registered dietitian who is a nutrition consultant and spokesperson for the American Dietetic Association. Most commonly associated with deficiency are fatigue and mental problems like depression or confusion. There is no nutritional deficiency that is diagnosed strictly on the basis of pain, she says.

Severe deficiencies are rare in the United States, but some doctors consider borderline deficiencies to be fairly common (and often overlooked). Among those persons at highest risk are alcoholics, people ages 60 and older, those with absorption problems, cancer patients, pregnant women, and teenagers. Studies show that the typical American diet is a Swiss cheese of nutritional lapses, with about 25 to 30 percent of Americans eating less than the Recommended Dietary Allowance (RDA) of one nutrient or another. Among the most common shortcomings: vitamin B_6 and other B-complex vitamins, iron (for women of childbearing age), and calcium.

Pain Demons of Deficiency

Pain from a nutritional deficiency develops because the body begins to malfunction or break down from lack of a particular building material.

Vague pain in the bones, joints, and muscles is among the early signs of scurvy, a rare vitamin C deficiency, for example. That's because without vitamin C, the body can no longer make collagen, a fibery tissue that helps form blood vessels, bone, cartilage, skin, and muscles. Early scurvy can be mistaken for arthritis, says Dr. Balch. A doctor who detects signs of capillary hemorrhage first in joints, then in other parts of the body, should make sure the condition is not being caused by a vitamin C deficiency, he says.

Pain in the leg bones when walking and in the back can

be a sign of osteomalacia, a bone-weakening vitamin D deficiency sometimes confused with osteoporosis, says Dr. Balch. Even if the body has plenty of calcium, it still needs vitamin D to make or maintain bones. People at highest risk for a vitamin D deficiency include those who don't drink much milk, those who have liver or kidney disease or adult-onset diabetes mellitus, those who are taking anticonvulsants, or those who avoid the sun, says Dr. Balch.

Thiamine, or vitamin B_1, deficiency is marked by burning, tingling pain in the feet and calves and muscle cramps in the legs, along with other symptoms, says Allan Bernstein, M.D., chief neurologist at the Kaiser-Permanente Medical Center, Hayward, California. That's because without thiamine, nerves in the feet and hands begin to deteriorate and can eventually die. Deficiencies of other B vitamins are also thought to make nerves vulnerable to erratic, painful "firings" and compression pain from nearby tendons or bones, says Dr. Bernstein. It's true that these nerve problems can be caused by other things, especially alcohol abuse, diabetes, and repetitive motions. But some doctors believe that even when the problem is not caused by a nutritional deficiency, certain B-complex vitamins can help. Doctors recommend up to 100 micrograms of B_{12} and up to 100 milligrams of thiamine, riboflavin, panthothenate, biotin, niacin, and B_6, says Dr. Bernstein. These nutrients should be used along with regular medical care and a well-balanced diet, he says.

But What About Pain Relief?

When it comes to the actual relief of pain—chronic, acute, or otherwise—few foods or nutrients stand out, unless they are being used to correct a painful condition caused by a nutritional deficiency or a metabolic disorder. Be especially cautious of any diet that seems unbalanced or that calls for large doses of nutritional supplements (especially amino acids).

The Fish Factor

One notable exception to this rule may be certain oils found in tasty cold-water fish like salmon and mackerel, says Joel M. Kremer, M.D., arthritis researcher and professor of medicine at Albany Medical College of Union University, in Albany, New York. The fatty acids in these fish oils may have inflammation-relieving effects, he says. (There is as yet no RDA for these oils.)

Several studies suggest that these oils, particularly eicosapaentenoic acid, change the chemical structure of two inflammation-causing substances produced in your body—prostaglandins and leukotrienes—making them less potent. The altered chemical structure apparently renders these substances inert, so they no longer can cause inflammation, says Dr. Kremer. And unlike anti-inflammatory drugs, fish oils work without inhibiting the helpful effects of prostaglandins in the body—protecting the stomach lining, for instance, or helping stop blood clots. In fact, fish oil, in the form of cod-liver oil, was used as early as the late 1700s to "lubricate" the "squeaky" joints of arthritis patients.

"I would not describe the study results as dramatic, but the effects are reproducible, which is saying something when you are talking about dietary intervention," says Dr. Kremer, who started his fourth study on fish oil and rheumatoid arthritis in September 1990. "In our studies so far, the majority of patients have had significant relief of joint tenderness, swelling, and morning stiffness," he says.

Dr. Kremer has found that beneficial effects start to appear after three months on a diet rich in fish oils and seem to reach their maximum at five to six months. He's also found that beneficial effects are more common when higher doses are used. In his latest study, the group of people receiving higher doses used 5 to 6 grams of fish oil a day (a combination of pure eicosapaentenoic acid and docosahexaenoic acid), or approximately 15 capsules.

Oils for the Skin

Doctors have used fish oils with some success in treating psoriasis—an itchy, scaly, inflammatory skin disease—and psoriatic arthritis—a rheumatoid-like form of arthritis associated with psoriasis. In preliminary studies, fish oils have also been used with some success for Raynaud's syndrome—a circulatory problem that constricts blood vessels in the hands and feet, making them cold—and ulcerative colitis. They've been used with mixed results for migraine headaches, says Dr. Kremer.

If you want to try fish-oil capsules, discuss it with the doctor who is treating your condition.

Break the Pain/Gain Cycle

The last thing you wanted to hear is that losing weight may help you say goodbye to your pain, but the latest scientific findings may give you new incentive to count those calories.

For most people in pain, doctors agree: The best nutrition plan is a commonsense, balanced diet that maintains proper weight. It's one that makes sure every calorie is jam-packed with nutrients, especially if you are temporarily confined to the couch as a result of your pain and so are using up fewer calories than normal.

Why is it so important to try to maintain your weight or to lose weight? Because extra pounds can lead to a vicious circle of pain, inactivity, despair, and . . . you guessed it . . . more pounds. That's true, at least, for people with backaches or pain in weight-bearing joints: the hip, knee, ankle, and foot.

In a study done at Vanderbilt University Medical Center's Pain Control Center in Nashville, Tennessee, researchers determined that patients who gained more than 15 pounds after the onset of their pain appeared more likely to have problems dealing with their pain than those who remained at the same weight.

Patients who gained tended to be those who "felt out of control of their situation, depressed, and anxious," says

Robert N. Jamison, Ph.D., the study's main author (now with the Pain Treatment Service at Brigham and Women's Hospital in Boston and an assistant professor at Harvard Medical School). "Their weight gain may feed into a sense of loss of control and lower self-esteem. Instead of seeing how they might change their situation, even in small ways, they let their pain dictate everything they do."

Both doctors and patients would like nothing better than to simply stop the pain, Dr. Jamison says. "Unfortunately, some of our patients are going to continue to have at least some pain no matter what we do." It's in those situations that he finds weight loss particularly helpful.

"If someone is able to drop 15 or 20 pounds and eat responsibly, he feels more in control of his body and himself," says Dr. Jamison. "He feels better about things, even if he still has pain and has to deal with the same problems as before."

Losing weight can be a major challenge to someone in pain. "If your back is killing you, and I say you need to exercise and that I am putting you on a 1,200-calorie diet and that you are going to feel great, initially that is rubbish," says Dr. Jamison. "You are going to hurt and you are going to feel lousy."

Dr. Jamison's seven years of experience with pain patients leads him to strongly recommend support groups for weight loss. "People who don't have the emotional support of others who've gone through the same thing are practically destined to fail in their attempts to lose weight. It's that hard," he says. "There is tremendous strength in being with those who have gone through the worst, who are now feeling better, and who can encourage and advise those who are following."

When Every Calorie Counts

Even with the best emotional support, you can't live on cottage cheese and black coffee—at least, not for long. People who go on such extreme diets tend to fall off the wagon in a bad way: When they go back to eating "normally," they regain their lost weight and then some. It's no wonder they give up. That's why nutritionists stress a balanced, commonsense diet.

These days, there's more agreement among nutritionists as to what exactly a commonsense diet includes, even though the typical meat-loaf-and-mashed-potatoes hospital meal may not reflect it.

The consensus is: You can't go wrong with a low-fat, high-fiber diet. It helps you shed pounds and restores good health at the same time. And it's filling, by sheer bulk.

"We don't make our pain patients count calories," says Karen Miller-Kovach, a registered dietitian and assistant director of nutrition for the Cleveland Clinic Foundation. "They have plenty to deal with as it is, so we try to keep their diet as simple and frustration-free as possible."

Instead, she concentrates on helping people trim fat from their regular diet, replacing it with carbohydrates or protein. Since many of the pain patients she sees also have constipation problems due to narcotics use, she's also intent on increasing their fiber and fluid intake.

In terms of daily rations, a typical high-fiber, low-fat diet translates this way: generous servings (1½ cups per meal) of whole grains like brown rice, oatmeal, millet, and cracked wheat; baked potatoes or yams; fresh corn; beans cooked with onions and other seasonings and only a small amount of oil; raw and lightly steamed vegetables; fruits; moderate amounts (5- to 7-ounce servings) of fish, shellfish, and lean meats like skinned chicken and turkey breast and some cuts of pork, veal, and beef; low-fat milk and cottage cheese or yogurt; and no more than a tablespoon or so a day of oil, butter, margarine, mayonnaise, or peanut butter. For dessert, it's fruit, yogurt, nuts, graham crackers, or some sponge cake with a dab of low-calorie whipped topping and some sliced strawberries.

How do people adjust to this diet?

"It may sound Spartan and does take a few days to get used to it; but most people find that because they can eat lots of low-calorie, high-fiber foods, they stay satisfied," Miller-Kovach says. After a few days without sugary des-

WHY BODY MASS + GRAVITY = PAIN

Extra weight leads to hip, knee, ankle, and foot pain for one reason: Each additional pound you pack piles more stress on these weight-bearing joints with every step, or even when you're standing still.

"Whenever you stand on one leg, you generate roughly three times your body weight on your hip, knee, and ankle; if you climb or descend stairs, you are putting roughly six times your body weight on these joints. So for every extra pound, the force goes up proportionately," explains Wilson Hayes, Ph.D., a professor of biomechanics at Harvard Medical School and director of the Orthopedic Biomechanics Laboratory at Beth Israel Hospital in Boston.

Knees are especially vulnerable to damage from extra weight, studies show. The joint is actually compressed, making the smooth, cartilage-lined bones grind against each other and causing wear and tear, pain, and eventually osteoarthritis. Heavy thighs can contribute to pain by forcing you to stand with your feet far apart and your toes pointed out. That stance throws your joints out of alignment and creates additional stress on your knees and hips.

Most overweight people also have foot pain. Their weight compresses the arch of their foot, exchanging its "spring" for a floppy, flat-footed stride. Compression of the many nerve endings found in the foot also causes pain.

Low back pain is linked with rotundity as well, especially when the extra weight hangs over your belt and is associated with a certain alcoholic beverage that comes in aluminum cans and is consumed in mass quantities during televised football games.

Dr. Hayes says, "If you have a big potbelly or are pregnant, you generate very large forces in your spine, and these forces can be associated with pain. You require much more muscle strength just to hold that weight up in front of you." Your body may be able to withstand this abuse when you're young, but with time you may pay the price, as stretched and weakened abdominal muscles and tight, shortened back muscles conspire to pull the spine out of whack.

"You are setting yourself up for all kinds of back pain—muscle spasms, degenerative disk disease, pinched nerves, you name it," says Carl Stoedefalke, Ph.D., a Pennsylvania State University professor of applied physiology.

It makes sense that losing weight would help to alleviate the pain from any one of these problems. And in fact, that's the case.

"There's no orthopedic surgeon who shouldn't suggest to their patients that they try to lose weight first, before they go for something like a hip or knee joint replacement," says Mervyn Deitel, M.D., a University of Toronto professor of surgery and nutritional sciences.

One of Dr. Deitel's studies shows the enormous benefit that weight loss can have on pain. Some 89 percent of his very overweight patients who shed weight reported complete pain relief from muscle and joint pain in their back, feet, or at least one joint (hips, knees, and ankles). "In many cases, losing weight was all they needed to do to ease their pain," Dr. Deitel says.

These people had good pain relief even if they lost less than 60 pounds (some lost 100 pounds or more). "From my experience," Dr. Deitel says, "losing just 20 pounds or so could be a tremendous benefit."

serts, for instance, they'll begin to find an orange or fresh ripe peach or banana wonderfully sweet.

Step One for Any Diet

Want to lose weight? Change your diet? Try nutritional supplements such as fish oil or vitamins C, E, and A?

If your goal is pain control, there is one thing you should always do first: Check with your doctor. He or she may agree that your plan is a good idea. He or she may also protect you from making the wrong dietary decision for your particular condition.

You also need to ask your doctor one very important question: Could the supplements you are taking or planning to take cause side effects or interfere with a medical treatment or a medication you are taking?

If you decide to go ahead and make changes in your diet and to take vitamins, find a doctor or nutritionist who can guide you. That's the best way to stay out of trouble.

INDEX

Page references in *italic* indicate illustrations.

Brain stimulation, electrical, 620–622

Breads, fiber in, 15

Breast pain, caffeine and, 568

Breathing
biofeedback and, 505
pain and, 519–520
pregnancy and, 378
sickle cell disease and, 486
sore throat and, 348
TENS and, 669–670

Bruxism, 167, 549–550

Buerger's disease, 333

Bunions, 297–301
contrast baths for, 298
description of, 297–298
exercise and, 299–300
moleskin for, 298
orthotics for, 300–301
removal of, 301
shoes for, 298–299

Burns, of eyes, 139–141

Bursitis, 269–279
arthritis vs., 270
description of, 270
exercise for, 273,
274–278
frozen shoulder, 270–271
ice for, 271, 275
instant relief from,
271–272
Milwaukee shoulder, 270
physical therapy for,
273–275
steroids for, 272
surgery for, 278–279
treatment of, 271–273

Bypass surgery, 100–101

C

Caffeine, 567–569
breast pain and, 568
headache and, 226, 568,
569
Raynaud's syndrome and,
195

Calcitonin, osteoporosis
and, 268

Calcium
absorption and depletion
of, 263–264, 267
for bone health, 262–265
leg cramps and, 310
vitamin D and, 264

Calcium channel blockers,
for angina, 95

Calcium tablets, 264

Calf cramps, from
intermittent
claudication, 331–335

Calf pain, in pregnancy,
378–379

Calf stretches, 307–309

Calories, exercise and,
530–531

Cancer pain, 460–466
altering perception of,
466
analgesics for, 464–465
imagery for, 687
instant relief from,
460–462
massage for, 460–461
narcotics for, 462–463,
464–465, 610, 611
in nerves, 465
nurse team treatment of,
463